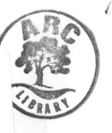

D0428970

UNDER THE INFLUENCE?

DRUGS AND THE AMERICAN WORK FORCE

Jacques Normand, Richard O. Lempert, and Charles P. O'Brien, editors

Committee on Drug Use in the Workplace
Commission on Behavioral and Social Sciences and Education
National Research Council/Institute of Medicine

NATIONAL ACADEMY PRESS
Washington, D.C.   1994

NATIONAL ACADEMY PRESS • 2101 Constitution Avenue, N.W. • Washington, D.C. 20418

NOTICE: The project that is the subject of this report was approved by the Governing Board of the National Research Council, whose members are drawn from the councils of the National Academy of Sciences, the National Academy of Engineering, and the Institute of Medicine. The members of the committee responsible for the report were chosen for their special competences and with regard for appropriate balance.

This report has been reviewed by a group other than the authors according to procedures approved by a Report Review Committee consisting of members of the National Academy of Sciences, the National Academy of Engineering, and the Institute of Medicine.

This study was supported by the National Institute on Drug Abuse, U.S. Department of Health and Human Services, under Contract No. 271-90-8203.

Library of Congress Cataloging-in-Publication Data

Under the influence? : drugs and the American work force / Jacques
    Normand, Richard O. Lempert, and Charles P. O'Brien, editors.
        p.   cm.
        Includes bibliographical references and index.
        ISBN 0-309-04885-0
        1. Drugs and employment—United States. 2. Alcoholism and
employment—United States. 3. Employee assistance programs—United
States. I. Normand, Jacques, 1954- . II. Lempert, Richard O.
III. O'Brien, Charles P.
    HF5549.5.D7U53   1994
    658.3'822—dc20   93-44292
                                                                CIP

Cover: Steelworkers at lunch more than 800 feet above street level during construction of the RCA building in Rockefeller Center, New York City, September 29, 1932. From UPI/Bettmann.

The National Academy of Sciences is a private, nonprofit, self-perpetuating society of distinguished scholars engaged in scientific and engineering research, dedicated to the furtherance of science and technology and to their use for the general welfare. Upon the authority of the charter granted to it by the Congress in 1863, the Academy has a mandate that requires it to advise the federal government on scientific and technical matters. Dr. Bruce M. Alberts is president of the National Academy of Sciences.

The National Academy of Engineering was established in 1964, under the charter of the National Academy of Sciences, as a parallel organization of outstanding engineers. It is autonomous in its administration and in the selection of its members, sharing with the National Academy of Sciences the responsibility for advising the federal government. The National Academy of Engineering also sponsors engineering programs aimed at meeting national needs, encourages education and research, and recognizes the superior achievements of engineers. Dr. Robert M. White is president of the National Academy of Engineering.

The Institute of Medicine was established in 1970 by the National Academy of Sciences to secure the services of eminent members of appropriate professions in the examination of policy matters pertaining to the health of the public. The Institute acts under the responsibility given to the National Academy of Sciences by its congressional charter to be an adviser to the federal government and, upon its own initiative, to identify issues of medical care, research, and education. Dr. Kenneth I. Shine is president of the Institute of Medicine.

The National Research Council was organized by the National Academy of Sciences in 1916 to associate the broad community of science and technology with the Academy's purposes of furthering knowledge and advising the federal government. Functioning in accordance with general policies determined by the Academy, the Council has become the principal operating agency of both the National Academy of Sciences and the National Academy of Engineering in providing services to the government, the public, and the scientific and engineering communities. The Council is administered jointly by both Academies and the Institute of Medicine. Dr. Bruce M. Alberts and Dr. Robert M. White are chairman and vice chairman, respectively, of the National Research Council.

Contents

PART III: EFFECTIVENESS OF
WORKPLACE INTERVENTIONS

APPENDIXES

Preface

The Committee on Drug Use in the Workplace was assembled in spring 1991 by the Commission on Behavioral and Social Sciences and Education of the National Research Council (NRC) and the Division of Health Promotion and Disease Prevention of the Institute of Medicine (IOM). The sponsor, the National Institute on Drug Abuse (NIDA), asked the NRC-IOM to gather and analyze the extant scientific knowledge on the prevalence and etiology of drug consumption by the U.S. work force, the impact of drug use on work performance, and the effectiveness of work site prevention and treatment programs. NIDA also requested that the committee provide, on the basis of its assessment of the available scientific evidence, recommendations for future research directions.

After carefully reviewing its charge, the committee adopted a more expansive yet explicit view of its task—a view that is reflected in the title of this volume: *Under the Influence? Drugs and the American Work Force.* To limit its examination to drug use in the workplace, if taken literally, would exclude issues the committee felt were germane to its charge. That is, the use of drugs away from the work site, hangover effects, and withdrawal effects—as well as use by those who are not currently employed but who are available for employment (e.g., job applicants)—are viewed as important issues that warranted the committee's attention. In addition, we make it clear throughout the report that our definition of drug use includes the use of alcohol.

Another point that should be clear at the outset relates to the committee's perspective in assessing workplace drug use research. This report is concerned with the implications of drug use for workplace productivity; it does not focus on the broader public health perspective. This emphasis on workplace outcomes rather than social consequences allowed the committee to focus on the issues specified in its charge.

Another matter that became apparent early in the committee's work was the need to concentrate on specific research areas. In an effort to provide a meaningful assessment of the scientific work performed to date, and given the diverse areas of drug use research that could feasibly be integrated into its report, the committee decided to rely primarily on the research literature that targets the work force as the population to be studied. In delineating the research areas for review, the committee focused on: (1) the etiology and epidemiology of alcohol and other drug use, (2) the impact of alcohol and other drug use on job-related behavior, and (3) the effectiveness of organizational drug intervention programs, with special emphasis on drug-testing programs. Although our review concentrates on the workplace literature, of necessity it relies from time to time on other research to address relevant issues. For example, epidemiological work on drug use abounds, but few surveys have been concerned with obtaining accurate estimates of the prevalence and trends of drug use by U.S. workers. Therefore, in the discussion of the epidemiological data, the report supplements work-force data with additional sources to better answer specific questions.

The committee wishes to acknowledge that ethical issues—including conflict of interest, confidentiality, fairness, and other concerns—have significant bearing on the work of occupational medicine practitioners, drug abuse professionals, personnel selection specialists, and a range of other human resources experts. Although the committee's charge and expertise precluded an in-depth treatment of these issues, a cursory discussion of ethics as it relates to drug testing is included in Appendix B of this report.

This report was written during a period of change in workplace policies toward alcohol and other drug abuse and change in the rate of their use in society, as well as during a period when the responsibility for medical care of substance abusers is being debated in the context of a national health care system. The report thus represents a 1993 snapshot of a complex picture in a state of flux.

During the course of this investigation, the committee was assisted by a number of individuals who took time to share their insights and expertise. On behalf of the committee, we extend sincere thanks and appreciation to those who volunteered to participate in the workshop the committee held on July 20, 1992: Joseph M. Cannella, Mobil Oil; Peter J. Eide, U.S. Chamber of Commerce; Roberta C. Mayer, National Highway Traffic Safety Administration; Vernon McDougall, International Brotherhood of Teamsters; Joel E. Miller, Health Insurance Association of America; John S. Oates, National Highway Traffic Safety Administration; Robert M. Tobias, National

Treasury Employee Union; and Ellen Weber, Legal Action Center. The committee also thanks Linda Kearney of the NRC and Dennis Crouch of the Center for Human Toxicology for their valuable assistance early in this project. Steven Gust and Linda Thomas of NIDA were critical in the successful completion of this complex undertaking.

This report is the collective product of the committee, and its contents reflect its deliberations. The committee is particularly indebted to one member, Richard O. Lempert, whose contributions of time, energy, and expertise to the crafting of the report were indeed extraordinary. In addition, Mary Ellen Marsden of Brandeis University and James W. Luckey of the Research Triangle Institute contributed substantially to the chapter on epidemiological evidence. To assist the committee further, several individuals were commissioned to provide background materials: Richard W. Foltin and Suzette M. Evans of the Substance Use Research Center, Columbia University; Michael T. French of Research Triangle Institute; Andrea Foote and John C. Erfurt of the University of Michigan; David Wasserman of the Institute for Philosophy and Public Policy, University of Maryland; and James Jacobs of New York University, School of Law.

The committee also benefited from the dedication and quality of the NRC and IOM staffs. These included Suzanne Woolsey, Susanne Stoiber, Rob Coppock, Gary Ellis, and Michael Stoto, who provided valuable insights and suggestions throughout the course of this study. Christine McShane and Eugenia Grohman provided constructive assistance through technical editorial work and coordination of the review, editing, and production processes of this report. Finally, special thanks are due to the committee staff. Carey Gellman, administrative assistant, coordinated all of our meetings, planned the workshop sessions, updated successive drafts of the report, kept track of the work flow, and generally kept our work team organized. Elaine McGarraugh, research associate, gathered and analyzed research materials, edited numerous drafts of the report, and was instrumental in preparing the report for production. The efforts of these talented people ensured the successful completion of this project.

Charles P. O'Brien, *Chair*
Jacques Normand, *Study Director*
Committee on Drug Use in the Workplace

UNDER THE INFLUENCE?

Summary:
Conclusions and Recommendations

This report is concerned with the implications of drug use for workplace safety and productivity. It examines the prevalence of alcohol and other drug use by the U.S. work force, the impact of such use on job-related behavior, and the effectiveness of workplace drug intervention programs. This emphasis on workplace productivity rather than social consequences affects the purpose, methods, and evaluation criteria used in this report, just as it often affects researchers investigating these issues.

THE COMMITTEE'S CHARGE

The committee was charged with: (1) analyzing the available research knowledge on the prevalence and etiology of drug consumption by the work force; (2) studying the impact of drug behavior on work performance, productivity, safety, and health; and (3) evaluating the effectiveness, costs, and benefits of organizational drug intervention programs at the work site.

DEFINITION OF TERMS

Three key terms in the committee's charge require clarification, because their definitions have a significant bearing on the committee's interpretation of the scope of its work.

Drug: The committee defines the term *drug* to include any psychotro-

1

pic substance that, if consumed, will affect a person's psychological status or physiological state or behavior. We consider only substances whose use is problematic enough to represent a meaningful threat to the welfare of individual users or others and whose prevalence is high enough among the work force to have the potential to affect business productivity. The report focuses its attention on general drug class categories, includes alcohol within its scope, and briefly addresses issues surrounding tobacco.

Use, Abuse, and Dependence: Drug taking can be classified into one of three categories: (1) use, (2) abuse, and (3) dependence. *Use* is defined as the limited, controlled consumption of a drug (in terms of frequency and quantity) without significant toxic, adverse physical, or psychological consequences to the user (Glantz, 1992). Regular use of prescribed medications, legal drugs such as nicotine, caffeine, and alcohol, and certain illegal drugs can lead to physiological dependence. This simply means that the abrupt cessation of drug taking produces a set of symptoms called a withdrawal syndrome. The presence of physiological dependence does not necessarily imply abuse or dependence in the behavioral sense. *Abuse* is defined as a level of drug use that typically leads to adverse consequences (physical or psychological). Drug use at this level is not necessarily associated with any particular frequency but is associated with use in quantities sufficient to result in some toxicity to the user, and the patterns of use usually have some characteristics of psychopathological behavior. *Dependence* in the behavioral sense is defined as a level of drug use that has significant adverse physical and psychological consequences. This level of use is characterized by the consumption of toxic doses of the drug that impair the user's ability to function and is also characterized by a compulsive desire to use a drug repeatedly.

Work Force: Although one might confine the question of alcohol and other drug use by the work force to the use of those substances by employees while at work, the committee believes its charge requires a more encompassing definition. By *work force* we mean to include any active member of the labor force, including those seeking or available for employment. Work force alcohol and other drug use is the use of those substances by any work force member, whether the use occurs on or off the job, so long as the use has potential workplace effects. Consequently, issues concerning hangover or residual effects of alcohol and other drugs taken when not at work, as well as correlates of individual alcohol and other drug use and work force participation, are all relevant.

CONCLUSIONS AND RECOMMENDATIONS

Part I: Scope of Alcohol and Other Drug Use

Chapter 2 Etiology of Alcohol and Other Drug Use: An Overview of Potential Causes

• The most vulnerable age and primary risk factors associated with drug use initiation typically precede an individual's entry into the work force. This fact has important implications for work-related prevention interventions designed to prevent the onset of drug use. This means that workplace interventions may have only limited effects on preventing initiation into most categories of drug use.

• Most alcohol and other drug users do not develop patterns of clinically defined abuse or dependence. The progression from use to abuse and dependence varies with drug type as well as with factors that are specific to individuals and their environments. It is not possible, however, to predict with great accuracy which alcohol and other drug users will become abusers or will eventually need treatment.

• If use and abuse have different causes, it follows that they are likely to benefit from different types of interventions, so it is important to further explore the hypothesis that any type of drug use at the work site in fact reflects abuse.

• Among illicit drug users, polydrug use, most often including the use of alcohol and tobacco, is the norm rather than the exception.

Recommendation: In evaluating the impact of alcohol and other drug use on behavior, specific attention should be paid to the actions of drugs in combination.

• Based on the sparse empirical evidence accumulated to date, alcohol and other drug use by the work force appears to be more a function of the personal qualities of individuals than of their work environments. However, most studies of why workers use alcohol and other drugs have serious methodological flaws. Hence, the work environment cannot be ruled out as a contributing or interactive factor in generating use among workers or protecting them from it.

Recommendation: Research is still needed to sort out the relative impact of the work environment and individual traits on workers' alcohol and other drug use. This research should test realistic theories involving such potential critical variables as drug availability,

local norms, work stress and attending to such complexities as interaction effects and reverse causation.

Chapter 3   Epidemiological Evidence: The Dimensions of the Problem

Data sources ranging from self-report questionnaires to urinalysis testing to emergency room visits provide important insights about the use of alcohol and other drugs among members of the general population and the work force. Taken together, the data indicate that, since the late 1970s:

(1)   The prevalence of illicit drug use among members of the general population and the work force has been decreasing, but continues to affect a sizable proportion of the population, especially young adults.

(2)   Illicit drug use may be decreasing among occasional users, but it may be stable or even increasing among hard-core users who are generally not well represented in surveys.

(3)   Heavy alcohol use has been relatively stable over the past several years; rates of heavy drinking have been notably high among young adult men, especially those in the military and among workers in such industries as construction, transportation, and wholesale goods.

(4)   Cigarette smoking has been declining during the past decade for those 18 and older, but has been relatively stable for youths ages 12 to 17.

(5)   Illicit drug use is more common among unemployed than employed persons, and weekly alcohol use is highest among young employed workers.

(6)   Illicit drug use is relatively high among male workers in certain industries such as construction and relatively low among professionals.

•   Given these long-term trends, we must be cautious in attributing short-term changes in alcohol and other drug use in either society or in the work force to specific national efforts to stem the use of drugs.

•   Few epidemiological studies are targeted directly at the work force, leaving researchers to rely on data sources designed for other uses.

Recommendation: More focused epidemiological studies, including longitudinal studies, are needed to assess the magnitude and severity of alcohol and other drug use among the work force. As a first step, the National Household Surveys on Drug Abuse should be modified to provide specific information about job characteristics, job-related behaviors, and alcohol and other drug use at work. Ultimately a national panel survey devoted to this topic should be instituted. In addition, other studies are needed that provide better

information about: (1) employment patterns among persons who use alcohol and other drugs; (2) patterns of alcohol and other drug use among workers; (3) patterns of use in heavily using populations to better understand the employment history and work experience of these individuals; and (4) the impact of illicit drug use and heavy alcohol use on work activity.

Although the workplace offers a unique opportunity to obtain leverage on the alcohol and other drug problems of some users, there are many serious alcohol and other drug abusers who are not regularly employed, if they are employed at all. In 1990, approximately 7 percent of workers reported having used an illicit drug and approximately 6 percent reported having drunk heavily in the past month, compared with 14 percent and 6 percent, respectively, for the unemployed.

• Given the relative low base rate of alcohol and other drug abusers in the employed segment of the work force compared with other selected populations, postemployment workplace alcohol and other drug interventions may help a limited number of abusers, but workplace-oriented interventions cannot solve society's problems with alcohol and other drugs.

• Alcohol and tobacco are the drugs most widely abused by members of the U.S. work force. The adverse health consequences of these drugs are well known. In terms of prevalence rates of work force use and perceived effects of use on performance, alcohol is more likely to have adverse consequences.

Recommendation: Any program that addresses drug use by the work force should include alcohol, the drug most associated with perceived detrimental job performance, as a priority.

Rates of self-reported alcohol and other drug use on the job vary according to occupation, age, gender, and ethnicity. Excluding tobacco and caffeine, most surveys find that fewer than 10 percent of workers report having used alcohol or other drugs while on the job during the prior year. Some studies, however, report significantly higher usage rates. Much of the difference in the reported rates appears attributable to differences in the samples surveyed and the questions asked.

Recommendation: It is important to investigate alcohol and other drug use in different well-specified samples and to develop benchmark measures to allow findings that are comparable across studies.

Part II: Effects of Use

Chapter 4 Impact of Alcohol and Other Drug Use: Laboratory Studies

•   Laboratory studies of the effects of alcohol and other drugs on behavior have shown inconsistent results. These differences may be due, in part, to differences in the populations tested, the measurements used, and the range of drug doses administered.

> **Recommendation: Benchmark measures should be included in laboratory studies to permit generalization across studies. Funding agencies should consider holding conferences to establish such benchmarks.**

Laboratory studies show small performance-enhancing effects of commonly used doses of cocaine and other stimulants. Commonly used doses of marijuana produce variable decrements in performance. Alcohol and prescribed sedatives produce decreases in performance depending on the dose, time of consumption, and the time-course of circulating concentrations of the drug's active metabolites, relative to the work schedule. All drug effects are influenced by dose and prior experience. The age of individuals and the presence of other drugs may also mediate the influence of particular drugs.

•   The use of alcohol and other drugs away from the work site, including prescription drugs and over-the-counter medication, may have detrimental effects during work, especially for those in safety-sensitive positions. Thus, a long-acting drug taken the night before work or alcohol taken at lunch away from the job may have on-the-job effects like those of drugs taken at the work site. In addition, cessation of drug use may produce either withdrawal or hangover effects that affect work site performance. To date there has been little research directed toward any of these issues.

> **Recommendation: Researchers and funding agencies should devote more attention to the ways in which prescription and over-the-counter medications affect job performance, especially for safety-sensitive positions.**

> **Recommendation: Studies of work site alcohol and other drug use should encompass off-site use that may have on-the-job effects. Hangover and withdrawal effects should also be considered in assessing the workplace implications of alcohol and other drug use.**

Chapter 5 Impact of Alcohol and Other Drug Use: Observational/Field Studies

•   Field studies have consistently linked alcohol and other drug use to higher rates of absenteeism; they also provide evidence of an association between alcohol (and perhaps other drug) use and increased rates of accidents, particularly in the transportation industry. Less consistent evidence exists linking alcohol and other drug use to other negative work behaviors, although the current research base is insufficient to support firm conclusions. When associations between alcohol and other drug use and counterproductive workplace behavior are found, relationships are most often of moderate or low strength even when they are statistically significant.

•   The empirical relationships found between alcohol and other drug use and job performance are complex and need not imply causation. Relationships may exist for some job performance outcomes like absenteeism but not for others. Alcohol and other drug use may be just one among many characteristics of a more deviant lifestyle, and associations between use and degraded job performance may be due not to drug-related impairment but to general deviance or other factors.

Recommendation: To intervene more effectively in improving job performance, we must develop a better research base from which to assess how alcohol and other drug use and other factors act alone and in combination to degrade job performance.

•   Widely cited cost estimates of the effects of alcohol and other drug use on U.S. productivity are based on questionable assumptions and weak measures. Moreover, these cost-of-drug-use studies do not provide estimates of potential savings associated with implementing particular public policies toward alcohol and other drugs.

Recommendation: Further research is needed to develop refined, defensible estimates of how much alcohol and other drug use costs specific organizations and society at large. Business decision makers and policy makers should be cautious in making decisions on the basis of the evidence currently available.

Part III: Effectiveness of Workplace Interventions

Chapter 6 Detecting and Assessing Alcohol and Other Drug Use

•   Methods approved by the National Institute on Drug Abuse (NIDA) for detecting drugs and their metabolites in urine are sensitive and accurate.

Urine collections systems are a critical component of the drug-testing process, but they are the most vulnerable to interference or tampering. Positive results, at concentrations greater than or equal to NIDA-specified thresholds, reliably indicate prior drug use. There is, however, room for further improvement along the lines of the recommendations emanating from the 1989 Consensus Report on Employee Drug Testing and the 1992 On-Site Drug Testing Study. Moreover, more could be learned about laboratory strengths and problems if data already collected in the Department of Defense and NIDA blind quality control and proficiency test programs were properly evaluated.

> **Recommendation: To obtain accurate test results, all work-related urine tests, including applicant tests, should be conducted using procedural safeguards and quality control standards similar to those put forth by NIDA. All laboratories, including on-site workplace testing facilities, should be required to meet these standards of practice, whether or not they are certified under HHS-NIDA guidelines.**

> **Recommendation: The extensive data on the reliability of laboratory drug-testing results that have been accumulated by the DoD and NIDA blind performance testing programs should be analyzed by independent investigators and the findings of their analyses published in the scientific literature.**

 • Government standards have improved the quality of laboratory practices; however, the inflexibility and the difficulty of making prompt changes to established government regulations may inhibit the development of new analytical techniques and better experimental-based procedures. Strict regulation of drug-testing procedures and the National Laboratory Certification Programs are nonetheless justified. High-volume, production-oriented drug-testing laboratory operations require the vigilant forensic quality control of routine repetitive procedures, rather than innovative experimental science. Strict regulation need not, however, mean bureaucratic inflexibility that pointlessly increases costs or retards progress, nor should it interfere with research designed to improve current urine testing procedures or efforts to develop reliable tests using specimens other than urine.

> **Recommendation: Within a regime of strict quality control, allowances should be made for variations in procedures so long as they do not compromise standards and they do reflect professional judgments of laboratory directors and forensic toxicologists about what is required to meet individual program needs. No laboratory should be penalized for any practice that is clearly an improvement on or**

beyond what is required by the HHS-NIDA guidelines. When such innovations are attempted, data on their performance should be systematically collected and shared with NIDA. NIDA should take the lead in disseminating to all laboratories information about such improvements and should provide advice promptly as problems, research results, and new data become available.

• At present, urine remains the best-understood specimen for evaluation of drug use, and it is the easiest to analyze. Thus, it must for the moment remain the specimen of choice in employee drug-testing programs. However, other specimens have potential advantages over urine in that they involve less intrusive collection procedures or have a longer detection period.

Recommendation: Researchers should be encouraged to evaluate the utility of using specimens other than urine, such as head hair and saliva, for the detection of drugs and their metabolites.

• There has been an unnecessary proliferation of drugs included in the urine test battery. Testing for LSD and sedative drugs, for example, is not always justified.

Recommendation: Additional drugs should not be added to the drug-testing panel without some justification based on epidemiological data for the industry and region. The analytical methods used to identify additional drugs should meet existing NIDA technical criteria.

• Preemployment drug testing may have serious consequences for job applicants. Applicants, unlike most employees, often do not enjoy safeguards commensurate with these consequences. A particular danger of unfairness arises because screening test data are often reported to companies despite the known possibility of false positive classification errors.

Recommendation: No positive drug test result should be reported for a job applicant until a positive screening test has been confirmed by GC/MS technology. If a positive test result is reported by the laboratory, the applicant should be properly informed and should have an opportunity to challenge such results, including access to a medical review officer or other qualified individual to assist in the interpretation of positive results, before the information is given to those who will make the hiring decision.

• Drug-testing results may reveal drugs taken legally for medical treatment that do not seriously affect an employee's job performance. These drugs may, however, be associated with conditions that the employee for good reasons wishes to keep private.

Recommendation: In the absence of a strong detrimental link to job performance, legally prescribed or over-the-counter medications detected by drug testing should not be reported to employers. Furthermore, such results should not be made part of any employment record, except confidential health records with the employee's permission.

• Alcohol and other drug use by work force members cannot be reliably inferred from performance assessments, since performance decrements may have many antecedents. Conversely, performance decrements are often not obvious despite alcohol and other drug use. More direct measures of the likely quality of worker performance hold promise for determining workers' fitness to perform specific jobs at specific times, regardless of the potential cause of impairment. Efforts to identify such measures, however, are still in their infancy.

Recommendation: If an organization's goal is to avoid work decrement (e.g., accidents, injuries, performance level) due to impairment, then research should be conducted on the utility of performance tests prior to starting work as an alternative to alcohol and other drug tests.

• Integrity testing and personality profiles do not provide accurate measures of individual alcohol and other drug use and have not been adequately evaluated as predictors or proxy measures of use. Using these tests to aid in employment decisions involves a significant risk of falsely identifying some individuals as users and missing others who actually use drugs. The accuracy of these tests is affected not only by their validity but also by the characteristics of the population being tested. Urine tests, by contrast, can be quite accurate in detecting recent drug use.

Recommendation: If an organization treats alcohol and other drug use as a hiring criterion, it should rely on urinalysis testing that conforms with NIDA guidelines to detect use rather than on personality profiles or paper-and-pencil tests.

Chapter 7   Impact of Drug-Testing Programs on Productivity

• The empirical evidence pertaining to the efficacy of preemployment drug testing indicates that such programs may be useful to employers in choosing wisely among job applicants. However, regardless of the magnitude of the correlations between drug use and dysfunctional job behavior measures, the practical effectiveness of any drug-testing program depends on other parameters, such as the prevalence of drug use in the population tested. The presence of significant relationships between drug use and workplace performance measures does not necessarily mean that an effective drug-testing program will substantially improve work force performance, and a program that substantially improves performance with some employees or in some job settings may do little to improve performance with other employees or in other job settings.

• Despite beliefs to the contrary, the preventive effects of drug-testing programs have never been adequately demonstrated. Although, there are some suggestive data (e.g., see the military data in Chapter 3) that allude to the deterrent effect of employment drug-testing programs, there is as yet no conclusive scientific evidence from properly controlled studies that employment drug-testing programs widely discourage drug use or encourage rehabilitation.

Recommendation: Longitudinal research should be conducted to determine whether drug-testing programs have deterrent effects.

• Many studies of alcohol and other drug use by the work force have been flawed in their designs and implementation. Organizations that conduct their own drug studies can, by encouraging their researchers to publish in professional journals, enhance quality control and contribute to a knowledge base that will enable them to deal more effectively with future alcohol and other drug problems.

• Different objectives have been suggested for work site drug testing and diverse alcohol and other drug intervention programs. These include improving workers' performance, preventing accidents, saving on health costs, and working toward a drug-free society by deterring drug use. The effectiveness of alcohol and other drug intervention programs cannot be adequately evaluated unless the goals of such programs are clear.

Recommendation: Organizations should clearly articulate their objectives prior to initiating alcohol and other drug intervention programs and should regularly evaluate their programs in light of these objectives.

Among job applicants and workers, testing for drugs other than alcohol is already common and generally accepted. Of young men in a 1991 general population survey of high school graduates, 33 percent reported that they had been tested, 61 percent reported that they approved of preemployment testing, and 60 percent reported that they approved of postemployment testing. Approval rates were even higher among those who had been tested.

• Very little is known about what happens to job applicants who are not hired or to employees who are fired as a consequence of a positive drug test.

Recommendation: Research should be conducted on the impact of drug-testing programs with attention to those who remain within the organization as well as to those who are not hired or are dismissed. In particular, more information is needed about the impact of drug-testing programs on the health and productivity of the work force.

Recommendation: In light of the relatively low rates of alcohol and other drug abuse among the work force (see Chapter 3), the moderate predictive validity of testing programs (see Chapter 7), and the fact that many factors other than drug use may cause performance deficiencies seen in drug users (see Chapter 5), drug-testing programs should not be viewed as a panacea for curing workplace performance problems. Nonetheless, drug testing for safety-sensitive positions may still be justified in the interest of public safety.

Chapter 8 Employee Assistance Programs

• Recovery from alcoholism and other drug use disorders is a process that can take months or years of continuing care. The continuing abuse of alcohol or other drugs is a chronic disorder, and the evidence suggests that the ameliorative effects of brief treatments without follow-up are seldom sustained over the long run. Employee assistance programs (EAPs) are well situated to oversee that follow-up, which is essential to a long-term recovery.

Recommendation: Because of high dropout rates in substance abuse treatment programs, EAPs should monitor treatment participation and provide for long-term follow-up.

• EAPs are not generic across work sites. EAPs should and do vary across work sites and over time. Thus, it is misguided to ask whether the generic EAP is an effective program.

Recommendation: EAPs should be evaluated in terms of the amount and quality (including process evaluation) of the services they provide and not just by patient count. Researchers should seek to understand how EAPs contribute to a range of different outcomes in a range of different settings. This requires more high-quality critical case studies of EAPs, perhaps with some common criteria of programmatic effectiveness. Care must be taken to secure adequate control groups, and, rather than attempting to evaluate the overall effectiveness of supposedly static programs, attention should be paid to the effects of particular EAP services and their dynamic nature.

•   Given the measurement limitations of drug test results in assessing drug abuse or dependence (see Chapter 6), not all individuals testing positive require or are likely to benefit from treatment, counseling, or other administrative actions that might be triggered by a positive drug test result. Blanket rules referring all positive-testing employees to treatment can be costly to employers without providing commensurate benefits to them or their employees. Care is required to determine the appropriate course of action in the event of a positive test.

Recommendation: Persons reviewing test results should be required to demonstrate expertise with respect to toxicology, pharmacology, and occupational medicine. Standards should be set and continuing education and certification should be required. Such individuals should be involved in the interpretation of the results of drug-testing programs, and in the case of positive postemployment tests, should assist other professional staff in interpreting the seriousness of revealed drug use and provide guidance in determining the best course of action for coping with any drug problems (e.g., evaluation referral to proper medical specialist if needed).

Appendix A   Methodological Issues

•   The most powerful methodology for evaluating the effectiveness of workplace alcohol and other drug intervention programs is the randomized field experiment. The implementation of new work site alcohol and other drug intervention programs or significant changes in existing programs provide propitious occasions for experimental assessment.

Recommendation: To enhance scientific knowledge, organizations instituting new work site alcohol and other drug intervention programs should proceed experimentally if possible. Funding agencies

should make field experiments a priority and should consider providing start-up aid to private companies that are willing to institute
programs experimentally and subject them to independent evaluation.

REFERENCE

Glantz, M.D.
  1992   A developmental psychopathology model of drug abuse vulnerability. Pp. 389-418
          in M. Glantz and R. Pickens, eds., *Vulnerability of Drug Abuse*. Washington, D.C.:
          American Psychological Association.

1

Introduction

Drug use and drug abuse are not new problems, but rather are ones that receive heightened attention at various points in time. The past 200 years have witnessed the gin epidemic in England, the opium wars in Asia, and the woefully forgotten cocaine patent medicine tragedies at the turn of this century. More recently, we have seen the end of prohibition in the 1930s, "reefer madness" in the 1940s, the drug culture of the 1960s, and the heroin epidemic of the 1970s. Currently—and for the second time in this century—cocaine has become a major problem in this country, particularly in its newest and more virulent form of rock or crack cocaine. The use of illegal drugs in recent years is thought to pose problems so severe as to justify a "war on drugs."

The current war on drugs overlooks, however, the abuse of alcohol and tobacco, which cause more deaths in the United States than all illegal drugs combined (Newcomb, 1992). Whereas illegal drugs are estimated to be responsible for approximately 30,000 premature deaths in the United States per year (Reuter, 1992), tobacco is responsible for nearly 400,000 premature deaths per year, and alcohol accounts for nearly 100,000 fatalities per year (Julien, 1992).

Drug use, and more specifically alcohol use, by U.S. workers has a long history. Fillmore (1984) argues that the acceptability of drug use on the job changed as a result of the industrial revolution and the temperance movement. She points out (p. 41) that ". . . prior to the industrial revolution, work and drinking appear to have been inseparable in the U.S. Although the drunken worker was disapproved, especially among the Puritans, drinking in the workplace was considered normal behavior. Drinking was long associated with hard work." The condemnation of alcohol and drug use in the workplace is a relatively recent reaction, arising largely over the past 100 years. Ames (1989), in her historical review of the influence of alcohol-related movements on drinking in the American workplace, points out, however, that many workplaces have been slow to integrate policies that reflect changes in society's views of alcohol. Indeed, in the past year, employees of a well-known Washington hotel were picketing the establishment over the management's attempt to abolish their contractual right to consume three beers per shift.

Recently, there has been increased awareness of the costs related to alcohol and drug abuse on the job. This may be due, at least in part, to the publicity given two recent tragic accidents, the Exxon Valdez oil spill in Alaska and the Amtrak train crash in Maryland, as well as to the "war on drugs" policies of the Reagan and Bush administrations. The effects of such events on perceptions of the alcohol and other drug abuse problem remind us that what constitutes unacceptable drug use varies not only across cultures but also within a culture. The perception of illicit drug use as a significant social problem in contemporary America is the product of social attitudes and perceptions that are shaped by policy makers and others in influential positions (Humphreys and Rappaport, 1993). Yet this does not mean that the problems associated with drug use lack reality. Drug use can have a devastating effect on the quality of life for both individuals and society. The problems associated with drug use, both licit and illicit, are complex and varied. They are not amenable to quick and easy solutions, for example, by simple slogans or by the appointment of a new drug czar.

A few scenarios illustrate the diversity of the problems associated with drug use by the U.S. work force:

> John's boss wanted him to make the sale. If the company could unload those extra parts, perhaps they could forestall a deficit for the quarter. John was given a liberal expense account; he was to wine and dine the prospective buyers before talking business. The restaurant was top of the line, and the liquor, expensive. When John woke up the next morning, he couldn't remember whether he made the sale, the terms of the bargain, or even how he got home.

> Hazel had worked hard to get where she was. She worked days and took cosmetology courses at night. She then worked in her girlfriend's beauty shop and finally was able to save and borrow enough to open her own shop. After three years, she had a thriving business. Hazel smoked marijuana from time to time, and it caused her no problems. So when she was offered cocaine by her cousin, she thought nothing of it. Within six months, she was using cocaine regularly; within a year, she was using it in the back

of the shop and taking money from the cash register to buy more; within a year and a half, she filed for bankruptcy.

George, an independent trucker, borrowed money to buy his own rig and now does transcontinental hauling. The longer he drives, the more money he makes to pay off those loans. Coffee, caffeine pills, and diet pills often allow him to drive 18 to 20 hours at a stretch, but they also make him an unsafe driver. Seventeen hours after leaving a truckstop, he ran a van off the road, killing three of its occupants.

Dr. S., a neurosurgical resident, was looking forward to a weekend off, especially since the past week had been stressful with difficult cases and learning new procedures. A former medical school classmate was coming to visit, and they had planned to relive the good old days by going out on the town. Unfortunately, the doctor assigned to take calls became acutely ill, and Dr. S. was forced to carry the emergency pager. Although a bit angered by this turn of events, Dr. S. did not let it spoil his plans. After having picked up his old buddy at the airport, they headed for the bar district. At the second bar, after his third beer, the pager went off. There was an auto accident, and Dr. S. was needed immediately at the hospital.

Sally felt a bit sick; she had a bad headache, nausea, and a mild tremor. She knew that she and Jim had too much to drink last night, but it was a great party, and he would be away for two weeks. Although she wanted to call in sick for work, she had been told that, if she called in one more time, she would be fired. She knew that a few cups of coffee would pull her together, and she felt relieved that she had to drive the school bus only for a couple of hours before returning home to get some sleep.

These scenarios are not intended to convey the idea that using alcohol or other drugs necessarily has negative consequences, but rather to illustrate the diversity in the nature, magnitude, and potential severity of the problems associated with alcohol and other drug use. The problems are serious, but there is no point in overstating or sensationalizing the difficulties associated with alcohol and other drug use in the workplace or by the U.S. work force. If we are to make wise policy decisions, we should be aware that much alcohol and other drug use consists of infrequent or moderate use that does not necessarily result in harmful consequences, and that most illicit drug-using careers are short-lived and end without requiring any treatment (Gerstein and Harwood, 1990).

The vignettes help to distinguish between two different perspectives concerning the consequences of alcohol and other drug use or abuse: (1) a concern for public health and social welfare and (2) a concern for workplace productivity. From a public health/social welfare perspective, the costs associated with drug abuse are exorbitant. They include the health care costs for treating AIDS patients, crack babies, victims of premature heart attacks, and others. They also include costs related to missed developmental opportunities that are linked to premature births, child abuse, and the like. Society must also absorb the costs of criminal drug activities (e.g., theft, court overload, incarceration) as well as the emotional and physical costs of the violence that often accompanies the trade in and use of illicit drugs. Researchers have estimated that illicit drug abuse results in the loss of approximately 38 years of life due to premature death (Rice et al., 1990).[1]

From the workplace perspective, productivity losses, employers' health costs, and workplace accidents are the principal harm caused by the use of alcohol and other drugs. These costs may result from alcohol and other drug use on or off the job and can be devastating to particular businesses.

This report is concerned with the implications of drug use for workplace safety and productivity. It looks at the prevalence of alcohol and other drug use by the U.S. work force, the impact of alcohol and other drug use on job-related behavior, and the effectiveness of workplace drug intervention programs. This emphasis on workplace outcomes rather than social consequences more generally affects the purpose, methods, and evaluation criteria used in this report and by researchers investigating these issues.

THE COMMITTEE'S CHARGE

The committee was charged with: (1) analyzing the available research knowledge on the prevalence and etiology of drug consumption by the work force; (2) studying the impact of drug behavior on work performance, productivity, safety, and health; and (3) evaluating the effectiveness, costs, and benefits of organizational drug intervention programs at the work site.

Three key terms in the committee's charge require clarification, because their definitions have a significant bearing on the committee's interpretation of the scope of its work. The first term is *drug*: how we define this term determines which substances are considered in the report. The second term is *use*: how the committee defines this term affects the degree of drug involvement considered (i.e., use, abuse, or dependence). And the

---

[1]Aside from accidents and auto fatalities, mortality associated with tobacco and alcohol abuse occur later in life than do fatalities associated with the abuse of such illicit drugs as heroin and cocaine, since deaths associated with the latter are largely attributable to the acute and immediate effects of the drug. Given that the average age of death attributed to illicit drugs is younger than that attributed to alcohol (Rice et al., 1990), illicit drug use results in higher average years of life lost (38) than alcohol (28). Nonetheless, when one takes into account the annual rate of these premature deaths (see Rice et al., 1990:135 and 136) and the relative frequency of heavy illicit drug, alcohol, and tobacco use, the social magnitude of the total premature death costs attributable to illicit drugs is still not at the level of those attributable to either alcohol or tobacco.

third term is *work force*: how the committee defines this term delineates the population of interest for this study.

Definition of the Term *Drug*

President Reagan's Executive Order 12564 in September 1986, which required all federal agencies to develop programs and policies to achieve a drug-free federal workplace, necessitated an agreed-on definition of the term *drugs*. Given the political climate at that time, the implication that *drugs* meant illicit drugs was clear. Consequently, in 1988 the U.S. Department of Health and Human Services (HHS) "Mandatory Guidelines for Federal Workplace Drug Testing Programs" limited the number of drugs to be tested for to the following commonly used illicit drug classes: (1) marijuana, (2) opiates (heroin, morphine), (3) cocaine, (4) amphetamine and methamphetamine, and (5) phencyclidine.

Of course, many other drugs in addition to these five groups are misused or abused, and, from the committee's point of view, this list is too narrow. As Dubowski and Tuggle (1990:74) argue: "If one . . . postulates that drug-use testing in its common current context is intended to identify and ultimately to eliminate or at least limit hazards to persons, operations, property, and the public at large arising from inappropriate use of drugs by the workforce, it becomes clear that the primary targets of the testing efforts should be those drugs that have mood-altering properties as either primary or secondary characteristics. Whether this mood-altering substance is licit or illicit should not be a factor." Consistent with this argument, Alleyne et al. (1991) find that, among work-related accident victims, alcohol is the most common drug involved in occupational fatalities, with 11 percent of industrial accident victims having alcohol in their system. This estimate is consistent with figures reported in earlier studies (Baker et al., 1982; Lewis and Cooper, 1989). In the trucking industry, a recent report from the National Transportation Safety Board (1990) showed that, for truck driver fatalities, the most prevalent drugs detected were alcohol and marijuana (both at a rate of 13 percent). Given that alcohol is considered the most commonly abused substance—from both the public health/social welfare and workplace perspectives—any intervention program that strives to have a meaningful impact on either the health of the general population or the productivity of a specific work force should not limit its efforts to the detection of a few illicit drug classes but should target alcohol as well.[2]

---

[2]One could argue that the long-term health effects of tobacco and caffeine and their more immediate withdrawal effects on behavior also warrant attention (Silverman et al., 1992; Hughes, 1992; Snyder et al., 1989; Snyder and Henningfield, 1989).

At the opposite end of the spectrum, some illicit drugs (such as LSD or synthesized substituted amphetamines) are used by so few individuals that they are unlikely to pose significant problems in the work force. The use of such drugs, however, may pose a risk under certain conditions and situations. For example, methamphetamine, which represented less than 2 percent of emergency room cases nationwide in 1988, accounted for 27 percent of emergency room cases in San Diego during that year (National Institute on Drug Abuse, 1989); methamphetamine might therefore have been a serious concern to the local business community in San Diego in 1988.

Although the committee judged that a consideration of prescribed medications was beyond the scope of its study, a short discussion is warranted. There are no accurate estimates of the prevalence of prescribed medications used by U.S. workers, but the fact that approximately 1.6 billion prescriptions are filled annually by outpatient pharmacies (U.S. Public Health Service, 1992) suggests that a substantial number of workers are using or are under the effect of therapeutic drugs while at work. Sales of over-the-counter medications that might be expected to affect safety or productivity (e.g., antihistamines, medication with significant alcohol content) run into the billions, which suggests that these drugs may also affect the workplace. More important, there is little scientific knowledge concerning the effects of medication on work productivity and safety (DeHart, 1990). Most of the scientific information on the effects of those drugs on performance have come from controlled laboratory studies, which are reviewed in Chapter 4 of this report. As pointed out in a recent issue of the *Journal of Occupational Medicine* (April 1990), better monitoring of the incidence of adverse effects of therapeutic drugs on workplace performance is needed (Tilson, 1990), as well as a better understanding of the interactive effects of the pharmacokinetics of therapeutic drugs, work activities, and the environment (DeHart, 1990) and proper evaluations of the interactive effects of various therapeutic drugs and worker performance (especially with the older worker). Nonetheless, as Potter (1990) concludes, one should keep in mind that, for many conditions, the lack of treatment is likely to cause more performance impairments than the side effects of such treatment.

Based on these considerations, the committee defines the term *drug* to include any psychotropic substance that, if consumed, will affect a person's psychological status or physiological state or behavior. We consider only substances whose use is problematic enough to represent a meaningful threat to the welfare of individual users or others and whose prevalence is high enough among the work force to have the potential to affect business productivity. The report focuses its attention on general drug class categories (see Table 1.1), includes alcohol within its scope, and briefly addresses issues surrounding tobacco.

TABLE 1.1 Drug Classes

Class	Examples
Opiates	Heroin, morphine, methadone, codeine
Depressants	Barbiturates, methaqualone, alcohol, benzodiazepine
Stimulants	Amphetamines, cocaine, caffeine, nicotine
Hallucinogens	LSD, mescaline, psilocybin, MDA
Phencyclidines	PCP, ketamine
Marijuana[a]	Hashish
Inhalants	Acetone, benzene, ethyl acetate, nitrous oxide, butyl nitrate

[a]The report uses the term marijuana as a drug class. For the purpose of this report, this drug class refers to any product containing the Δ^9-THC cannabis metabolite.

SOURCE: Gerstein and Harwood (1990).

Definitions of Use, Abuse, and Dependence

Drug taking can be classified into one of three categories: (1) use, (2) abuse, and (3) dependence. *Use* is defined as the limited, controlled consumption of a drug (in terms of frequency and quantity) without significant toxic, adverse physical, or psychological consequences to the user (Glantz, 1992). Regular use of prescribed medications, legal drugs such as nicotine, caffeine, and alcohol, and certain illegal drugs can lead to physiological dependence. This simply means that the abrupt cessation of drug taking produces a set of symptoms called a withdrawal syndrome. The presence of physiological dependence does not necessarily imply abuse or dependence in the behavioral sense. *Abuse* is defined as a level of drug use that typically leads to adverse consequences (physical or psychological). Drug use at this level is not necessarily associated with any particular frequency but is associated with use in quantities sufficient to result in some toxicity to the user, and the patterns of use usually have some characteristics of psychopathological behavior. *Dependence* in the behavioral sense is defined as a level of drug use that has significant adverse physical and psychological consequences. This level of use is characterized by the consumption of toxic doses of the drug that impair the user's ability to function and is also characterized by a compulsive desire to use a drug repeatedly.

Dependence is associated with an overwhelming involvement in drug-seeking and drug-taking activities. It typically leads to drug tolerance, which means that increasing doses of the drug are needed to obtain the same physiological effect. Each of these terms describe points along a continuum of drug involvement. Of those who use a drug, some never try it again, others continue their use on an irregular or regular basis and take it in doses that amount to abuse, and some continue to the stage of addiction and dependence.[3] As depicted in Chapter 3 of this report, with the exception of users of nicotine and caffeine which are associated with physiological dependence, most workers who have taken drugs can be classified as users of alcohol or other drugs, rather then as abusers or as individuals who are dependent (in either sense) on them.

The clinical diagnostic criteria used to determine an individual's location on the use-dependence continuum are to some extent subjective—the diagnostic process is open to influences from culture, society, and individual diagnosticians. Furthermore, applications of these definitions can vary according to the type of substance taken, the dose taken, the route of administration, prior health history, vulnerability factors, and the environmental context of use. It is safe to say, however, that in the workplace, with the exception of nicotine and caffeine (which are associated with dependence), the majority of those experienced with drugs are *users* of alcohol and other drugs, rather than abusers or dependent. Thus, when we refer without additional qualification to alcohol or other drug use among the work force, we mean to encompass any degree of drug use, ranging from casual use to dependence. Whenever appropriate we acknowledge the special problems caused by abuse and dependence.

Definition of the Work Force

Although one might confine the question of alcohol and other drug use by the work force to the use of those substances by employees while at work, the committee believes its charge requires a more encompassing definition. By *work force* we mean to include any active member of the labor force, including those seeking or available for employment. Work force alcohol and other drug use is the use of those substances by any work force member, whether the use occurs on or off the job, so long as the use has potential workplace effects. Consequently, issues concerning hangover or residual effects of alcohol and other drugs taken when not at work, as well as correlates of individual alcohol and other drug use and work force participation, are all relevant.

---

[3]Standard clinical criteria for diagnoses of use, abuse, and dependence are found in the *International Classification of Diseases* (ICD-10), which is the official classification system of the World Health Organization (WHO, 1990) and the *Diagnostic and Statistical Manual* (DSM-III-R), which is published by the American Psychiatric Association (1987). For a more thorough discussion of the idiosyncracies and commonalities across these two classification systems, the reader is referred to Babor (1992).

SCOPE OF THE REPORT

This report examines a wide range of studies concerning the magnitude and severity of alcohol and other drug use among the work force as well as the probable effects of alcohol and other drugs on the work force. These studies include laboratory experiments, field studies, epidemiological surveys, organization-specific prevalence reports, and descriptive accounts as well as empirical evaluations of drug intervention programs. As is typical in other areas of behavioral research, the results of no single study are definitive (Lempert, 1989). Consider, for example, studies of the effects of drug testing on employee job performance. Studies examining this question suffer from a variety of flaws, including inadequate samples, problematic measures, and incomplete analyses. But the flaws differ across studies, so that when the results of a number of studies converge, the convergent results are likely to be valid. For this reason, whenever possible in this report, we ground our conclusions in the accumulated results of multiple studies. In some areas, however, this was impossible and the committee's efforts to answer certain questions were hampered by the lack of adequately sound research.

There are a number of mechanisms that are used by the scientific community to ensure the scientific adequacy of studies, including the peer review process used in scientific and professional journals, the use of scientific advisory panels and review groups, and the use of external reviews of research prior to its execution and/or publication. Many of the studies reviewed in this report failed to incorporate any of these mechanisms, and they frequently failed to employ the research methods most likely to yield interpretable and valid results or failed to report their results in ways that allowed us to adequately evaluate their findings. One conclusion we reached after examining the body of relevant research was that much of it was methodologically weak, and that future research in this area should incorporate such mechanisms as peer review, which will help improve the quality of both the research itself and the research reports that appear in the scientific literature on the effects of alcohol and other drug use on the U.S. work force.

This report is organized into three parts. Following this introduction, Part I first summarizes current knowledge concerning the primary causes and the severity and magnitude of alcohol and other drug use. Chapter 2 provides some insight into the etiology of alcohol and other drug use. Chapter 3 examines the latest prevalence estimates and trends in alcohol and other drug use behavior.

Part II addresses the critical issue of the impact of alcohol and other drug use on behavior. Chapter 4 summarizes a substantial body of literature that has evaluated the effects of various classes of drugs on performance within controlled laboratory settings, including effects of stimulants (e.g., amphetamines, cocaine), sedatives (e.g., benzodiazepines, alcohol), and marijuana. Chapter 5 reviews applied research on the potential causal relationship between alcohol and other drug use and various work-related outcome measures, such as job performance and productivity indicators.

Part III addresses the effectiveness of intervention programs with special emphasis given to drug-testing programs. Given that drug-testing programs are commonplace in American corporations today, the committee felt that special attention to this form of drug use intervention program was imperative.[4] Chapter 6 describes current analytical methods used to test biologic specimens for drugs and discusses the strengths and weaknesses associated with the procedures and techniques for analyzing biological specimens (e.g., urine, hair, saliva). It also reviews indirect methods of assessing drug use, including attitude questionnaires and others. Chapter 7 provides a critical review of studies that have attempted to evaluate the effectiveness of workplace drug-testing programs. Chapter 8 reviews the scientific evidence on the effectiveness of employee assistance programs (EAPs) and workplace prevention programs.

Appendix A addresses basic but critical measurement, methodological, and design issues, and Appendix B addresses relevant drug-testing legal issues.

REFERENCES

Alleyne, B.C., P. Stuart, and R. Copes
  1991   Alcohol and other drug use in occupational fatalities. *Journal of Occupational Medicine* 33(4):496-500.

American Psychiatric Association
  1987   *Diagnostic and Statistical Manual of Mental Disorders*, 3rd ed., revised. Washington, D.C.: American Psychiatric Association.
Ames, G.M.
  1989   Alcohol-related movements and their effects on drinking policies in the American workplace: an historical review. *The Journal of Drug Issues* 19(4):489-510.
Babor, T.F.
  1992   Nosological considerations in the diagnosis of substance use disorders. Pp. 53-74 in

---

[4]Of the 24 million tests performed annually in the United States, 18 million are performed by the approximately 100 NIDA-certified laboratories, 6 million by noncertified laboratories. Cost per test is estimated at approximately $50 (includes laboratory fees, collection site costs, medical review officers costs, and quality control costs). Using these numbers, it is estimated that approximately $1.2 billion per year is spent on drug testing (Michael Walsh, personal communication, 1993).

M. Glantz and R. Pickens, eds., *Vulnerability to Drug Abuse*. Washington, D.C.: American Psychological Association.

Baker, S., J.S. Samkoff, R.S. Fisher, et al.
1982   Fatal occupational injuries. *Journal of the American Medical Association* 248:692-697.

DeHart, R.L.
1990   Medication and the work environment. *Journal of Occupational Medicine* 32(4):310-312.

Dubowski, K.M., and R.S. Tuggle, III
1990   *Drug-Use Testing in the Workplace: Law and Science*. Eau Claire, Wis.: Professional Education Systems, Inc.

Fillmore, K.M.
1984   Research as a handmaiden of policy: an appraisal of estimates of alcoholism and its cost in the workplace. *Journal of Public Health Policy* March:40-64.

Gerstein, D.R., and H.J. Harwood
1990   *Treating Drug Problems*, Vol. 1. Washington, D.C.: National Academy Press.

Glantz, M.D.
1992   A developmental psychopathology model of drug abuse vulnerability. Pp. 389-418 in M. Glantz and R. Pickens, eds., *Vulnerability to Drug Abuse*. Washington, D.C.: American Psychological Association.

Hughes, J.
1992   Clinical importance of caffeine withdrawal—editorial. *New England Journal of Medicine* 327(16):1160-1161.

Humphreys, K., and J. Rappaport
1993   From the community mental health movement to the war on drugs. *American Psychologist* 48(8):892-901.

Journal of Occupational Medicine
1990   Medication-induced performance decrements. *Journal of Occupation Medicine* 32(4):309-370.

Julien, R.M.
1992   *A Primer of Drug Action*, 6th ed. New York: Freeman and Co.

Lempert, R.
1989   Humility is a virtue: on the publicization of policy-relevant research. *Law and Society Review* 23:145-161.

Lewis, R.J., and S.P. Cooper
1989   Alcohol and other drugs, and fatal work-related injuries. *Journal of Occupational Medicine* 31(1):23-28.

National Institute on Drug Abuse
1989   *Annual Emergency Room Data: 1988*. Data from the Drug Abuse Warning Network (DAWN). Rockville, Md.: National Institute on Drug Abuse.

National Transportation Safety Board
1990   *Safety Study: Fatigue, Alcohol, Other Drugs, and Medical Factors in Fatal-to-the-Driver Heavy Truck Crashes*, Vol. 1. NTSB/SS-90-01. Washington, D.C.: National Transportation Safety Board.

Newcomb, M.D.
1992   Substance abuse and controls in the United States: ethical and legal issues. *Social Science and Medicine* 35:471-479.

Potter, W.Z.
1990   Psychotropic medications and work performance. *Journal of Occupational Medicine* 32(4):355-361.

Reuter, P.
   1992   Hawks ascendant: the punitive trend of American drug policy. *Daedalus* 121(3):15-
           52.
Rice, D.P., S. Kelman, L.S. Miller, and S. Dunmeyer
   1990   *The Economic Costs of Alcohol and Drug Abuse and Mental Illness: 1985.* Wash-
           ington, D.C.: U.S. Department of Health and Human Services.
Silverman, K., S.M. Evans, E.C. Strain, and R.R. Griffiths
   1992   Withdrawal syndrome after the double-blind cessation of caffeine consumption. *New
           England Journal of Medicine* 327(16):1109-1114.
Snyder, F.R., and J.E. Henningfield
   1989   Effects of nicotine administration following 12 h of tobacco deprivation: assess-
           ment on computerized performance tasks. *Psychopharmacology* 97:17-22.
Snyder, F.R., F.C. Davis, and J.E. Henningfield
   1989   The tobacco withdrawal syndrome: performance decrements assessed on a comput-
           erized test battery. *Drug and Alcohol Dependence* 23:259-266.
Tilson, H.H.
   1990   Medication monitoring in the workplace: toward improving our system of epidemiologic
           intelligence. *Journal of Occupational Medicine* 32(4):313-319.
U.S. Public Health Service
   1992   *Prevention Report* August/September. Washington, D.C.: U.S. Department of Health
           and Human Services.
World Health Organization
   1990   *International Classification of Diseases, Injuries, and Causes of Death*, 10th ed.
           Geneva: World Health Organization.

I
SCOPE OF ALCOHOL AND OTHER DRUG USE

2

Etiology of Alcohol and Other Drug Use: An Overview of Potential Causes

The underlying causes of alcohol and other drug use and abuse are many, varied, and not well understood. Hundreds of variables have been studied as potential predictors of the onset of alcohol and other drug use. While most alcohol and other drug use initiation occurs with friends or peers who are also using drugs, the stage for this event has been set much earlier by parents, the community, and society.

OVERVIEW

This chapter provides some insight into the causes of alcohol and other drug use and proceeds to focus on the potentially different causes of off- and on-the-job alcohol and other drug use. Finally, it examines the potential influence of environmental factors on workers' alcohol and other drug use.

The individual and social influences that have been investigated can be classified into four categories: (1) the cultural/societal environment, (2) the immediate community, (3) interpersonal forces such as school, peers, and family, and (4) individual factors, including genetics, personality, and attitudes. An individual can be considered "at risk" because of factors or forces within each of these areas. Considerable theoretical and empirical attention has been devoted to each of these possible influences (e.g., Glantz and Pickens, 1992; Galizio and Maisto, 1985; Lettieri, 1985; Lettieri et al., 1980). Hawkins et al. (1992) reviewed the possible risk factors for youth-

TABLE 2.1   Summary of Risk Factors for Drug Use

Domain	Risk Factor
Culture and Society	Laws favorable to drug use Social norms favorable to drug use Availability of drugs Extreme economic deprivations Neighborhood disorganization
Interpersonal	Family use Positive family attitudes toward drug use Poor/inconsistent family management practices Family conflict and disruption Peer rejection Association with drug-using peers
Psychobehavioral	Early/persistent problem behavior Academic failure Low commitment to school Alienation Rebelliousness Favorable attitudes toward drug use Early onset of drug use
Biogenetics	Inherited susceptibility to drug use Psychophysiological vulnerability to drug effects

SOURCE: Adapted from Hawkins et al. (1992).

ful alcohol and other drug use and identified 20 potential causes reflecting the 4 general areas listed above (see Table 2.1). Cultural/societal factors include laws and norms favorable to drug use, the availability of drugs, extreme economic deprivation, and neighborhood disorganization. Interpersonal factors include family alcohol and drug use behavior and attitudes, poor and inconsistent family management practices, family conflict, peer rejection in elementary grades, and association with drug-using peers. Psychobehavioral influences include early and persistent problem behaviors, academic failure, a low degree of commitment to school, alienation and rebelliousness, attitudes favorable to drug use, and early onset of drug use. And biogenetic factors include the possible heritability of a vulnerability to drug abuse and a psychophysiological susceptibility to the effects of drugs. In a comprehensive review of the "risk factor" literature, Clayton (1992) provides a tabulation of the primary topologies and concludes that there is an emergent consensus on the most important risk factors for drug use and abuse.

Within the behavioral sciences it is often stated that the best predictor of future behavior is past behavior. The study of alcohol and other drug use behavior is no exception to this rule. For any given individual, the strongest predictor of current use is past use. Other potential predictors are relatively more important in predicting the initiation of use or the progression of alcohol and other drug abuse. If, however, the question is whether a particular individual is likely to use or abuse drugs in the future, the individual's past history of use and abuse will tell us more about future prospects than the incremental contributions of other variables related to alcohol and other drug use.

The risk for initiating alcohol and other drug use increases for most drugs to a peak during mid- to late adolescence and decreases thereafter (Kandel and Logan, 1984). Tobacco has the youngest age of highest vulnerability, usually in early adolescence. Increased likelihood for beginning alcohol, marijuana, and psychedelics typically occurs in mid-adolescence. Interestingly, the most hazardous age for experimenting with cocaine has typically been young adulthood—about the mid-twenties; however, this pattern for cocaine may be changing due to the emergence of crack, the inexpensive and smokable form of cocaine, which may be more available and alluring to teenagers.

Some types of alcohol and other drug abuse appear to have a genetic component (Cadoret, 1992; Merikangas et al., 1992; Vaillant and Milofsky, 1982), although environmental, social, and psychological factors have received primary attention as causes of the initiation of alcohol and other drug use and progression to abuse (e.g., Sadava, 1987; Zucker and Gomberg, 1986). Attention to the latter factors is appropriate, for biogenetic influences are shaped and modified by personal attributes and environmental conditions (e.g., Marlatt et al., 1988). An important question concerns what precisely is inherited if there is a genetic influence for alcoholism or other drug abuse. Research evidence, primarily but not exclusively based on animal models, suggests at least two mechanisms (e.g., Bardo and Risner, 1985). Those at genetic risk for alcohol and other drug abuse may inherit a biological vulnerability to the hedonic effects of the drug, so for them drug effects are more attractive than for others. They may also not experience the withdrawal effects as severely as those not at risk (i.e., less likelihood of hangover). However, these proposed mechanisms and perhaps others (e.g., inherited behavioral traits; Tarter, 1988) must be evaluated more conclusively in further research (Schuckit, 1987).

Some have suggested that involvement with alcohol and other drugs progresses in a fixed sequence, moving from licit drugs to illicit substances (e.g., Kandel, 1975; Kandel and Faust, 1975). An individual's drug-using career might start with beer, wine, or cigarettes, move to hard liquor, then to marijuana, and subsequently to other illicit drugs, such as amphetamines, cocaine, and heroin. Desistance may occur at any point (O'Donnell and Clayton, 1982), meaning that involvement at one stage does not necessarily lead to involvement at the next stage, but rather that involvement at the next stage is unlikely without prior involvement in the previous stage. Results in various cross-sectional and longitudinal studies have generally confirmed the stage hypothesis with some variations (e.g., Hays et al., 1987; Mills and Noyes, 1984; Newcomb and Bentler, 1986a). Donovan and Jessor (1983), for example, found that problem drinking occurred higher in the progression than general alcohol use, and Newcomb and Bentler (1986a) found that, when the role of cigarettes and nonprescription medications was included, several mini-sequences accounted for drug involvement from early adolescence to young adulthood.

Social factors that determine the availability and the attractiveness of alcohol and other drugs to particular individuals are important to this progression, and highly addictive drugs, such as crack cocaine, may alter this sequence of drug progression. Thus it may be that the severe addictive potential and wide and inexpensive availability of crack may lead to its being used earlier in the sequence than other less addictive illicit drugs or even licit drugs. There are, however, few data currently available to test this notion. The mechanism that drives staging, such as availability, anxiety reduction, peer groups norms, and physiological vulnerability, are not known, but these factors may not be the same at all stages. Peer group norms, for example, might be of vital importance to initiation, while individual psychopathology may figure more in shifts toward the end of the involvement sequence.

Some research suggests that the reasons people begin using alcohol and other drugs are different from the reasons they continue or escalate their use, which is to say, the factors that influence initiation are different from those that influence progression to more serious use. Several researchers have found that initiation is often strongly tied to social and peer influences, whereas biological and psychological processes appear to be associated with abuse (Carman, 1979; Kandel et al., 1978; Newcomb and Bentler, 1990; Paton et al., 1977). Even though data may as yet be too sparse to establish firmly that the causes of use are different from the causes of abuse, the evidence consistent with this hypothesis is accumulating (Glantz and Pickens, 1992).

A wide range of correlates with the initiation of alcohol and other drug use have been identified. They tend to overlap substantially with predictors of general problem behavior or deviance, which is not surprising given the correlation of other problem behaviors with alcohol and other drug use. The primary mechanism for establishing unique predictors of alcohol and other drug use has been longitudinal studies, controlling statistically for other deviant behaviors and attitudes using structural equation modeling methods (Bentler, 1980; Newcomb, 1990). These studies suggest that peer influences (such as modeling use, providing drugs, and encouraging use) are the most consistent and strongest predictors. In addition to the role of prior behavioral experience with alcohol and other drugs and peer influences, other factors associated with initial involvement with drugs include social structural variables, such as socioeconomic status (with heavier use among more disadvantaged groups), family role and socialization variables (with greater use in families with adult drug users, dysfunctional family structures), educational variables (with poor school attachment and performance associated with greater drug use), psychological variables (such as a high need for stimulation), attitudinal variables such as tolerance for deviance (with nontraditionalism associated with greater drug use), behavioral variables such as deviant behaviors and low law abidance (implying greater substance use), emotional variables (such as anxiety and need for excitement), psychopathology (with greater depression and antisocial personality related to higher drug use), temperament and exposure to stressful life events (see Hawkins et al., 1992; Clayton, 1992).

While influences like these have been related to involvement with alcohol and other drug use or abuse, none has ever been found to be a single primary factor that causes alcohol and other drug use or abuse. Indeed, it seems highly unlikely that any one factor or even a few factors will ever be found to account fully for all variations in drug involvement. Because the range of variables leading to initial involvement in alcohol and other drug use is so large, recent views of this phenomenon have emphasized the risk factor notion that is often used in medical epidemiology (Bry et al., 1982; Schreier and Newcomb, 1991a,b). Risk factors include environmental, behavioral, psychological, and social attributes.

Viewing alcohol and other drug involvement as multiply determined suggests that the more risk factors someone is exposed to that encourage use, the more likely he or she is to use or abuse alcohol and other drugs. Exposure to a greater numbers of risk factors is not only a reliable correlate of use, but it also influences the increase in alcohol and other drug use over time, implying a true causal role for those variables that together make for increased risk (Schreier and Newcomb, 1991b). It appears from this approach that the presence of particular factors that can encourage drug use are not as important as the accumulation and interaction of such factors in a person's life.

Protective factors, in contrast to risk factors for alcohol and other drug use, reduce the likelihood and level of drug use and abuse. Protective factors are those psychosocial influences that limit or reduce drug involvement (Newcomb, 1992). Only recently has the risk factors approach to drug use and abuse been expanded to test for multiple protective factors as well (Newcomb, 1992; Newcomb and Felix-Ortiz, 1992). Protective factors may operate through mechanisms other than simply by a direct reduction of alcohol and drug involvement. For example, protective factors have been shown to buffer or moderate the association between risk factors and drug use and abuse (Brook et al., 1992). Recent examples of protective factors that have been found to mitigate the risk of alcohol and other drug use or abuse involve aspects of the environment (e.g., maternal affection—Brook et al., 1989) and the individual (e.g., introversion or self-acceptance—Stacy et al., 1992).

ALCOHOL AND OTHER DRUG USE ON THE JOB

As we discussed in Chapter 1, the definition of terms can significantly shape the problem under study. More specifically, with respect to on-the-job versus off-the-job drug use, Chapter 1 indicates the importance of such a distinction in the study of alcohol and other drug use by the work force. The term *on-the-job drug use* is ambiguous and can mean different things in different studies. Taken literally, the phrase refers only to drugs used at the work site while work is or should be going on. By this definition, a three-martini lunch or a two-joint break would not be considered drug use on the job. Yet many drugs affect work performance for hours, if not days, after consumption. Several self-report measures of workplace drug use ask respondents whether they have used a particular drug on the job. It is unclear whether employees interpret this question to include alcohol and other drugs used just before work, during breaks, or at lunch. Alcohol and other drugs used at these times could lead to workplace impairment even though they do not involve "drug use on the job" if the term is taken literally. The more relevant question might be whether employees have ever been drunk, high, or stoned at work, but this is rarely asked. It is well known that small differences in question wording or even question order can affect survey responses, and attention should be paid to this dynamic in future surveys of workplace drug use.

Patterns of Alcohol and Other Drug Use on the Job

Employers have often been plagued by the occasional alcoholic employee who is frequently absent or tardy or may drink or be drunk on the job. Some employers believe that such behavior is increasing and extends to drugs other than alcohol. However, no large-scale surveys of adult workers exist to substantiate such conclusions.

Alcohol is believed to be the most frequently used drug in the workplace (apart from nicotine and caffeine), but precise comparisons with other drugs and evaluations of their relationship to alcohol cannot be made (Cohen, 1984, 1986). The few surveys that attempt to assess the prevalence of alcohol and other drug use in the work site typically report estimates from management or union sources rather than from employees (e.g., Schreier, 1987; Steele, 1981). Such surveys report the perceptions of knowledgeable observers who are close to the problem, but as a measure of actual alcohol and other drug use they are obviously flawed.

Nevertheless, as discussed in more detail in Chapter 3, a few studies designed specifically to estimate rates of alcohol and other drug use on the job provide tentative estimates of work force alcohol and other drug use. Those studies vary greatly in terms of methods used to assess alcohol and other drug use and when similar methods are used, they often define their measures of alcohol and other drug use differently (e.g., on-the-job drug use).

Although these studies do not provide precise estimates of the rate of alcohol and other drug use by the work force, they do, however, provide information concerning which members of the work force are more likely to use drugs and what drugs are most likely to be used. Rates of self-reported alcohol and other drug use on the job vary according to occupation, age, gender, and ethnicity. Excluding tobacco and caffeine, most surveys find that fewer than 10 percent of workers report having used alcohol or other drugs while on the job during the prior year. Some studies, however, report significantly higher use rates. Much of the difference in the rates reported appears attributable to differences in samples surveyed and questions asked.

It appears that a sizable number of people use alcohol or other drugs regularly, but not at work; others use alcohol or other drugs both at work and away from work. Some use alcohol or other drugs only when they are away from the workplace, and others use alcohol or other drugs only when they are at work. There may also be a group of individuals who use one drug at work and other drugs at home or away from the work site. Researchers have only begun to confront the degree of correspondence between a general proclivity to use alcohol and other drugs and the use of alcohol or other drugs on the job. Often implicit is the yet unproven assumption that the association is quite high, if not perfect. For instance, many discussions of on-the-job drug use cite statistics of general drug use of various populations and argue that alcohol and other drug use in the workplace must be rampant (e.g., Backer, 1987). Since people can choose where to use alcohol and other drugs and what drugs to use, heavy off-the-job use of specific drugs does not mean that those drugs will be used at work. The "weekend drunk" is an example. It is, however, reasonable to assume that at least some general drug use must precede on-the-job use for most people.

Newcomb (1988) found that alcohol and other drug use at work and general alcohol and other drug use were highly, but not perfectly, related (i.e., high general use of drugs did not mean drugs would necessarily be used in the workplace, but the two were clearly associated). In most cases, knowing the extent of general alcohol and other drug use among a sample of individuals predicted less than 50 percent of the variance of on-the-job alcohol and other drug use. Thus the propensity to use alcohol and other drugs on the job varied with the degree of off-the-job alcohol and other drug involvement, but the relationship was not so strong as to justify treating overall alcohol and other drug use prevalence rates as indicators of the likely extent of different types of drug use on the job.

The association that Newcomb found between the use of drugs at and away from work varied by drug combination. For instance, those who reported using marijuana off the job were twice as likely to use alcohol and seven times more likely to use cocaine on the job than those who did not report off-the-job marijuana use (Newcomb, 1988:72-73). Similarly, cigarette smokers were twice as likely to use alcohol on the job and over three times as likely to use marijuana, cocaine, or other hard drugs on the job, as those who did not smoke cigarettes.

Moreover, previous research has revealed that a person's drug use is typically not limited to one specific substance, but often involves the use of various drugs, sometimes more or less simultaneously. This is particularly true for teenagers and for those who use illicit drugs (i.e., marijuana, cocaine), but it has been documented among young adults (Newcomb and Bentler, 1988a,b) and adults (Newcomb, 1992) as well. Clayton and Ritter (1985:83), after examining many studies, concluded that "more often than not, the persons who are using drugs frequently are multiple drug users." Cocaine users, for example, reported significantly higher rates of use for all other types of drugs, including cigarettes, alcohol, marijuana, over-the-counter medications, hypnotics, stimulants, psychedelics, inhalants, narcotics, and PCP, compared with those who had never used cocaine. These large differences were found for both men and women and were prevalent during adolescence as well as young adulthood (e.g., Newcomb and Bentler, 1986b). The association between various types of drug use is so high that common underlying constructs of general polydrug use (Newcomb and Bentler, 1986b) and polydrug use in the workplace (Newcomb, 1988; Stein et al., 1988) have been distinctly and reliably identified.

In an extensive series of analyses of alcohol and other drug use, one of the overriding conclusions reached by Newcomb (1988) was that alcohol and other drug use in the workplace was not typically restricted to single drugs but was highly related to the use of other drugs of both similar and different types. Thus someone caught using marijuana at work is more likely than a random worker to have also used alcohol on the job and far more likely to have used harder drugs. Indeed, Newcomb's study suggests that substance use in the workplace is best characterized as polydrug use at work. The use of one substance at work increases the likelihood of using other drugs in that context.

As we already noted, it appears that alcohol and other drug involvement progresses by stages (Kandel, 1975; Kandel and Faust, 1975). Newcomb (1988) reports data suggesting that using alcohol and other drugs at work reflects a relatively high level of drug involvement. Newcomb's data indicate that using drugs at work is located after both alcohol and marijuana use on the drug involvement continuum for men and subsequent to cocaine use for women. Thus it appears that workplace alcohol and other drug use implies a degree of drug involvement somewhere between that implied by marijuana and cocaine use, on one hand, and cocaine and harder drug use, on the other. The different scaling results for men and women suggest that using alcohol and other drugs at work occurs earlier in the sequence of drug involvement for men than women. This may help explain the gender differences in the prevalence of alcohol and other drug use in the workplace that is reported in Chapter 3. The polydrug use concept is consistent with the view of drug involvement as a staged process defined in large measure by the types of drugs used (e.g., Newcomb and Bentler, 1986b). Those who have tried drugs high in the progression of drug involvement may also continue to use the drugs that do not by themselves characterize high involvement. Indeed, a more elaborate stage model might identify certain configurations of polydrug use as separate stages in the progression of drug involvement.

Predictors of Alcohol and Other Drug Use on the Job

Evidence of social-environmental influences on drug use have led many to believe that job conditions constitute important risk or protective factors with respect to alcohol and other drug use. Among the characteristics of the work environment that have been posited to influence employee alcohol and other drug use are organizational frustration and job stress (Milbourn, 1984), distancing forces, attractions, and constraints (Gupta and Jenkins, 1984), occupational and coworker norms (Shore, 1986), and alcohol and other drug use "enabling" aspects of the work environment (Ames, 1990; Roman et al., 1992).

In empirical tests of these expectations, the primary focus has been on correlates with alcohol and other drug use in general and not specifically with alcohol and other drug use on the job. Markowitz (1984), for example, found that indicators of general alcohol misuse were significantly correlated with less responsibility and autonomy in the workplace. Martin et al. (1992) found that some form of alcohol use was significantly associated with more pressure and fewer extrinsic rewards, although demographic factors (divorced and urban residence) were far more important than these job characteristics.

A few studies have directly examined the relationship of job characteristics as they relate to actual alcohol and other drug use on the job. Lehman and Simpson (1992) found that alcohol and other drug use at work was directly correlated with male gender, depression, not working in an office, job dissatisfaction, job tension, accidents, and absences; it was inversely correlated with age, education, faith in management, job involvement, and organizational commitment. Some of these correlations appear to be causally related to alcohol and other drug use (e.g., age); others are the likely results of use (e.g., accidents); and for still others the relationship is likely to be bidirectional (e.g., organizational involvement). In a different analysis of this data set, Lehman et al. (1991) found seven significant predictors of alcohol and other drug use at work: (1) not being married, (2) having been arrested, (3) low self-esteem, (4) high peer drug use, (5) working alone or in a small group, (6) having a high-risk job, and (7) low job involvement.

Mensch and Kandel (1988) examined various job dimensions as possible correlates of on-the-job marijuana use for men and women. They found eight small, but significant correlates of using marijuana at work among men: (1) low skill discretion, (2) low decision authority, (3) high job insecurity, (4) low supervisor support, (5) high physical demands, (6) high hazardous exposure, (7) low substantive complexity, and (8) high motor skills. Among women, marijuana use on the job was significantly correlated with five job characteristics: (1) low skill discretion, (2) low decision authority, (3) high coworker support, (4) low substantive complexity, and (5) high physical demands.

Mangione and Quinn (1975) examined relationships between alcohol and other drug use on the job and job satisfaction among men and women above and below age 30. There were no significant correlations between alcohol and other drug use in the workplace and job satisfaction for either group of women. The only significant correlation was found for men 30 years or older—but it was small (r = −.12).

Using ethnographic methods, Ames (1990) found that certain aspects of the work environment, as well as ambiguous or conflicting responsibilities of supervisors, encouraged drinking on the job. They characterized these aspects of the working environment as enabling influences for on-the-job alcohol use.

Newcomb (1988) has presented a comprehensive set of both cross-sectional and prospective survey findings on the correlates and predictors of alcohol and other drug use in the workplace. He examined many personal, social, and work-related factors in terms of their associations with using alcohol and other drugs on the job. Demographically, Newcomb found that those most likely to use alcohol and other drugs in the workplace were male, either black (for use of marijuana) or white (for use of other drugs), had few educational plans, had cohabited sometime in their life, had no children, and were not currently married. Higher income was related to greater use of cocaine and harder drugs. A wide range of personality, emotional functioning, social support, and problem variables were examined as possible correlates of alcohol and other drug use in the workplace. Several small, but significant, effects were found. Using alcohol or other drugs at work was slightly but significantly related to relationship and family problems and emotional distress. Alcohol and other drug use at work was most highly related to having drug and alcohol problems, being low in law abidance, being liberal, feeling powerless, and lacking fear of injury. In other words, alcohol and other drug use in the workplace typically does not appear to result from life problems or general unhappiness (although a few small associations in these variables were found). It was most related to general nonconformity, low fearfulness, having some trouble with an intimate relationship, off-the-job drug or alcohol problems, and feeling powerless.

Workplace alcohol and other drug use was not highly related to such work-related variables as income, collecting public assistance, hours worked, and support for work problems. It was most strongly related to job instability (frequently being fired), committing vandalism at work, and somewhat less strongly to job dissatisfaction. Alcohol and other drug use in the workplace was only slightly but significantly related to problems and unhappiness in the workplace.

To summarize, Newcomb's studies indicate that alcohol and other drug use in the workplace appears to be more a function of the personal qualities of individuals, rather than functions of their work environments. Alcohol and other drug use on the job is strongly related to such personality characteristics as rebelliousness, nonconformity, deviance, and perhaps acting out; the prospective studies reveal that people with such traits are more likely than others to use alcohol and other drugs at work at later points in time. Based on Newcomb's studies, it appears that alcohol and other drug use on the job is neither largely nor generally situationally determined, but is a manifestation of a general syndrome of problem behaviors, both related to and separate from alcohol and other drug use. But some of the other studies reviewed by the committee do show small but not always consistent workplace environment effects.

Several reviews of the literature reach conclusions similar to those of Newcomb. For instance, Harris and Heft (1992:241) concluded that "though statistically significant in some cases, the relationship between work conditions and drug/alcohol consumption appears to be quite small." Over a decade earlier, Herold and Conlon (1981:337) reached the same conclusion regarding the association between work factors and alcohol abuse, stating that "unequivocal evidence of such linkages is scarce."

There are, however, problems with this general conclusion, which mean that the work environment cannot be ruled out as a contributing or interactive factor for generating alcohol and other drug use among workers or protecting them from it. All the studies that find that personality variables dwarf work environment variables are biased by an imbalance in the use of individual and job condition and attitude measures. Some studies measure many individual traits but have relatively few measures of job conditions; in a few others, the imbalance is reversed. One might expect that the more variables used to measure a domain, the greater the amount of variance attributable to a domain and the more likely some significant relationships will be revealed. These complexities are confounded by the fact that no existing study has been designed to test directly and explicitly whether alcohol and other drug use on the job is associated more or less with personal qualities (i.e., traits) or job characteristics (e.g., role ambiguity, stress, shift work) when appropriate and thorough measures of both domains have been gathered.

Moreover, most existing studies employ models that assume only direct or main effects of work environment on alcohol and other drug use. This perspective is too narrow. As several reviews have noted, the associations between work environment and on- or off-the-job alcohol and other drug use are likely to be far more complex (e.g., Martin et al., 1992). They may involve intervening variables (e.g., Violanti et al., 1983), generalization processes (e.g., Martin et al., 1992), influence by individual differences (Conway et al., 1981), as well as interactions or moderated relationships between personal characteristics and job conditions (e.g., Brief and Folger, 1992). For example, a poor work environment may lead to family stresses that promote alcohol and other drug use, or those with low self-esteem may be prone to use alcohol and other drugs on the job, but only on those jobs in which supervisors are authoritarian and seldom give positive feedback. Because of possibilities like these and the shortcomings of the extant research, we cannot conclude that the work environment does not affect worker alcohol and other drug use both on and off the job to an important extent. More comprehensive analyses and tests of more realistic theories are necessary to sort out the relative impact of work environment and individual traits on worker alcohol and other drug use and the ways in which variables in these domains relate to each other.

Nature Versus Nurture in Alcohol and Other Drug Use on the Job

Data on different levels of alcohol and other drug use across occupations that are discussed in Chapter 3 raise an important issue. That is, are these occupational differences explained in part by the social dynamics of particular occupations, or are they the result of the individual characteristics of those who gravitate toward certain occupations? Okinuora (1984) and

Plant (1981) identified several risk factors that were related to the connection between occupation and alcoholism. These included the availability of alcohol at work, social pressure to drink on the job, separation from normal social relationships, freedom from supervision, very high or very low income, collusion by colleagues, strains, stresses, and hazards, and self-selection for high-risk occupations.

The association between job type and alcohol or other drug use may be because those with a propensity to use drugs are attracted to particular positions/occupations (e.g., alcoholics may find brewery jobs enticing), because particular job conditions are conducive to drug use (e.g., brewery workers may find it hard to resist social pressures to drink), or to some combination of causal possibilities. Plant (1978, 1979) attempted to tease apart these possibilities by studying new recruits to the liquor or brewery trade (a very high-risk occupation) and comparing them with those applying for jobs at low risk for alcohol problems. He found that those who sought liquor and brewery jobs had poorer employment records and were heavier drinkers prior to their employment than were applicants to lower-risk occupations. This supports the self-selection hypothesis. He also found, however, that those in the liquor industry increased their drinking behavior (including on-the-job drinking) in conformity to perceived social norms. Thus it appears that self-selection and environmental pressures combine to account for the high rates of alcoholism that are found in the alcoholic beverage industry.

In a study of prevalence rates for lifetime cocaine use (Trinkoff et al., 1990) reported that among 6 job categories studied, the skilled labor category had the highest level of lifetime cocaine use (12 percent) followed by management professionals (8 percent), technical/sales/support (8 percent), service (7 percent), farm/forest/fishing (7 percent), and unskilled labor with the lowest rate of 6 percent. The authors point out that such rates were strongly related to education level and varied substantially across age groups with the highest reported rates observed among respondents below age 35. In another prevalence study Trinkoff et al. (1991) analyzed a different subset of data from the Epidemiologic Catchment Area Program to estimate rate of alcohol and other drug use among nurses and compared those rates to a matched control group of employed non-nurses. Their results showed that nurses were no more likely to have engaged in illicit drug use than non-nurses. However nurses were found to be less likely to have experienced problems with alcohol abuse than non-nurses. Unfortunately, prevalence estimates on specific drug types, other than alcohol, were unstable with large confidence intervals due to the missing data and the small size of the samples studied.

Cosper (1979) and Cosper and Hughes (1982) challenged the notion that occupations associated with heavy drinking are disproportionately characterized by alcohol abuse or alcoholism. They suggested that the frequency, but not the quantity, of drinking is higher in certain occupations, and that the frequency of drinking may not reflect problem levels. They suggest that conformity to the unique norms of an occupation may generate differences in drinking behavior and thus may not indicate deviance or low social conformity. Although this may be true in certain jobs (they studied naval officers and journalists), it does not account for the differential treatment rates for alcohol and other drugs nor for mortality differences observed in other studies.

Alcohol and Other Drug Use by Occupation and Context

Several recent studies have identified industries or job categories that have different risks for on-the-job alcohol and other drug use. Lehman et al. (1990) found the highest rates of alcohol and other drug use in the workplace for skilled, technical, paraprofessional, and service occupations (ranging from 3 to 4 percent) and the lowest for professional and clerical positions (from 0 to 1 percent). Mensch and Kandel (1988), in exploring similar occupations, found interactions between job sector, drug type, and gender. Among men, the recreation, entertainment, and construction industries were associated with the highest rates of alcohol, marijuana, and cocaine use on the job. Among women, alcohol use at work was most likely in the agriculture, forestry, and fishery industries; marijuana use on the job most often occurred in construction jobs, and cocaine was most prevalent on the job in the transportation sector. Gleason et al. (1991) found that the highest prevalence rates of drug use on the job were in the construction and entertainment/recreation industries, whereas the lowest rates were found in the professional services and public administration industries.

Results from the High School Senior survey presented in detail in Chapter 3 indicate that military and protective services occupational groups (e.g., police, fire fighters) had very low rates of use at work. Reported alcohol use at work (at least once in the previous 12 months) was highest for men in professional, skilled, and managerial or semiskilled jobs. Women were only slightly lower than men in their rate of using alcohol. The High School Senior follow-up survey revealed greater variation in marijuana use at work. Between 9 and 10 percent of skilled and semiskilled male workers had smoked marijuana at work, compared with less than 5 percent in any of the other gender-occupation categories. Skilled and semiskilled male workers were also more likely to report having used cocaine at work; 2 to 4 percent said they had done so. The situation was different for the nonmedical use of psychotherapeutic drugs. Amphetamine use was highest among female skilled workers, with prevalence rates of 4 percent, while male and female semiskilled workers and men in the military had rates of around 3 percent. About 3 percent of female skilled workers had taken tranquilizers at work; no other group much exceeded 1 percent.

CONCLUSIONS AND RECOMMENDATIONS

- The most vulnerable age and primary risk factors associated with drug use initiation typically precede an individual's entry into the work force. This fact has important implications for work-related prevention interventions designed to prevent the onset of drug use. This means that workplace interventions may have only limited effects on preventing initiation into most categories of drug use.

- Most alcohol and other drug users do not develop patterns of clinically defined abuse or dependence. The progression from use to abuse and dependence varies with drug type as well as with factors that are specific to individuals and their environments. It is not possible, however, to predict with great accuracy which alcohol and other drug users will become abusers or will eventually need treatment.

- If use and abuse have different causes, it follows that they are likely to benefit from different types of interventions, so it is important to further explore the hypothesis that any type of drug or alcohol use at the work site in fact reflects abuse.

- Among illicit drug users, polydrug use, most often including the use of alcohol and tobacco, is the norm rather than the exception.

Recommendation: In evaluating the impact of alcohol and other drug use on behavior, specific attention should be paid to the actions of drugs in combination.

- Based on the sparse empirical evidence accumulated to date, alcohol and other drug use by the work force appears to be more a function of the personal qualities of individuals than of their work environments. However, most studies of why workers use alcohol and other drugs have serious methodological flaws. Hence, the work environment cannot be ruled out as a contributing or interactive factor in generating use among workers or protecting them from it.

Recommendation: Research is still needed to sort out the relative impact of the work environment and individual traits on workers' alcohol and other drug use. This research should test realistic theories involving such potential critical variables such as drug availability, local norms, and work stress and attending to such complexities as interaction effects can reverse causation.

REFERENCES

Ames, G.M.
  1990   The workplace as an enabling environment for alcohol problems. *Anthropology of Work Review* 11:12-16.
Backer, T. E.
  1987   *Strategic Planning for Workplace Drug Abuse Problems.* Rockville, Md.: National Institute on Drug Abuse.
Bardo, M.T., and M.E. Risner
  1985   Biochemical substrates of drug abuse. Pp. 65-99 in M. Galizio and S.A. Maisto, eds., *Determinants of Substance Abuse: Biological, Psychological, and Environmental Factors.* New York: Plenum Press.
Bentler, P.M.
  1980   Multivariate analysis with latent variables: Causal modeling. *Annual Review of Psychology* 31:419-456.
Brief, A.P., and R.G. Folger
  1992   The workplace and problem drinking as seen by two novices. *Alcoholism: Clinical and Experimental Research* 16:190-198.
Brook, J.S., C. Nomura, and P. Cohen
  1989   Prenatal, perinatal, and early childhood risk factors and drug involvement in adolescence. *Genetic, Social, and General Psychology Monographs* 115:223-241.
Brook, J.S., P. Cohen, M. Whiteman, and A.S. Gordon
  1992   Psychosocial risk factors in the transition from moderate to heavy use or abuse of drugs. Pp. 359-388 in M.D. Glantz and R. Pickens, eds., *Vulnerability to Drug Abuse.* Washington, D.C.: American Psychological Association.
Bry, B.H., P. McKeon, and R. Pandina
  1982   Extent of drug use as a function of number of risk factors. *Journal of Abnormal Psychology* 91:273-279.
Cadoret, R.J.
  1992   Genetic and environmental factors in initiation of drug use and the transition to abuse. Pp. 99-114 in M.D. Glantz and R. Pickens, eds., *Vulnerability to Drug Abuse.* Washington, D.C.: American Psychological Association.
Carman, R.S.
  1979   Motivations for drug use and problematic outcomes among rural junior high school students. *Addictive Behaviors* 4:91-93.
Clayton, R.R.
  1992   Transitions in drug use: risk and protective factors. Pp. 15-52 in M. Glantz and R. Pickens, eds., *Vulnerability to Drug Abuse.* Washington, D.C.: American Psychological Association.
Clayton, R.R., and C. Ritter
  1985   The epidemiology of alcohol and drug abuse among adolescents. *Advances in Alcohol and Substance Abuse* 4:69-97.
Cohen, S.
  1984   Drugs in the workplace. *Journal of Clinical Psychiatry* 45:4-8.
  1986   Drug urinalysis: selected questions. *Drug Abuse and Alcoholism Newsletter* 15:10.
Conway, T.L., R.R. Vickers, H.W. Ward, and R.H. Rahe
  1981   Occupational stress and variation in cigarette, coffee, and alcohol consumption. *Journal of Health and Social Behavior* 22:155-165.
Cosper, R.
  1979   Drinking as conformity. *Journal of Studies on Alcohol* 40:868-891.
Cosper, R., and F. Hughes
  1982   So-called heavy drinking occupations. *Journal of Studies on Alcohol* 43:110-118.

Donovan, J.E., and R. Jessor
1983   Problem drinking and the dimensions of involvement with drugs: a Guttman scalogram analysis of adolescent drug use. *American Journal of Public Health* 73:543-552.

Galizio, M., and S.A. Maisto, eds.
1985   *Determinants of Substance Abuse: Biological, Psychological, and Environmental Factors.* New York: Plenum Press.

Glantz, M.D., and R.W. Pickens
1992   Vulnerability to drug abuse: introduction and overview. Pp. 1-14 in M. Glantz and R. Pickens, eds., *Vulnerability to Drug Abuse.* Washington, D.C.: American Psychological Association.

Gleason, P.M., J.R. Veu, and M.R. Pergamit
1991   Drug and alcohol use at work: a survey of young workers. *Monthly Labor Review* August:3-7.

Gupta, N., and G.D. Jenkins, Jr.
1984   Substance use as an employee response to work environment. *Journal of Vocational Behavior* 24:84-93.

Harris, M.M., and L.L. Heft
1992   Alcohol and drug use in the workplace: issues, controversies, and directions for future research. *Journal of Management* 18:239-266.

Hawkins, J.D., R.F. Catalano, and J.Y. Miller
1992   Risk and protective factors for alcohol and other drug problems in adolescence and early adulthood: implications for substance abuse problems. *Psychological Bulletin* 112:64-105.

Hays, R.D., K.F. Widaman, M.R. DiMatteo, and A.W. Stacy
1987   Structural equation models of current drug use: are appropriate models so simple? *Journal of Personality and Social Psychology* 52:134-144.

Herold, D.M., and E.J. Conlon
1981   Work factors as potential causal agents of alcohol abuse. *Journal of Drug Issues* 11:337-356.

Kandel, D.B.
1975   Stages in adolescent involvement in drug use. *Science* 190:912-914.

Kandel, D.B., and R. Faust
1975   Sequence and stages in patterns of adolescent drug use. *Archives of General Psychiatry* 32:923-932.

Kandel, D.B., and J.A. Logan
1984   Patterns of drug use from adolescence to young adulthood: I: Periods of risk for initiation, continued use, and discontinuation. *American Journal of Public Health* 74:660-666.

Kandel, D.B., R.C. Kessler, and R.Z. Margulies
1978   Antecedents of adolescent initiation into stages of drug use: a developmental analysis. In D.B. Kandel, ed., *Longitudinal Research on Drug Use: Empirical Findings and Methodological Issues.* Washington, D.C.: Hemisphere.

Lehman, W.E.K., and D.D. Simpson
1992   Employee substance use and on-the-job behaviors. *Journal of Applied Psychology* 77:309-321.

Lehman, W.E.K., D.J. Farabee, M.L. Holcom, and D.D. Simpson
1991   Prediction of Substance Use in the Workplace: Unique Contributions of Demographic and Work Environment Variables. Unpublished manuscript, Institute of Behavioral Research, Texas Christian University, Fort Worth.

Lehman, W.E.K., M.L. Holcom, and D.D. Simpson
1990   Employee Health and Performance in the Workplace: A Survey of Municipal Em-

ployees of a Large Southwest City. Unpublished manuscript, Institute of Behavioral Research, Texas Christian University, Fort Worth.

Lettieri, D.J.
1985   Drug abuse: a review of explanations and models of explanations. *Advances in Alcohol and Substance Abuse* 4:9-40.

Lettieri, D.J., M. Sayers, and H.W. Pearson, eds.
1980   *Theories on Drug Abuse: Selected Contemporary Perspectives.* Rockville, Md.: National Institute on Drug Abuse.

Mangione, T.W., and R.P. Quinn
1975   Short note: job satisfaction, counter-productive behavior, and drug use at work. *Journal of Applied Psychology* 60:114-116.

Markowitz, M.
1984   Alcohol misuse as a response to perceived powerlessness in the organization. *Journal of Studies on Alcohol* 45:225-227.

Marlatt, G.A., J.S. Baer, D.M. Donovan, and D.R. Kivlahan
1988   Addictive behaviors: etiology and treatment. *Annual Review of Psychology* 39:223-252.

Martin, J.K., T.C. Blum, and P.M. Roman
1992   Drinking to cope and self-medication: characteristics of jobs in relation to workers' drinking behavior. *Journal of Organizational Behavior* 13:55-71.

Mensch, B.S., and D.B. Kandel
1988   Do job conditions influence the use of drugs? *Journal of Health and Social Behavior* 29:169-184.

Merikangas, K.R., B.J. Rounsaville, and B.A. Prusoff
1992   Familial factors in vulnerability to substance abuse. Pp. 75-98 in M.D. Glantz and R. Pickens, eds., *Vulnerability to Drug Abuse.* Washington, D.C.: American Psychological Association.

Milbourn, G.
1984   Alcoholism, drug abuse, job stress: what small business can do. *American Journal of Small Business* 8:36-48.

Mills, C.J., and H.L. Noyes
1984   Patterns and correlates of initial and subsequent drug use among adolescents. *Journal of Consulting and Clinical Psychology* 52:231-243.

Newcomb, M.D.
1988   *Drug Use in the Workplace: Risk Factors for Disruptive Substance Use Among Young Adults.* Dover, Mass.: Auburn House.
1990   Losing the War on Drugs: Are We Too Addicted to the Quick Fix to Seek the Ultimate Fix. Paper presented to United States Congress sponsored by the Federation of Behavioral, Psychological, and Cognitive Sciences, Washington, D.C.
1992   Understanding the multidimensional nature of drug use and abuse: the role of consumption, risk factors, and protective factors. Pp. 255-297 in M.D. Glantz and R. Pickens, eds., *Vulnerability to Drug Abuse.* Washington, D.C.: American Psychological Association.

Newcomb, M.D., and P.M. Bentler
1986a   Cocaine use among adolescents: longitudinal associations with social context, psychopathology, and use of other substances. *Addictive Behaviors* 11:263-273.
1986b   Cocaine use among young adults. *Advances in Alcohol and Substance Abuse* 6:73-96.
1988a   *Consequences of Adolescent Drug Use: Impact on the Lives of Young Adults.* Beverly Hills, Calif.: Sage Publications.

1988b Impact of adolescent drug use and social support on problems of young adults: a longitudinal study. *Journal of Abnormal Psychology* 97:64-75.

1990 Antecedents and consequences of cocaine use: an eight-year study from early adolescence to young adulthood. Pp. 158-181 in L. Robins, ed., *Straight and Devious Pathways from Childhood to Adulthood.* Cambridge, Mass.: Cambridge Press.

Newcomb, M.D., and M. Felix-Ortiz

1992 Multiple protective and risk factors for drug use and abuse: cross-sectional and prospective findings. *Journal of Personality and Social Psychology* 63:280-296.

O'Donnell, J.A., and R.R. Clayton

1982 The stepping-stone hypothesis: marijuana, heroin, and causality. *Chemical Dependencies: Behavioral and Biomedical Issues* 4:229-241.

Okinuora, M.

1984 Alcoholism and occupation. *Scandinavian Journal of Work and Environmental Health* 10:511-515.

Paton, S., R.C. Kessler, and D.B. Kandel

1977 Depressive mood and illegal drug use: a longitudinal analysis. *Journal of Genetic Psychology* 131:267-289.

Plant, M.A.

1978 Occupation and alcoholism: cause or effect? A controlled study of recruits to the drink trade. *International Journal of the Addictions* 13:605-626.

1979 Occupations, drinking patterns and alcohol-related problems: conclusions from a follow-up study. *British Journal of Addiction* 74:267-273.

1981 Risk factors in employment. In B.D. Hore and M.A. Plant eds., *Alcohol Problems in Employment.* London: Croom Helm.

Roman, P.M., T.C. Blum, and J.K. Martin

1992 Enabling of male problem drinkers in work groups. *British Journal of Addiction* 87:275-298.

Sadava, S.W.

1987 Interactional theories. In H.T. Blane and K.E. Leonard, eds., *Psychological Theories of Drinking and Alcoholism.* New York: Guilford.

Schreier, J.W.

1987 *Substance Abuse in Organizations, 1971-1986: Realities, Trends, Reactions.* Milwaukee, Wis.: Far Cliffs Consulting.

Schreier, L.M., and M.D. Newcomb

1991a Differentiation of early adolescent predictors of drug use versus abuse: a developmental risk factor model. *Journal of Substance Abuse* 3:277-299.

1991b Psychosocial predictors of drug use initiation and escalation: an expansion of the multiple risk factors hypothesis using longitudinal data. *Contemporary Drug Problems* 18:31-73.

Schuckit, M.A.

1987 Biological vulnerability to alcoholism. *Journal of Consulting and Clinical Psychology* 3:301-309.

Shore, E.R.

1986 Norms regarding drinking behavior in the business environment. *Journal of Social Psychology* 125:735-741.

Stacy, A.W., M.D. Newcomb, and P.M. Bentler

1992 Interactive and higher-order effects of social influences on drug use. *Journal of Health and Social Behavior* 33:226-241.

Steele, P.D.

1981 Labor perceptions of drug use and drug problems in the workplace. *Journal of Drug Issues* 11:279-292.

Stein, J. A., M.D. Newcomb, and P.M. Bentler
   1988   Structure of drug use behaviors and consequences among young adults: multitrait-multimethod assessment of frequency, quantity, work site, and problem substance use. *Journal of Applied Psychology* 73:595-605.

Tarter, R.E.
   1988   Are there inherited behavioral traits that predispose to substance abuse? *Journal of Consulting and Clinical Psychology* 56:189-196.

Trinkoff, A.M., C. Ritter, and J.C. Anthony
   1990   The prevalence and self-reported consequences of cocaine use: an exploratory and descriptive analysis. *Drug and Alcohol Dependence* 26:217-225.

Trinkoff, A.M., W.W. Eaton, and J.C. Anthony
   1991   The prevalence of substance abuse among registered nurses. *Nursing Research* 40(3):172-175.

Vaillant, G., and E. Milofsky
   1982   The etiology of alcoholism: a prospective viewpoint. *American Psychologist* 37:494-503.

Violanti, J., J. Marshall, and B. Howe
   1983   Police occupational demands, psychological distress and the coping function of alcohol. *Journal of Occupational Medicine* 25:455-458.

Zucker, R.A., and E.S.L. Gomberg
   1986   Etiology of alcoholism reconsidered: the case for a biopsychosocial approach. *American Psychologist* 41:783-793.

3

Epidemiological Evidence:
The Dimensions of the Problem

This chapter presents epidemiological evidence regarding drug use from a number of sources and different populations and discusses its implications for the workplace. The studies reviewed provide data on prevalence and trends in alcohol and other drug use by the U.S. work force, including use in general—for which there is considerable information—and use on the job—for which there is relatively little information.

There is a wide array of studies that examine the prevalence and impact of drug use in the workplace; some of the more recent work is summarized in two NIDA monographs, edited by Gust et al. (1990) and Gust and Walsh (1989). The most informative data come from four sources that are reviewed in this chapter: large-scale surveys conducted over the last two decades, large-scale drug testing among employed people, organization-specific studies, and other studies assessing on-the-job drug use.

Three large-scale survey series have closely examined issues that concern this study: the High School Senior surveys (HSS) and their follow-up component on college-age youth and young adults; the National Household Surveys on Drug Abuse (NHSDA); and the Worldwide Surveys of Substance Abuse and Health Behaviors Among Military Personnel (MWS). These surveys provide several perspectives about drug use and the work force. The HHS surveys, with their follow-up components, furnish data about youth who are prospective workers, who have just recently entered the work force, or who are relatively young members of the work force. The NHSDA surveys offer data on drug use among the general household population and about the subset of this population who constitute the mainstream workers in the nation. The MWS surveys contribute data on a large but distinctive work force, the U.S. military. The self-report data from these studies are compared with data obtained from a large-scale drug-testing monitoring project across work sites. The chapter also examines organization-specific studies that have assessed the prevalence of alcohol and other drug use within specific organizations based on self-reports and/or urinalysis. Finally, the chapter looks at studies that have attempted to assess the prevalence rates of on-the-job drug use.

Over the past 15 years, there has been substantial epidemiological research conducted on drug abuse. This chapter does not exhaustively review all of this work, but looks at those studies that best allow us to provide sound estimates of prevalence and trends of alcohol and other drug use by the work force. From time to time we call on other sources of data (e.g., the National Longitudinal Survey, the Drug Abuse Warning Network data [DAWN], the Drug Use Forecasting system data [DUF]) to complement the primary data sources.

In reviewing research in this area, we highlight some of the strengths and limitations of self-report and urinalysis data. Specific methodological and measurement weaknesses associated with the primary data sources relied on in this chapter are addressed in their respective sections. More general limitations associated with epidemiological research are addressed in Appendix A (e.g., self-report measures).

SURVEY AND DRUG-TESTING APPROACHES: STRENGTHS AND LIMITATIONS

The methodological differences between data obtained from surveys and from work site drug testing mean that one can expect to gain from these sources somewhat differing pictures of alcohol and other drug use. Surveys designed to estimate the prevalence of drug use suffer from that very fact; their purposes are transparent and sensitive, and respondents may not give candid answers. Drug-testing programs, in contrast, have not been developed to provide prevalence estimates, but the widespread implementation of testing programs may allow aggregate test results to serve as a broad barometer of drug use among the work force. Using results of urine testing as an epidemiologic tool serves a complementary role to studies based on self-reports such as the three large-scale survey series we examine.

Urine testing, done with appropriate quality control procedures, provides an objective indicator of recent drug use, which complements the subjectivity of survey studies. Drug-testing results are readily available in large numbers. Approximately 100 laboratories certified by the National Institute on Drug Abuse conduct much of the work site drug testing. These laboratories typically store test results in computer files, a procedure that allows large numbers of test results to be easily accumulated.

At the same time, drug test results do have limitations as epidemiologic indicators. Applicants and employees are selected for testing for corporate rather than statistical sampling reasons. Consequently, those tested are not a random sample of the work force population, and drug use estimates based on test results are likely to be biased. Most drug testing is designed to detect between five and eight drugs. Most work site urine testing protocols, for example, do not test for alcohol; thus, no reliable test-based information can be provided about this drug. Moreover, positive urine test results indicate only that a person has recently used a particular drug, typically, in the past 2 to 7 days, varying with the drug tested. Heavy marijuana use, however, can produce positive results for up to a month after cessation of use. Moreover, positive rates at NIDA-certified laboratories will be inflated due to the required blind-spiked quality control samples that are submitted to all certified laboratories as part of the NIDA certification process. Furthermore, test results, either positive or negative, also provide no information on patterns of use such as frequency, amount or place of use (e.g., off or on the job). In contrast, studies based on self-reports generally inquire into alcohol and other drug use over an extended period of time, frequently the previous month, year, or lifetime. Self-report studies typically ask about the amount and frequency of use to distinguish casual from regular or heavy users and occasionally inquire about the context or social setting in which the drug was used.

Changes in drug-testing programs, usually to encompass new situations or new groups of workers or applicants, hamper longitudinal comparisons of drug use unless specific information on reasons for testing and types of people tested is linked to test results in the computerized data base. Even then, labs and industries perceive little reason to link wide-ranging demographic or attitudinal information to test results, although such information would allow for a far richer analysis of the types of people who use drugs and a more comprehensive study of trends in drug use over time. Currently available work site drug-testing data banks can provide valuable information on differences in prevalence rates across types of industries and on the relative frequency of use of specific drugs, but much more could be learned if additional data were systematically collected.

Survey data, such as those from the three studies that are the focus of much of this chapter's discussion, often use sophisticated sampling techniques that allow for precise estimates of drug use for well-defined populations. They also collect demographic information that allows for estimates of alcohol and other drug use within population subgroups. Survey results, however, are subject to the potential bias of self-reports as well as to the ambiguities caused by questions that are subject to varying interpretations.

The populations they represent often exclude groups, like high school dropouts, who are part of the work force. In addition, surveys are relatively expensive to conduct, so sample sizes even in large-scale studies may have too few members of particular subgroups or users of particular drugs to allow for the computation of reliable estimates.

Thus, in investigating trends in alcohol and other drug use, both surveys and drug test data have their uses and limits. When the implications of the two types of data converge, we may have increased confidence in the jointly suggested conclusions. But because of the nature of these two data sources, far more could be learned if individual survey data designed to capture demographic traits and worker attitudes could be combined with drug test results of the millions of people tested for drugs each year.

Interestingly, both demographic and attitudinal/personality data are often routinely collected in the preemployment setting, in which most job-related drug testing occurs. Employers typically require personal background information from job applicants and often give applicants additional personality and other tests. Those data, however, are rarely accessible for research, since they are not usually linked to drug test results. If a link could be made, considerably more could be learned about trends in and correlates of drug use.

LARGE-SCALE SURVEYS

The three survey series we review are similar in that they provide estimates of illicit drug use based on self-reports of representative samples of the populations under study. Illicit drug use, as measured in these surveys, involves the use of illegal drugs and the nonmedical use of prescription-type psychotherapeutic drugs. Respondents are typically asked about their use of such drugs in the month or year preceding the survey.

The surveys all asked about use of marijuana (including hashish); hallucinogens (including phencyclidine or PCP and lysergic acid diethylamide or LSD); cocaine (including crack); heroin and other opiates; inhalants such as lighter fluids, aerosol sprays, glue, paint thinners, and cleaning fluids; and the nonmedical use of prescription-type psychotherapeutic drugs (i.e., stimulants, sedatives, tranquilizers, and analgesics used without a doctor's prescription or for purposes other than intended). In addition, the surveys gathered information about alcohol use and cigarette smoking.

The different surveys, however, define "heavy drinking" somewhat differently. For the HSS, heavy drinking refers to 5 or more drinks in a row at least once in the prior 2 weeks. For the NHSDA, heavy drinking refers to the consumption of five or more drinks on the same drinking occasion on 5 or more days in the last 30 days. For the MWS, the definition of heavy drinking is similar to that of the NHSDA and refers to consumption of 5 or more drinks of beer, wine, or liquor per typical drinking occasion at least once a week.

Definitions of cigarette smokers are similar with some slight variations. All of the surveys asked respondents about smoking cigarettes during various time periods (lifetime, past year, past month). The HHS and the NHSDA define smokers as those who have smoked one or more cigarettes during those periods. The MWS definition is similar, but for past month use, which is the primary measure (i.e., current smokers), it incorporates an additional criterion that individuals must have smoked at least 100 cigarettes (i.e., five or more packs) during their lifetime.

High School Senior Surveys

The High School Senior surveys are an ongoing study of young Americans, conducted by the Institute for Social Research at the University of Michigan (Johnston et al., 1992). The studies began with the high school class of 1975, and follow-up surveys began with the class of 1976. Thus, through 1991, the population surveyed consists of young American men and women ages 18 to 33 who were not high school dropouts. For present purposes, high school seniors and high school graduates ages 19 to 28 are discussed in this report (because sufficient trend data exist for the latter). The HSS respondents who are in the work force are young workers, members of the age group most likely to be involved with alcohol and other drug use, particularly illicit drug use.

Prevalence and Trends in Illicit Drug Use

Over the past 10 years there have been appreciable declines in the use of a number of illicit drugs among high school seniors and over the past 5 years (for which data are available) among young adults more generally. Figure 3.1 shows trends for any illicit drug use and heavy alcohol use along with marijuana use and cocaine use among high school seniors: more than half of the high school classes of 1977 through 1981 had used an illicit drug during their senior year, a proportion peaking at 54 percent for the class of 1979; this statistic fell gradually, reaching 29 percent for the class of 1991. The decline in recent years is also evident among young adults ages 19 to 28, as shown in Figure 3.2. In 1991, 27 percent of these young adults reported having used an illegal drug at least once in the past 12 months; that statistic was over 40 percent as recently as 1986 (the first year for which the data are available for this age range). Clearly, new workers entering the work force in the 1990s are likely to have substantially less experience with illicit drugs than did their counterparts in the 1980s and the late 1970s.

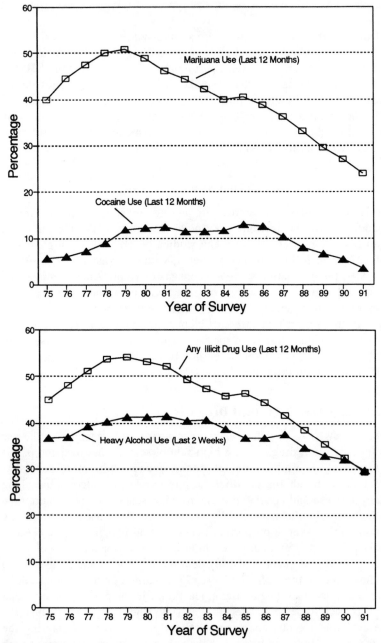

FIGURE 3.1 Trends in alcohol and other drug use among high school seniors, past 12 months, 1975-1991. SOURCE: Unpublished data from the High School Senior Surveys (1992).

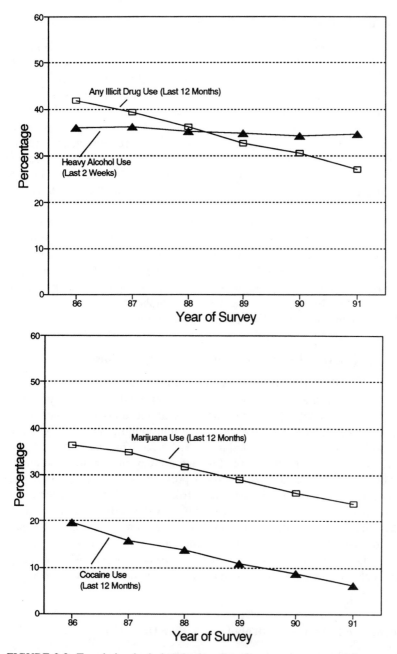

FIGURE 3.2 Trends in alcohol and other drug use among young adults ages 19-28, past 12 months, 1975-1991. SOURCE: Unpublished data from the High School Senior Surveys (1992).

Alcohol and Cigarettes

Most high school seniors use alcohol, even though there is now a minimum purchase age of 21 in all 50 states. Heavy drinking is the behavior of most concern (5 or more drinks in a row almost surely result in inebriation), and it is strikingly prevalent. In 1991, some 30 percent of seniors reported having had 5 or more drinks in a row at least once in the prior 2 weeks; young adults up to about age 22 report such binge drinking even more frequently. Although heavy drinking is distressingly common, the prevalence of such behavior among high school seniors has steadily decreased from about 41 percent in the early 1980s (Figure 3.1). The trend among young adults ages 19 to 28 is not so encouraging: in the last 6 years, prevalence has stayed at about 35 percent (Figure 3.2).

Cigarette use changed surprisingly little during the 1980s. An estimated 28 percent of 1991 seniors smoked cigarettes in the month prior to the survey and 19 percent were daily smokers. In 1981, the figures were 29 and 20 percent, respectively. In addition, some of the lighter smokers become heavy smokers after high school. For example, more than 1 in every 5 young adults ages 19 to 28 is a daily smoker (22 percent), and one in six (16 percent) smokes a half-pack a day or more.

National Household Surveys on Drug Abuse

The National Household Surveys on Drug Abuse (NHSDA) provide national data about the prevalence, correlates, and trends in the use of illicit drugs, alcohol, and tobacco among members of the household population age 12 and older, including members of the household population who are employed. Surveys were conducted in 1971, 1972, 1974, 1976, 1977, 1979, 1982, 1985, 1988, 1990, 1991, and 1992 and are currently conducted annually. The 1988, 1990, and 1991 NHSDAs provide the basis of much of the discussion here because more recent data from the 1992 NHSDA have not yet been fully analyzed. Some trend data from 1979 to 1991 are presented.

The surveys reveal that there has been a decline in the use of illicit drugs and alcohol since the late 1970s; they also report a longer-term decline in tobacco use. These trends for the household population are likely to be reflected in the employed population, as some data from the NHSDAs indicate.

Prevalence and Trends in Alcohol and Other Drug Use

The percentage of the household population who were current (past month) users of any illicit drug, alcohol, or cigarettes has steadily declined over the past decade. In 1979, approximately 14 percent of the total house-

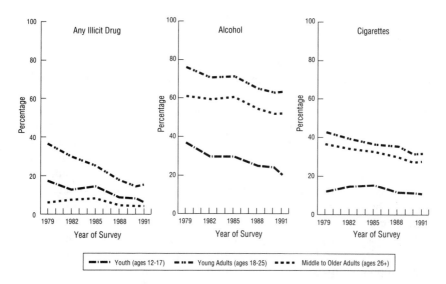

FIGURE 3.3 Trends in the percentage reporting use of all illicit drugs, alcohol, and cigarettes in the past month, by age group, 1979-1991. SOURCE: Data from the National Household Survey on Drug Abuse (Substance Abuse and Mental Health Services Administration, 1993).

hold population had used one or more illicit drugs in the past month compared with 6 percent in 1991 (Substance Abuse and Mental Health Services Administration, 1993). The decreases were more rapid in the earlier part of this period and have since leveled off. Illicit drug use has historically been highest among young adults, and dramatic decreases in the percentage of this group using any illicit drugs in the past month were observed between 1979 and 1991. Intermediate rates of use were found for youth; these rates also decreased, but not as rapidly. Use rates among older adults were the lowest of the three age groups, and more modest decreases were observed (Figure 3.3).

Alcohol use has also declined over the past 15 years: although prevalence of any alcohol use has decreased for all three age groups since the late 1970s, rates of heavy alcohol use have been more stable. In 1988, 1990, and 1991, about 5 percent of the total household population were heavy alcohol users. Decreases in current cigarette use have been steadier over the period, diminishing from a prevalence rate of 32 percent in 1985 to 27 percent in 1991 for the total household population. Related decreases in current cigarette use were observed for young adults and middle to older adults, but current cigarette use has remained relatively stable among youth ages 12 to 17 (see Figure 3.3).

Demographic Correlates of Alcohol and Other Drug Use

Current use of illicit drugs was more common among those ages 18 to 25 than among other age groups and more common among men, blacks, residents of large metropolitan areas, and residents of the West than among other groups (Figure 3.4). For alcohol use in the past month, rates were significantly greater among those ages 18 to 25 and 26 to 34 than among other age groups, among men than among women, among whites than among blacks and Hispanics, among residents of large and small metropolitan areas than among residents of nonmetropolitan areas, and among residents of the Northeast, North Central, and West regions than among residents of the South (Substance Abuse and Mental Health Services Administration, 1993). Rates of cigarette smoking were significantly higher among adults aged 18 to 25 and 26 to 34 than among other age group, among men than women, among whites and blacks than among Hispanics, among residents of nonmetropolitan areas. There were no differences among the four regions of the country (Substance Abuse and Mental Health Services Administration, 1993).

Alcohol and Other Drug Use by the Work Force

Relatively few analyses of the prevalence of the use of illicit drugs, alcohol, and tobacco among employed and unemployed persons or among occupational groups have been conducted. The NHSDA surveys have some data that bear on these issues. Although the surveys do not gather information specific to alcohol and other drug use at work (i.e., on the job), they do nonetheless, provide valuable estimates of the extent of alcohol and other drug use by various segments of the work force (regardless of where the use took place). Kopstein and Gfroerer (1990), using data from the 1988 NHSDA, found that illicit drug use was substantially higher among unemployed (18 percent) than among full-time (8 percent) or part-time (9 percent) employed persons. In contrast, weekly alcohol use was higher among full-time employed persons (40 percent) than among those in other employment statuses (33 percent), whereas heavy alcohol use showed little variation among employment groups. Age and sex differentials in rates of alcohol and other drug use among employed persons were similar to those for all adults.

To explore alcohol and other drug use among the work force further, the Kopstein and Gfroerer analyses were replicated using data from the 1990 NHSDA. These data examine the prevalence of current use of selected illicit drugs and heavy alcohol among employed and unemployed persons age 18 and older. Findings from the 1990 NHSDA substantiate many of the findings from the 1988 analyses. As shown in Table 3.1, illicit

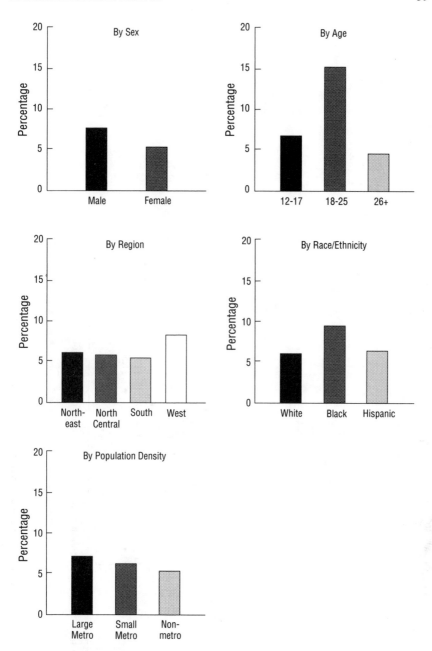

FIGURE 3.4 Prevalence of any illicit drug use in the past month, by demographic characteristics, 1991. SOURCE: Data from the National Household Survey on Drug Abuse (Substance Abuse and Mental Health Services Administration, 1993).

TABLE 3.1 Prevalence of Alcohol and Other Drug Use, by Selected Type of Use, Employment Status, Sex, and Age, 1990

Employment Status and Age Group	Percent of Population							
	Past Month Use of Any Illicit[a]		Past Month Use of Marijuana		Past Year Use of Cocaine		Heavy Use of Alcohol[b]	
	Male	Female	Male	Female	Male	Female	Male	Female
Full-Time Employed								
18-25 years	17.1	10.1	15.1	9.2	9.5	6.4	20.7	4.4
26-34 years	10.1	5.8	8.9	4.9	8.5	4.0	12.6	1.5
35+ years	4.0	4.3	2.6	3.3	1.3	1.6	5.1	2.2
All ages 18+	7.8	5.7	6.3	4.8	4.7	3.1	9.6	2.4
Part-Time Employed								
18-25 years	17.6	14.7	14.7	10.1	7.3	c	14.8	5.2
26-34 years	25.0	11.6	23.3	10.2	17.2	4.8	22.9	c
35+ years	c	c	c	c	c	c	c	c
All ages 18+	12.0	6.5	10.3	5.8	5.8	1.1	11.7	2.6
Unemployed								
18-25 years	24.2	14.3	22.4	11.8	20.2	11.1	10.7	c
26-34 years	20.0	24.9	19.6	21.5	18.3	9.9	c	4.5
35+ years	14.1	c	c	c	c	c	c	c
All ages 18+	19.3	17.0	17.0	9.0	15.0	5.3	10.8	3.7

[a]Includes use of marijuana, hashish, inhalants, hallucinogens, cocaine, heroin, and nonmedical use of stimulants, sedatives, tranquilizers, or analgesics.

[b]Heavy drinking is having 5 or more drinks on the same occasion 5 or more times in the past 30 days.

[c]Low precision; no estimate reported.

SOURCE: Data from the National Household Survey on Drug Abuse (National Institute on Drug Abuse, 1991).

drug use is substantially higher among the unemployed (14 percent) than among the full-time (7 percent) or part-time (8 percent) employed. The highest rate of illicit drug use was among unemployed persons ages 26 to 34 (23 percent). Weekly alcohol use was somewhat higher among full-time employed persons (27 percent) than among part-time employed persons (22 percent) or the unemployed (20 percent). Overall, heavy alcohol use showed similar rates among employment groups (5 to 7 percent). Both weekly alcohol use (34 compared with 21-25 percent) and heavy alcohol use (14 compared with 9 percent) were highest among full-time employed people ages 18 to 25 relative to their part-time employed and unemployed counterparts.

The prevalence of illicit drug use diminished between 1988 and 1990 for most drugs and employment groups, as shown in Table 3.2. The exception to the general downward trend in rates of use was an increase in past-year cocaine use among the full-time employed, from 6 to 7 percent. Alcohol use decreased for most comparisons, and decreases of more than 10 percent were observed in the rates of weekly alcohol use for all three employment groups. Rates of heavy alcohol use were more stable.

Among full-time employed male workers, rates of marijuana, cocaine, heavy alcohol, and any illicit drug use varied inversely with income level, as shown in Table 3.3. Among women, the reported use of these substances was lower and an association with income was not found. Rates of any illicit drug use were higher among blacks than among whites or Hispanics for both men and women. Cocaine use was also higher among black men than white or Hispanic men, whereas cocaine use was relatively low among women with little variation among racial or ethnic groups. There were no racial or ethnic differences in heavy alcohol use for men, and because of sample size constraints an estimate of heavy alcohol use was available only for white women.

Among full-time employed persons, rates of illicit drugs and heavy alcohol use varied across industries and for men and women, as shown in Table 3.4. Many of the estimates for women are unreliable due to small sample sizes, but the available data show few differences for women across industries. Among men, current use of illicit drugs and heavy alcohol use were highest among construction workers. Some 20 percent of male construction workers reported using one or more illicit drugs in the past month, 18 percent used marijuana, 14 percent used cocaine, and 26 percent were heavy drinkers. Rates of illicit drug use were relatively low among male professional, manufacturing, and transportation workers. Intermediate levels of any illicit drug use were found among male retail trade, repair services, and wholesale trade workers. More than 20 percent of men employed full time in construction, transportation, and wholesale trade were heavy drinkers.

TABLE 3.2 Prevalence of Alcohol and Other Drug Use, by Selected Type of Use, and Employment Status, Age 18 and Older, 1988 and 1990

Employment Status	Past Month Use of Any Illicit[a]		Past Month Use of Marijuana		Past Year Use of Cocaine		Weekly Use of Alcohol[b]		Heavy Use of Alcohol	
	1988	1990	1988	1990	1988	1990	1988	1990	1988	1990
Full-Time Employed	8.2	7.0	6.8	5.7	5.7	7.2	39.9	27.4	6.4	6.8
Part-Time Employed	9.4	8.0	7.5	6.2	4.5	2.4	32.9	21.6	5.6	5.1
Unemployed	18.2	14.0	14.8	12.3	9.5	9.3	32.9	19.7	7.9	6.6

[a]Includes use of marijuana, hashish, inhalants, hallucinogens, cocaine, heroin, and nonmedical use of stimulants, sedatives, tranquilizers, or analgesics.

[b]Heavy drinking is having 5 or more drinks on the same occasion 5 or more times in the past 30 days.

SOURCE: Data from the National Household Survey on Drug Abuse (National Institute on Drug Abuse, 1991).

TABLE 3.3 Prevalence of Alcohol and Other Drug Use Among Full-Time Employed Persons Ages 18-34, by Selected Type of Substance, Sex, Personal Income, and Race/Ethnicity, 1990

| | Percent of Full-Time Employed | | | | | | | |
| Personal Income and Race/Ethnicity | Past Month Use of Any Illicit[a] | | Past Month Use of Marijuana | | Past Year Use of Cocaine | | Heavy Use of Alcohol[b] | |
	Male	Female	Male	Female	Male	Female	Male	Female
Annual Income								
Less than $12,000	21.7	7.8	19.5	6.9	11.1	6.0	19.1	3.2
$12,000 to $19,999	11.7	5.8	10.4	5.4	9.3	5.4	17.2	2.2
$20,000 to $29,999	11.0	9.7	9.8	8.2	9.7	c	11.8	3.5
$30,000 or over	7.8	6.2	6.3	5.0	5.7	4.4	13.9	c
Race/Ethnicity								
White	12.2	7.2	10.7	6.2	8.0	5.0	15.5	2.9
Black	17.8	10.1	17.3	9.6	14.5	3.9	14.3	c
Hispanic	11.1	6.4	8.4	5.3	11.3	4.2	14.8	c

[a]Includes use of marijuana, hashish, inhalants, hallucinogens, cocaine, heroin, and nonmedical use of stimulants, sedatives, tranquilizers, or analgesics.
[b]Heavy drinking is having 5 or more drinks on the same occasion 5 or more times in the past 30 days.
[c]Low precision; no estimate reported.

SOURCE: Data from the National Household Survey on Drug Abuse (National Institute on Drug Abuse, 1991).

TABLE 3.4 Prevalence of Alcohol and Other Drug Use Among Full-Time Employed Persons Ages 18 to 34, by Selected Industries, Selected Type of Substance, and Sex, 1990

Percent of Full-Time Employed

Selected Industry	Past Month Use of Any Illicit[a]		Past Month Use of Marijuana		Past Year Use of Cocaine		Heavy Use of Alcohol[b]	
	Male	Female	Male	Female	Male	Female	Male	Female
Construction	20.0	c	18.1	c	14.0	c	26.4	c
Manufacturing	9.7	5.0	7.7	5.0	8.9	c	12.7	c
Transportation	10.5	c	6.9	c	9.5	c	20.4	c
Wholesale Trade	13.8	c	11.0	c	12.7	c	20.5	c
Retail Trade	16.8	7.3	15.2	5.2	9.8	7.3	14.3	4.3
Finance	11.3	7.0	c	c	13.6	c	16.7	c
Repair Services	16.1	c	15.8	c	5.7	c	9.3	c
Professional	9.0	5.5	9.0	4.1	4.5	5.6	9.9	3.9

[a]Includes use of marijuana, hashish, inhalants, hallucinogens, cocaine, heroin, and nonmedical use of stimulants, sedatives, tranquilizers, or analgesics.
[b]Heavy drinking is having 5 or more drinks on the same occasion 5 or more times in the past 30 days.
[c]Low precision; no estimate reported.

SOURCE: Data from the National Household Survey on Drug Abuse (National Institute on Drug Abuse, 1991).

Similar variations across occupational groups in alcohol consumption were recently reported by Parker and Harford (1992). These investigators provided estimates of the prevalence of alcohol use, alcohol dependence, and severe alcohol dependence among working men and women in both blue-collar and white-collar occupations. Self-report interview data obtained from 26,738 employed respondents who participated in the National Health Interview Survey revealed that rates of drinking (i.e., respondents reporting the consumption of 12 drinks or more during the year preceding the interview) were higher among people in white-collar occupations such as managerial, professional, technical, and sales. Although fewer current drinkers were found among blue-collar workers, those who were current drinkers were found to have higher average daily consumption levels, alcohol dependence, and severe dependence rates than members of white-collar occupations. Their analysis indicated that the prevalence of dependence and severe dependence on alcohol was especially high among food service workers, farmers, mechanics, construction workers, machine operators, and laborers.

In summary, the percentage of the work force population who are using illicit drugs, alcohol, or cigarettes has decreased over the past decade. However, rates of use remain relatively high among young workers ages 18 to 25. Rates of illicit drug use are higher among unemployed than employed persons. Also potentially affecting the workplace are the relatively higher rates of weekly and heavy alcohol use among full-time employed workers ages 18 to 25, compared with the part-time employed or unemployed. Some industries are more likely to be affected by high rates of alcohol and other drug use. Among the full-time employed, rates of illicit drug use and heavy alcohol use are highest among male construction workers. Rates of heavy drinking are also relatively high among male transportation workers, a fact that has obvious public safety implications.

Military Worldwide Surveys

The U.S. Department of Defense worldwide surveys of military personnel provide data comparable to the High School Senior surveys and the National Household Surveys on Drug Abuse for active-duty military personnel stationed across the world. Surveys were conducted in 1980, 1982, 1985, 1988, and 1992.

The military is a distinctive workplace, however, in that members have a special mission to preserve and defend the nation and consequently are often subject to a strictly controlled environment, including a well-established substance abuse policy aimed at preventing the misuse of alcohol and other drugs.

Trends in Alcohol and Other Drug Use

Figure 3.5 presents trends over the five surveys in the proportions of the total active military force who engaged in illicit drug use, heavy drinking, and cigarette smoking between 1980 and 1992. As shown, there are significant declines in all three measures, although the rate of decline varied for each. The percentage of military personnel admitting to having used any illicit drug within the past 30 days declined significantly and markedly from 28 percent in 1980 to 3 percent in 1992.

The prevalence of heavy drinking among military personnel also declined significantly between 1980 and 1992, although the decrease was less dramatic than for illicit drug use. In 1980, 21 percent of military personnel reported heavy drinking, compared with 15 percent in 1992. Although heavy drinking does not by itself constitute alcohol abuse, it does indicate drinking levels that are likely to have detrimental consequences, particularly in a group that works with weapons, vehicles, and other dangerous equipment. The percentage of military personnel who were cigarette smokers also decreased during the 12-year period, from 51 percent in 1980 to 35 percent in 1992.

The question arises whether these decreases in alcohol and other drug use are an artifact of changes in the demographic composition of the armed forces during the 1980s and early 1990s, a reflection of general population trends, or the result of military policy. Recruiting and reenlistment suc-

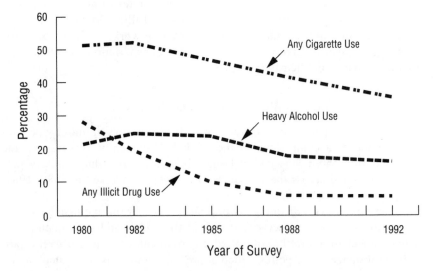

FIGURE 3.5 Trends in alcohol and other drug use, past 30 days, total U.S. Department of Defense, 1980-1992. SOURCE: Bray et al. (1992).

cesses during this time resulted in a military work force in 1992 that was somewhat older, had more married personnel, and was better educated than in 1980, characteristics that are associated with a lower likelihood of alcohol and other drug use. For example, nearly 63 percent of the military force in 1992 were married compared with 53 percent in 1980; moreover, 61 percent were over age 25 in 1992 compared with 43 percent in 1980.

To assess the effect of the changing demographic characteristics on rates of alcohol and other drug use, the 1982, 1985, 1988, and 1992 surveys were standardized to the age, education, and marital status distribution of the military population in 1980. Significant declines in any illicit drug use and cigarette smoking remained after adjusting for demographic changes in the military population. In contrast, much of the decline in heavy drinking observed between 1980 and 1992 was attributable to changes in the demographic composition of the armed forces. After the data were adjusted to reflect demographic changes, the rate of heavy drinking in 1992 (19 percent) did not differ significantly from the rate in 1980 (21 percent).

Demographic Correlates of Alcohol and Other Drug Use

Table 3.5 presents data on reported illicit drug use during the past year and on heavy drinking and cigarette smoking for the past 30 days among various demographic subgroups. Overall, illicit drug and heavy alcohol use occurred among those who were younger, single, and less educated. In addition, men were much more likely to drink heavily than women. The common patterns observed for age, marital status, and educational status were not surprising because marriage and higher educational attainment generally occur with increasing age. Data on marital status indicate that the presence of a spouse was associated with reduced alcohol and other drug use. Among military personnel whose spouses were not with them, illicit drug use rates were similar to what they were among unmarried personnel, and rates of heavy alcohol use were above what they were for those who had spouses present.

Cigarette smoking was also associated with education and marital status. More educated military personnel were less likely to smoke than those with less education, and married personnel accompanied by a spouse were somewhat less likely to smoke than those who were unmarried or married but unaccompanied by a spouse. Blacks and Hispanics were less likely to smoke than whites, and women were less likely to smoke than men, but the differences were not large. Smoking prevalence declined with increasing age, but less dramatically than did illicit drug and alcohol use.

TABLE 3.5 Prevalence of Alcohol and Other Drug Use Among Military Personnel by Sociodemographic Characteristics (in percent)

Sociodemographic Characteristic	Any Illicit Drug Use	Heavy Alcohol Use	Cigarette Smoking
Age			
20 and under	12.9	24.5	40.8
21-25	10.3	22.5	36.4
26-34	3.8	12.3	34.4
35 and older	1.9	7.0	32.0
Sex			
Male	6.7	17.1	35.7
Female	3.4	4.4	31.5
Race/ethnicity			
White	6.6	16.5	37.4
Black	4.2	10.3	29.0
Hispanic	8.9	17.9	31.6
Other	4.4	13.7	32.9
Education			
High school graduate/GED	9.0	22.4	44.2
Some college	5.5	13.2	35.5
College graduate or higher	1.9	4.7	14.9
Marital status			
Not married	9.9	23.7	37.6
Married, unaccompanied by spouse	7.1	15.8	35.4
Married, accompanied by spouse	3.6	9.5	33.3
Total	6.2	15.2	35.0

NOTE: Prevalence of any illicit drug use is measured for the past 12 months; heavy alcohol use and cigarette smoking are measured for the past 30 days.

SOURCE: Data from Bray et al. (1992).

Effects of Alcohol and Other Drug Use at Work

Two measures from the MWS were used to examine selected aspects of alcohol and other drug use on work behavior. The first focused on productivity loss attributed to alcohol and other drug use, and the second examined alcohol use at work, during lunch breaks, or shortly before going to work. Five items on the MWS sought to measure productivity losses attributed to alcohol and other drug use: being late, leaving work early, not coming to work, performing below normal, and aftereffects or illnesses. Figure 3.6 presents trends in self-perceived productivity losses due to any illicit drug or alcohol use. Overall, the data indicate that military personnel are more likely to experience work-related deficits because of alcohol use than because of illicit drug use. In the 1992 survey, about one in six military personnel reported some productivity loss due to alcohol use during the past year. As might be expected, the probability of a productivity loss is directly related to the level of use.

Table 3.6 presents information about alcohol use by military personnel immediately before or during work hours. As shown, 6 percent of military personnel reported drinking at these times. The percentage using alcohol was slightly lower among officers than enlisted personnel, indicating that the former had a somewhat lower exposure to the risk of alcohol-related problems at work. Taken together, the findings in Figure 3.6 and Table 3.6 suggest that alcohol use has some negative effects on the productivity and

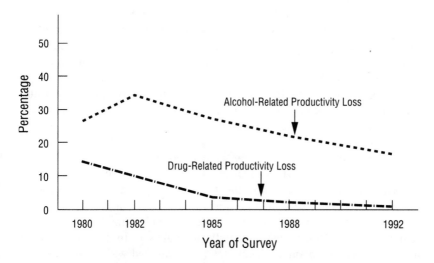

FIGURE 3.6 Trends in drug- and alcohol-related productivity loss, past 12 months, total U.S. Department of Defense, 1980-1992. SOURCE: Bray et al. (1992).

TABLE 3.6 Alcohol Use Among Military Personnel on
Workdays, Past 30 Days (in percent of total personnel)

	Grade		
Drinking Occasion	Enlisted	Officers	Total
Within 2 hours of going to work	3.4	0.5	2.9
During lunch break	4.1	3.7	4.0
During work or work break	1.6	0.7	1.4
Total	6.5	4.4	6.2

SOURCE: Data from Bray et al. (1992).

work behaviors of military personnel, but drug use is now affecting the
work of relatively few.

Comparing Military and Civilian Alcohol and Other Drug Use

Because of the unique mission of the military, the armed forces impose
rather strict controls over the lives of their members in a number of areas,
including alcohol and other drug use. To help gauge the relative magnitude
of alcohol and other drug use patterns among military personnel, it is useful
to have a civilian comparison group to serve as a benchmark.

In a recent study, Bray et al. (1991) conducted standardized comparisons of illicit drug use, heavy alcohol use, and smoking among military
personnel and civilians. Military data were drawn from the 1985 MWS and
civilian data from the 1985 NHSDA. The two data sets were equated for
age and geographic location of respondents, and civilian alcohol and other
drug use rates were standardized to reflect the sociodemographic distribution of the military. Standardized comparisons showed that military personnel were significantly less likely than civilians to report having used any
illicit drugs during the past 30 days (8 compared with 24 percent), but they
were significantly more likely to be heavy drinkers (21 compared with 11
percent) and to be cigarette smokers (44 compared with 39 percent).

More recently, similar analyses were conducted using data from the
1992 MWS and the 1991 NHSDA (Bray et al., 1992). Findings showed the
same basic pattern of results as in the 1985 data: military personnel were
still significantly less likely than civilians to engage in any illicit drug use
(3 compared with 10 percent), but more likely than civilians to drink heavily
(15 compared with 10 percent), especially men ages 18 to 25 (26 compared
with 14 percent) and to smoke cigarettes (34 compared with 30 percent).

The fact that the proportion of illicit drug users is lower among military
personnel than among civilians does not in itself constitute evidence of the

effectiveness of military policies and practices concerning illicit drug use. Nonetheless, it does make it a plausible hypothesis worth evaluating according to scientific methods. The military surveys point to the potential preventive effects of a clearly articulated and well-advertised policy against illicit drug use that is supported by drug testing with serious consequences for violations. However, the military is so different from most work settings that it is not clear to what extent military practices can be generalized to the civilian work force.

Is Heavy Illicit Drug Use Declining?

Although the overall prevalence of illicit drug use is declining, there is some question as to whether heavy use of illicit drugs is also declining. Some researchers believe that there may be a population of hard-core users whose numbers are not declining (Wish, 1990-1991). A 1993 National Research Council report (Gerstein and Green, 1993:2) vividly describes two worlds of drug use:

> In one world, that of relatively low-intensity consumption (drug *use*) among individuals who can be found in schools and households, drug experience is self-reported more frequently by the wealthy than the less wealthy and by whites than Hispanics or blacks. In this world, there have been steady and cumulatively very marked declines in the prevalence of marijuana use since the late 1970s and of cocaine since the middle 1980s, and heroin use is so rare as to be barely measurable. In another world, that of emergency rooms, morgues, drug clinics, juvenile detention centers, jails, and prisons, in which indicators of intensive drug consumption (*abuse* and *dependence*) are collected: the poor predominate, blacks and Hispanics appearing in numbers much higher than their household or school proportions; marijuana and heroin use are common (though less so in some areas than in the 1970s); and cocaine use increased explosively throughout the 1980s and simply leveled off at high levels in the 1990s.

As Gerstein and Green suggest, trend data from the HSS and the NHSDA indicate that current (past 30 days) as well as heavy use of marijuana has declined (Table 3.7). The declines have been substantial for high school seniors as well as young adults ages 18 to 25—those for whom drug use tends to be highest. But these surveys of the general population do not capture large enough numbers of addicts or very heavy users of cocaine or heroin to provide reliable estimates of such drug users. Thus, to examine hard-core users, alternative sources of data should be investigated.

Perhaps the best information available to examine the extent and trends in the use of heroin and cocaine among hard-core users is the Drug Abuse Warning Network (DAWN) data from hospital emergency rooms. Prior to

TABLE 3.7 Comparison of Trends in Current Use and Daily Use of
Marijuana from the High School Senior Surveys and the National
Household Surveys on Drug Abuse, Past 30 Days (in percent)

| | Year of Survey | | | | | | |
Use Level/Survey	1985	1986	1987	1988	1989	1990	1991
Current Marijuana Use							
HHS, seniors	25.7	23.4	21.0	18.0	16.7	14.0	13.8
NHSDA, young adults[a]	21.8			15.5		12.7	13.0
Daily Marijuana Use							
HHS, seniors	4.9	4.0	3.3	2.7	2.9	2.2	2.0
NHSDA, young adults[a]	4.7			2.4		2.0	1.7

[a]Young adults aged 18-25.

SOURCES: Data from the National Household Survey on Drug Abuse (Substance Abuse and
Mental Health Services Administration, 1993); unpublished data from the High School Senior
Survey (1992).

1989, these data were obtained from a set of hospitals that were not statistically representative of any defined population, making it difficult to assess
the validity of trends. Since 1989, however, participating hospitals are
representative of defined areas, so trend data can be more reliably assessed.
These data, which are reported quarterly, showed upward trends in the first
three quarters of 1991 and the first quarter of 1992 in the number of persons
treated in emergency rooms for cocaine use. These increases do not, however, necessarily indicate increased use among the hard-core population.
There are many possible alternative explanations. For example, there could
be changes in the extent to which emergency room personnel correctly
ascertain the presence of cocaine in a presenting patient; changes in the
purity of cocaine may have increased the effective dosage; added adulterants could have increased toxicity; lower prices may have resulted in people
taking higher doses; or more new users may be taking cocaine, resulting in
"over" reactions to its effects. Nevertheless, the recent increases in emergency room mentions of cocaine suggest that cocaine use may not be declining among all subgroups. The data for heroin use also show similar
trends: increases in the first three quarters of 1991 and again in the first
quarter of 1992 (HHS *News*, October 23, 1992).

Other less reliable indicators than the DAWN data corroborate the sug-
gestion that illicit drug use may not be declining among all subgroups of the
population. One such indicator comes from the Drug Use Forecasting (DUF)
system (Wish, 1990-1991). This system assesses illicit drug use among
recent arrestees in selected metropolitan areas. Because of the nature of the
data collection procedures, as well as aspects of the design of the system, it

is difficult to know what these data reflect about the larger society. However, the data do show that there are very high levels of illicit drug use among recent arrestees, approaching or even exceeding 50 percent in some locations. And there is no evidence of any consistent decline in such proportions since the data were first collected in 1986.

Treatment facilities could, in theory, provide additional information on trends in illicit drug use among the general population. However, there are no data that can be reliably used to assess such trends in treatment facility utilization. Factors such as cost of treatment, availability, preferred modality, referral sources, and length of treatment all vary tremendously, and each can have major effects on treatment utilization.

Despite the fact that there may be some hard-core illicit drug users whose numbers are not declining, it seems clear that there are declining numbers of experimental and casual users among the general population. It is these latter users who have been most likely to be members of the work force. Although some, if not many, hard-core illicit drug users are employed at various times, their numbers in recent years have been relatively low compared with the number of experimental or casual users, most of whom are regular members of the work force.

Summary

All three survey series indicate that illicit drug use has declined over the past decade or more. The decline is evident among the populations of young people, households, and military personnel. Use has similarly declined both among the working-age population and among people who are currently working. Nevertheless, despite these declines, alcohol and other drug use continues to affect significant proportions of the work force and selected industries. Heavy alcohol use also affects performance negatively and, unlike illicit drug use, survey findings suggest that its prevalence has not been decreasing. Although surveys of the general population do not provide meaningful estimates of hard-core use of illicit drugs, findings from alternative sources suggest that rates of heavy use of cocaine and heroin may be stable or even increasing. The implications of such trends for the work force are largely unknown. Heavy drug use is likely to prevent hard-core users from becoming productive workers, so such users may not be actively employed in the work force.

WORK SITE DRUG TESTING

Increasing proportions of the work force have undergone urine tests for drug use in recent years. The most common reason for conducting the tests was as part of job application procedures.

The data from work site drug testing reviewed here consist of urinalysis results obtained from a monitoring project of laboratories certified by the National Institute on Drug Abuse (NIDA). The labs tested large numbers of urine samples for organizations with drug-testing programs. Urine testing done with appropriate quality control procedures provides an objective indicator of recent drug use that is not subject to problems of underreporting, as are self-reports of use. However, because this kind of testing measures only a subset of drugs and detects only very recent drug use, the results may not be directly comparable with self-reported data, which are typically based on longer reference periods such as a month or a year. Furthermore, drug test findings are not based on probability samples, hence estimates of drug use prevalence derived from them may be subject to unknown biases. An inherent source of bias of NIDA-certified laboratory test results is a direct consequence of the blind quality control programs. That is, spiked samples will be reported as positive and will inevitably inflate the estimated positive rate.

Background

The most comprehensive and up-to-date source of information on work site drug-testing results is a study funded by NIDA[1] that summarizes test results collected quarterly from a sample of seven NIDA-certified laboratories that currently report on over 300,000 tests per quarter. For each test, laboratories provide information on the drugs included in the test protocol along with screening and confirmatory levels used in the testing procedure.[2] Along with information on the testing protocol, data are collected on geographic location, type of industry, and reason for testing. (No information that can link a test result to a company or an individual is submitted to the project.)

These test situations vary with the group to be tested and whether the person has any forewarning that testing will occur. The latter is important, as prior notification provides an opportunity for a drug user to temporarily suspend use to avoid a positive test result. The testing categories used include:

- **Preemployment**—testing of job applicants, typically announced.

---

[1]NIDA Contract No. 271-89-8525, "Drug Testing Laboratories Data Analysis" performed by Research and Evaluation Associates, Chapel Hill, N.C.

[2]Chapter 6 of this report deals extensively with the procedures and protocols of testing, in both NIDA-certified and other laboratories.

- **Random**—unannounced testing of current employees unrelated to suspicion about a specific individual.
- **Periodic medical**—announced testing of current employees, often part of a regularly scheduled physical, again unrelated to suspicion about a specific individual.
- **Reasonable cause**—unannounced testing of current employees suspected of drug use.
- **Post-accident**—testing of employees involved in an accident or incident.
- **Return-to-duty**—unannounced testing of employees who are returning to work after a leave related to drug use.

Findings

Of the nearly 2 million test results obtained from October 1990 through March 1992, almost 4 percent[3] or nearly 70,000 were positive for one or more illicit drugs. Marijuana was the most commonly detected drug, with 2 percent of the specimens testing positive for its metabolites, followed by cocaine (1 percent), opiates (0.6 percent), and benzodiazepines (0.5 percent) (Figure 3.7).

As discussed in more detail in Chapter 6, the standard test protocol, commonly referred to as the "NIDA-5," includes testing for marijuana, cocaine, phencyclidine (PCP), opiates, and amphetamines, using standard cutoff levels for screening and confirmatory results. The advantage of examining results from the NIDA-5 panel is that any variations observed reflect differences in rates of drug use rather than in testing procedures. The disadvantage of limiting the discussion to this testing protocol is that it does not include findings on drugs such as alcohol, benzodiazepines, and barbiturates.

Using the NIDA-5 panel, the positive rate for detecting any illicit drug was 3 percent; using any test protocol, the rate was 4 percent. Part of the difference between the two percentages is that the NIDA-5 protocol tests for only five drugs, and most of the other protocols test for six to eight different drugs. The additional drugs included in the testing protocol do not, however, account for all of the observed difference in positive rates. The positive rates for specific drugs are typically 20 percent lower with the

---

[3]The positive rates are inflated by an unknown amount. Along with regular specimens, some employers submit blind quality control samples to the testing laboratories, typically with some 20 percent containing one or more drugs in the specimen. It is not possible to determine what percentage of tests were quality control specimens, so the data cannot be adjusted for this upward bias.

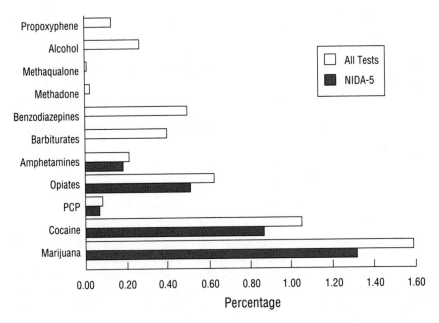

FIGURE 3.7 Positive rates for work site urine testing by type of drug, October 1990-March 1992. SOURCE: Unpublished data from the NIDA Drug Testing Laboratories analysis.

NIDA-5 panel compared with all testing. One factor is that many private employers have set up drug-testing programs that have lower cutoff levels than the NIDA-5 protocol for either the initial screening test, the confirmation test, or both. The use of a lower cutoff would result in a higher detection rate. Another factor that might account for this difference is the type of work settings that use the NIDA-5 panel. Many of the employers using the NIDA-5 panel are under a mandate, such as the U.S. Department of Transportation (DOT) regulations, to have an antidrug program. Organizations that are required to have a program may be more aggressive in their efforts to deter drug use with programs involving a range of antidrug activities, not just urine testing. From an epidemiologic perspective, the advantage of the NIDA-5 test panel is that it is a standardized measure of drug use. Any differences in positive rates by reason, over time, or across regions or industries will not reflect variations in the test methods. For this reason, the remaining comparisons we make are limited to testing done using the NIDA-5 panel.

Reasons for Testing

For the NIDA-5 test results, the reasons for testing reported to the project were preemployment (44 percent), random (27 percent), and periodic medical (26 percent) testing. Of these three types of testing, preemployment tests for job applicants have the highest positive test rate, with one or more drugs detected in 3 percent of the specimens. With current employees, the positive rate for random testing was almost 3 percent and for periodic medical testing it was 2 percent (see Figure 3.8). The figure for periodic medical testing, although low, is striking, since employees are typically aware that testing will occur. In spite of forewarning, nearly 2 percent test positive. One possible explanation is that some employees are not capable or

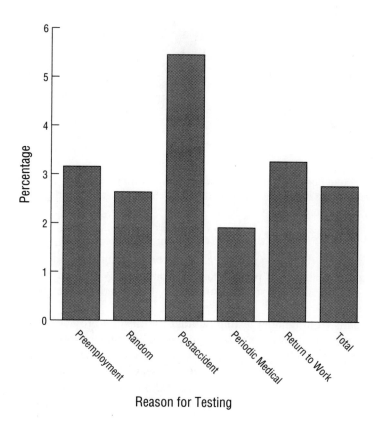

FIGURE 3.8 Positive rates for work site urine testing by reason for testing, October 1990-March 1992. SOURCE: Unpublished data from the NIDA Drug Testing Laboratories analysis.

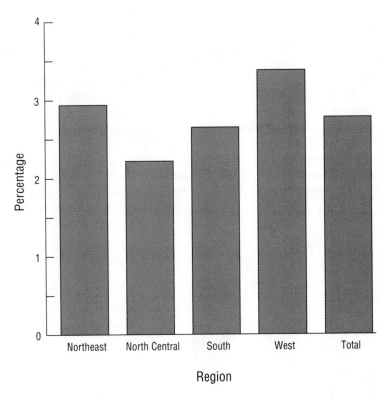

FIGURE 3.9 Positive rates for work site urine testing by region of the country, October 1990-March 1992. SOURCE: Unpublished data from the NIDA Drug Testing Laboratories analysis.

willing to stop their drug use, even for the brief period necessary to produce a "clean" specimen. It is also possible, particularly with respect to marijuana, that use was not stopped soon enough to eliminate metabolites from the urine.

Results from random testing without notification provide the best indicator of the actual prevalence of regular drug use among workers. Approximately 1 in 40 employees tested positive (3 percent) on random tests. Among all categories of testing, the highest rate was observed for post-accident testing, with 5 percent of more than 12,000 tests positive.[4]

---

[4]Results for reasonable cause testing are not reported because of the small number of tests.

Region and Type of Industry

As shown in Figure 3.9, there were small but significant regional differences in positive rates, with the West having the highest rate (3.36 percent), followed by the Northeast (2.94 percent), the South (2.65 percent), and the lowest in the North Central (2.22 percent). All differences between regions were statistically significant. The rate for the West is over 50 percent higher than the one observed in the North Central region. Except for cocaine, positive rates for particular drugs were also highest in the West. The highest positive rate for cocaine has consistently been in the Northeast.

Consistent with data from self-reports based on the 1990 National Household Surveys on Drug Abuse (NHSDA) cited earlier in this chapter, differences were also observed across industry types. As was the case with the NHSDA, the highest rate of drug use was observed in the construction industry (see Figure 3.10). However, a much lower positive rate for urine tests (6 per-

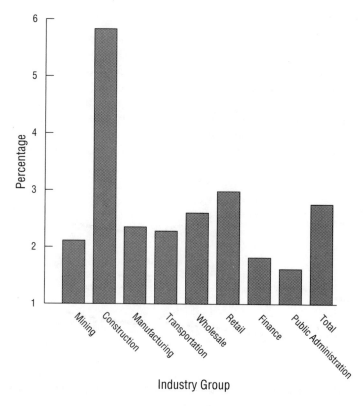

FIGURE 3.10 Positive rates for work site uring testing by industry groups, October 1990-March 1992. SOURCE: Unpublished data from the NIDA Drug Testing Laboratories analysis.

cent) was observed among construction workers than from self-reports in
the 1990 NHSDA (20 percent). This lower rate from urine testing is to be
expected for several reasons. First, testing yields information only on recent use, whereas the NHSDA is based on self-reported use in the past 30
days. Second, the NHSDA asks about the use of a larger number of drugs
than in the NIDA-5 test panel. Third, the NHSDA includes responses from
casual construction workers working for small companies; those tested were
more likely to be working on government projects or for larger organizations. Despite the difference in absolute values between questionnaire data
and the urine test data, there is a concordance in the relative rankings
between the 1990 NHSDA results for men aged 18 to 34 and the results of
urine testing data. Moreover, among the industries common to the two
studies, rank ordering of the top three was the same (construction, retail
sales, and wholesale trade).

Time Trends

Quarter-to-quarter variations were observed in the positive rate for any
illicit drug, ranging from 2.53 to 2.95 percent (Figure 3.11). The most
striking fluctuations were in the rates for marijuana and cocaine. Positive
rates for marijuana, the most frequently detected drug, ranged from 0.93
percent to 1.65; with cocaine, the low was 0.71 percent and the high was
1.07 percent. Changes in positive rates for the two drugs were inversely
related, with cocaine increasing when marijuana declined and visa versa.
As data from additional quarters become available, it may be possible to

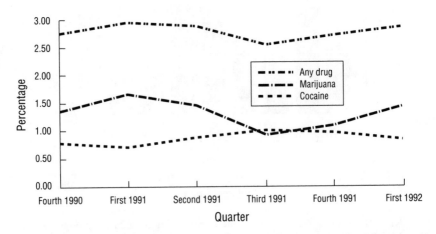

FIGURE 3.11 Positive rates by quarter for work site drug testing. SOURCE:
Unpublished data from the NIDA Drug Testing Laboratories analysis.

identify factors, such as variations over time, related to changes in illicit drug use patterns.

Summary

As with survey findings, drug-testing results indicate that the vast majority of the work force does not use the illicit drugs that are included in the test protocol. Alcohol is generally not included in employment drug test panels. Random testing results, which provide the best indicator of recent worker illicit drug use suggest that approximately 1 in 40 workers uses illicit drugs at a given point in time. Among those who do, marijuana is the most commonly detected drug, followed by cocaine; although the relative prevalence of marijuana use may be overstated because its metabolites are detectable for a longer period than those of most other drugs, this finding is consistent with survey results and so appears reliable. Variations in the positive rate were observed across regions of the country (with the highest in the West) and type of industry (with construction highest).

ORGANIZATION-SPECIFIC PREVALENCE STUDIES

Another source of data about drug use in the work force is a set of recent studies of the prevalence of alcohol and other drug use within single organizations. However, these studies as a group have significant limitations. Because many private corporations do not want to publicize information on alcohol and other drug use within their organizations, the published research involves mainly government employees (Postal Service, military, and municipal employees) and employees of utility companies. Moreover, these studies have seldom been designed to estimate prevalence of employee alcohol and other drug use or the characteristics of employees using alcohol and other drugs. Rather they report results from company drug-testing programs from which it is possible to make certain inferences regarding the extent of employee alcohol and other drug use, the kinds of drugs used, and the characteristics of at-risk employees. Because these data are less than ideal, the inferences are limited and most must be put forth tentatively.

A brief list of organization-specific studies and a summary of each study's results is provided in Table 3.8.

U.S. Postal Service

Normand and others (Normand and Salyards, 1989; Normand et al., 1990) studied drug test results of 5,465 job applicants to the U.S. Postal Service and followed the careers of those who were hired. The drug tests

TABLE 3.8 Organization-Specific Prevalence Studies

Study	Sample	Measures	Results
Normand et al. (1990)	Applicants to U.S. Postal Service from 21 sites	Preemployment urine test	9.4% positive for illicit drug; 6.2 % for marijuana, 2.6% for cocaine, 0.2% for other drugs; blacks, males, aged 25-35 more likely to test positive
Zwerling et al. (1990)	Applicants to U.S. Postal Service in Boston	Preemployment urine test	8% positive for marijuana, 2% for cocaine, 2% for other drugs; males more likely to test positive for marijuana but less likely for cocaine and other drugs; blacks more likely to test positive for marijuana and cocaine
Parish (1989)	Hospital hires	Preemployment urine test	12% positive for drug use; clerical/aide positions more likely to test positive; young males more likely to test positive
Lehman et al. (1990a)	Municipal employees	Self-report substance use on and off the job and voluntary urine test	12.6% tested positive; 9.6% for marijuana, 2.8% for cocaine, 2.8% for other drugs; 38% reported last year alcohol use, 14% reported getting drunk weekly; 7% drink at work, 17% report alcohol-related problems; 22% report lifetime marijuana use, 6% lifetime cocaine; 7% report last year marijuana use, 3% last year cocaine use; 2% report use at work

Lehman et al. (1990b)	Municipal Housing Authority employees	Self-report substance use on and off the job	38% report weekly use of alcohol in last year, 15% get drunk weekly; 11% report alcohol use at work, 13% report alcohol-related problems; 13% report lifetime marijuana use, 7% other illicit drug use; 4% report last-year marijuana use, 3% other illicit drug use
Rosenbaum et al. (1992)	Municipal employees	Self-report substance use on and off the job	25% report weekly use of alcohol in last year, 8% get drunk weekly; 19% report alcohol-related problems, 6% drink at work; 27% report lifetime marijuana use, 10% lifetime cocaine use; 5% report last year marijuana use, 2% cocaine use
Blank and Fenton (1989)	Navy recruits	Preemployment urine test	Recruits testing positive for THC less likely to be high school graduates, more likely to be black, and test lower on intelligence tests
McDaniel (1988)	Navy recruits	Self-report drug use	40% report lifetime marijuana use, 13% more than 10 times, 5% 50 or more times; 13% report stimulant use, 3% 10 or more times; 5% report cocaine use, 5% report depressant use
Taggert (1989)	Railroad applicants and employees	Preemployment, scheduled, for cause, and postaccident urine testing	Overall positive rates from 22% in 1984 falling to 5.8% in 1987; 12.3% positive for marijuana in 1984, 2.5% in 1987; 4.6% for cocaine in 1984, less than 1% in 1987
Sheridan and Winkler (1989)	Power company employees	Preemployment, scheduled, and for cause urine testing	In 1986, 13.4% positive, 4.8% for THC, 2.2% for cocaine, 6.5% for other drugs; in 1987, 14.8% positive, 5.2% for THC, 1.6% for cocaine, 7.9% for other drugs

continued

TABLE 3.8 *(Continued)*

Study	Sample	Measures	Results
Osborn and Sokolov (1989)	Nuclear plant employees	Employee urine tests	3% drug test failure in November, 1988, less than 2% per month thereafter; higher for contract than for permanent employees; 40% of positives for marijuana, 31% for amphetamines, 29% for cocaine
Crouch et al. (1989)	Power company applicants	Preemployment, for cause, and for promotion urine tests	2.8% positive, all but 1 for marijuana; positives more likely to be skilled/technical and male
Cook and Bernstein (1991)	Manufacturing plant employees	Self-report and voluntary urine test	10.3% reported illicit drug use last 6 months, 12.1% when interviewed at work, 6.4% in group administration, 11% for telephone interview, 11% for offsite interview; 8.1% for drug tests; 4.2% who denied drug use tested positive, 14.5% overall prevalence rate; 9.5% prevalence rate for marijuana, 1.6% for cocaine, 1.9% for amphetamines

were conducted strictly for research purposes and the results were known only to research staff.

Overall, 10 percent of applicants tested positive for at least one illicit drug; 7 percent were positive for marijuana, 3 percent for cocaine, and 1 percent for one of the other drugs. The odds of being positive were higher for blacks, men, and applicants between the ages of 25 and 35. Blacks were more than twice as likely as whites (15 compared with 7 percent) to test positive: they were more than six times as likely to test positive for cocaine and almost twice as likely to test positive for marijuana. Men were about 1.5 times as likely to test positive for marijuana than were women, but there were no gender differences for cocaine.

Zwerling et al. (1990) also report on a prospective study of Postal Service applicants, although their study was limited to applicants in the Boston, Massachusetts, area. As in the Normand et al. (1990) study, applicants submitted a urine specimen that was tested for drugs, the results of which, with the exception of opiates, were confined to the research team and not used in making hiring decisions. Of 4,764 applicants, 7 percent tested positive for marijuana, 2 percent for cocaine, and 3 percent for other drugs. Men were more likely than women to test positive for marijuana but less likely than women to test positive for cocaine and other drugs. Blacks were more likely than whites to test positive for marijuana and cocaine.

Hospital Employees

A study of research-oriented preemployment urine testing is reported by Parish (1989). All employees (N = 180) hired at a large teaching hospital over a 6-month period were included in the study: 12 percent tested positive for drug use. Because of the small number of employees testing positive, no breakdown by drug type was provided. Employees in clerical/aide positions were more likely than others to test positive. Drug-positive employees were also more likely to be young and male.

Municipal and Housing Authority Workers

In a study of 1,795 municipal employees in a large city in the southwest United States, Lehman et al. (1990a) administered a paper-and-pencil questionnaire to obtain self-reports of alcohol and other drug use. In addition, 500 urine specimens were collected from randomly chosen work groups. The urinalysis data indicated that 13 percent of participants tested positive for at least one drug. This included 10 percent for marijuana, 3 percent for cocaine, and 3 percent for other drugs such as opiates, amphetamines, and benzodiazepines. Two or more drugs were detected in specimens of 3 percent of the sample. Some 77 percent reported using alcohol during the past year, 38 percent admitted to drinking at least weekly, 49 percent re-ported getting drunk in the last year, and 14 percent reported getting drunk at least weekly.

A study of 343 employees of a housing authority from the same south-west U.S. city as the municipal worker study, using the same methods and questionnaire, showed similar results (Lehman et al., 1990b). Overall, 75 percent of the housing authority employees reported using alcohol in the last year, 38 percent reported weekly use or more, and half reported getting drunk in the last year, with 15 percent getting drunk at least weekly.

Reports of illicit drug use were generally lower than they were for municipal employees: 13 percent reported any marijuana use in their life-time, and 7 percent reported lifetime use of other illicit drugs. Only 4 percent reported marijuana use in the past year, with 3 percent reporting other illicit drug use; 4 percent of the sample reported illicit drug use in the past month.

A survey of 1,081 municipal workers from a second large city in the Southwest showed similar patterns of drug use (Rosenbaum et al., 1992). Overall, 74 percent reported alcohol use in the past year, with 25 percent using it at least weekly; 32 percent reported getting drunk in the last year, with 8 percent getting drunk at least once per week.

Naval Recruits

Blank and Fenton (1989) examined urinalysis results for 1,052 Navy recruits who were tested at the Great Lakes Recruit Training Center be-tween January 2 and March 4, 1985. There were significant differences between the groups testing positive and negative for marijuana on educa-tion, race, and scores on the Armed Forces Qualification Test (AFQT). The group testing positive for marijuana included 13 percent who did not gradu-ate from high school, compared with 6 percent of the group testing nega-tive. The positive-testing group included 23 percent blacks; the negative-testing group was 13 percent blacks. On AFQT scores, positive-testing recruits scored significantly lower than the negative-testing groups. There were no differences on age (due perhaps to a limited age range), marital status, or geographic region.

McDaniel (1988) examined self-reported drug use among 10,188 appli-cants who completed the Educational and Biographical Information Survey within a year of entering the Navy. A series of questions on the survey asked about previous use of marijuana and other illicit drugs and frequency of use. Overall, about 40 percent of the recruits admitted to having used marijuana before entering the Navy, 13 percent having used it at least 10 times and 5 percent admitting to marijuana use on at least 50 different occasions. Use of stimulants was reported by 13 percent, with 3 percent having used them at least 10 times. Finally, both cocaine and depressant use was revealed by 5 percent of the respondents with less than 1 percent in each case admitting to use at least 10 times.

Utility Employees

Taggert (1989) described the results of a drug-testing program at the Southern Pacific Railroad. Testing was conducted for all applicants for employment in conjunction with regularly scheduled physical exams, for reasonable suspicion, and for personnel involvement in accidents regardless of obvious cause. Of those tested, 23 percent were positive in 1984, 12 percent in 1985, 5 percent in 1986, and 6 percent in 1987. No breakdown by demographic characteristics were provided.

Sheridan and Winkler (1989) examined data from the drug-testing program at the Georgia Power Company, which included preemployment testing, testing for cause, and regular testing of nuclear plant and security personnel, both as part of the security clearance process and as part of annual physical examinations. In 1986, in a work force of about 15,000, 463 drug tests were conducted. Of these, 13 percent were positive, with 5 percent positive for marijuana, 2 percent for cocaine, and 6 percent for other drugs. In 1987, 366 tests were conducted, resulting in 15 percent positives (5 percent for marijuana, 2 percent for cocaine, and 8 percent for other drugs). Those in skilled and technical job classes were more likely than others to test positive, as were younger employees and employees hired after 1983.

Results from the drug-testing program at Southern California Edison's San Onofre Nuclear Generating Station (SONGS) are provided by Osborn and Sokolov (1989, 1990) for the period November 1988 to November 1989. During the first months, positive drug tests initially occurred at a rate of 3 percent, but the rate quickly fell to less than 2 percent per month for the remainder of the study. Rates of positive test results were considerably higher for contract workers than for SONGS employees. Positive rates for SONGS employees remained under 2 percent for the entire study period but were more variable among the contract workers, reaching a high of 5 percent. Osborn and Sokolov suggest that the difference exists because contract workers generally have less to lose from positive tests, as they can often find work at another site, but SONGS employees face a 14-day suspension and 1-year mandatory treatment program.

Crouch et al. (1989) examined the drug-testing and employee assistance programs at the Utah Power and Light Company in order to evaluate the cost-benefit ratios of the programs. Data from 1986 and 1987 were examined. A total of 1,036 drug tests were conducted during the period that included preemployment, for-cause, and promotion tests. There were 28 positive tests, for a prevalence rate of 3 percent. All but one of the positive tests involved marijuana. Demographically, those testing positive were likely to be male (75 percent), to have a mean age between 32 and 37, and to have worked as a laborer, operator, or craftsman.

Manufacturing

Cook and Bernstein (1991) reported on a study of a large manufacturing facility in the western United States with a work force of 2,400 primarily male blue-collar employees. Their study's goal was to assess the validity of different self-report methods for measuring employee illicit drug use. Four different self-report conditions were studied, and 200 employees were randomly selected and assigned to each of the four conditions: (1) individual interview in the workplace, (2) questionnaire administration in small groups, (3) telephone interviews away from work, and (4) individual interviews off the work site. Urine samples were also collected from all subjects at the time of the self-report data collection.

By condition, the prevalence rates were 12 percent for individual interviews at work, 6 percent for group administration, 11 percent for telephone interviews, and 12 percent for off-site interviews. These results indicate little difference between the three individual interview conditions, but lower reporting of illicit drug use in the group administration condition. Urinalysis indicated an 8 percent positive rate across all four conditions. The combination of self-report and urinalysis produced the most complete picture of the overall level of illicit drug use among the work force.

Summary

The reported literature on organization-specific studies of alcohol and other drug use prevalence provides a very sketchy picture of use within organizations. Few studies were designed specifically to examine prevalence or include both self-report and urinalysis data. Most of the other studies were designed for some other purpose, such as assessing the validity of preemployment selection or assessing the effectiveness of drug-testing programs. However, reports from these programs often did not differentiate between preemployment, random, and for-cause testing, so it is virtually impossible to compare results from organization to organization or to assess drug use prevalence. Programs that include a higher proportion of for-cause testing will have higher rates of positives, but they do provide some information about the types of drugs most likely to be detected. Data from random testing programs are also suspect because selection for testing is typically confined to certain job categories, it is often not done truly at random, and in practice employees are often aware of impending tests before they are officially informed they must take them.

OTHER PREVALENCE STUDIES OF ALCOHOL AND OTHER DRUG USE IN THE WORKPLACE

Few businesses have systematically studied the problem of on-the-job alcohol and other drug use. As was mentioned in Chapter 2, it is often assumed rather than proven that those who use alcohol and other drugs away from work will also do so on the job or in close enough proximity to affect workplace performance. Studies showing the prevalence of alcohol and other drug use by workers and job applicants are thought to shed light on alcohol and other drug use in the workplace, although they do not specifically or necessarily relate to this problem. Thus, the actual extent of alcohol and other drug use at work remains debatable.

Some articles in the popular press suggest that "everyone's doing it," but there are personnel experts who believe that the furor about alcohol and other drug use on the job reflects exaggerations by the media and other sources (e.g., Gordon, 1987). But it is not just the media estimates that may be excessive. For instance, Backer (1987) reports that "experts estimate that between 10 and 23 percent of all U.S. workers use dangerous drugs on the job." Such estimates are, however, based on best guesses rather than reliable assessment of alcohol and other drug use on the job. Furthermore, such estimates are typically based on two types of data, which, if not adequately discounted, overstate the problem (Alden, 1986): (1) information from addicted individuals seeking treatment who admit to having used alcohol or other drugs on the job and (2) estimates of the prevalence of alcohol or other drug problems among individuals in various occupations.

Washton and Gold (1987), for example, found that 75 percent of the callers to the national cocaine hotline (800-COCAINE) had used some drugs on the job. Not surprisingly, cocaine was the most prevalent drug used in the workplace by the callers, and 92 percent had done their job while under the influence of some drug. Similarly, Levy (1973) found that all but 2 of a group of 95 former addicts had used some drugs on the job. In both cases, the figures tell us only what a small group of severe abusers have done, and there is no simple way to generalize findings from such respondents to workers in general.

We were able to find only 15 studies that report rates of on-the-job alcohol and other drug use among specialized, general, and community samples. These studies cannot be readily compared because they vary greatly with respect to samples, job types, periods of assessment, definitions of *at work*, and type of substance. At best, these studies provide only preliminary estimates of the extent of alcohol and other drug use on the job or being high at work. Table 3.9 summarizes their results. We describe each briefly below.

Canadian Facts (1991) reported that 22 percent of 13,234 Canadian employees reported using alcohol on the job or having their job affected by alcohol use in the past month prior to the survey. Decima (1990) examined self-reports of on-the-job alcohol and illicit substance use during the past month for four types of Canadian mariners (private and public shore workers and private and public fleet workers). Findings showed that: (1) 12 percent of private shore workers reported using alcohol and 1 percent acknowledged using an illicit drug; (2) 5 percent of private fleet workers reported using alcohol and 1 percent reported using an illicit drug; (3) 8 percent of public shore workers admitted using alcohol and less than 0.5 percent reported using an illicit drug; and (4) 7 percent of public fleet employees reported using alcohol and 2 percent admitted using an illicit drug.

Gleason et al. (1991) analyzed data from 12,069 individuals from the National Longitudinal Survey of Youth regarding drug use on the job during the past year. Their findings indicate that in 1984, 7 percent of the U.S. work force aged 19-27 had used illicit drugs on the job. Men were more likely to report a higher use (10 percent) than women (4 percent), and white respondents were substantially more likely to report using drugs in the workplace than blacks or Hispanics. Moreover, this study reports that illicit drug use among young workers varies considerably by occupational group, with blue-collar workers reporting a much higher rate of on-the-job illicit drug use than white-collar workers. Specifically, craftworkers, operatives, and laborers all had rates of more than 9 percent compared to 5 percent for professional workers. By industry type their analyses show that the entertainment/recreational (14 percent) and construction industries (13 percent) had the highest rates of illicit drug use on the job, whereas professional services and public administration industries had the lowest, 3 percent and 2 percent, respectively. With regard to alcohol use at work, these researchers asked respondents whether they ever got drunk on the job. The difference between the percentage of men who reported having got drunk was significantly larger that the percentage of women who reported doing so (4 compared to 2 percent). Unfortunately most of the alcohol questions contained in this survey dealt with subjective judgments concerning the effects of alcohol use rather than actual on-the-job alcohol use.

Guinn (1983) studied self-reports from 112 long-distance truckers and found that over 80 percent had used some drug (excluding over-the-counter medications) to stay awake and alert while trucking during the past year. Holcom et al. (1991) found that 13 percent of 367 workers in safety-sensitive jobs reported using a psychoactive drug on the job compared with 8 percent of 687 workers in low-risk positions. Hollinger (1988) examined the use of any drug on the job during the past year for large samples

TABLE 3.9 Prevalence of Drug Use on the Work Site

Study	Type of Sample	N	Reporting Period	Any Drug	Alcohol	Any Illicit Drug	Marijuana	Cocaine
Canadian Facts (1991)	Canadian employees	13,234	Past month	—	22.0	—	—	—
Decima (1990)	Canadian mariners		Past month					
		Private						
		243 (share)		—	12.0	1.0	—	—
		1,645 (fleet)		—	5.0	1.0	—	—
		Public	Past month					
		550 (share)		—	8.0	0.0	—	—
		828 (fleet)		—	7.0	2.0	—	—
Gleason et al., (1991)	National youth	12,069	Past year					
		men		9.5	—	—	—	—
		white		10.1	—	—	—	—
		black		6.7	—	—	—	—
		Hispanic		6.5	—	—	—	—
		women		4.2	—	—	—	—
		white		4.5	—	—	—	—
		black		2.8	—	—	—	—
		Hispanic		2.9	—	—	—	—
Guinn (1983)	Long-distance truckers	112	Past year	80.4	—	—	—	—

continued

TABLE 3.9 (*Continued*)

Study	Type of Sample	N	Reporting Period	Any Drug	Alcohol	Any Illicit Drug	Marijuana	Cocaine
Holcomb et al. (1991)	Municipal employees	367 (high risk)	Past year	13.0	—	—	—	—
		687 (low risk)	Past year	8.0	—	—	—	—
Hollinger (1988)	Retail employees	3,512	Past year	7.6	—	—	—	—
	Manufacturing employees	1,484	Past year	12.8	—	—	—	—
	Hospital employees	4,040	Past year	3.2	—	—	—	—
O'Malley (1992)	High school seniors	c.8,000 men	Past year	—	8	—	5	—
	Women	c.8,000	Past year	—	5	—	1	—
Lehman and Simpson (1992)	Municipal workers	1,325	Past year	10	—	—	—	—
Lehman et al. (1990)	Municipal employees	1,239 (men)	Past year	—	8.0	3.0	—	—
		556 (women)	Past year	—	3.0	1.0	—	—

Study	Sample	N	Subgroup	Time period					
Martin et al. (in press)	National youth	not given	men[a]	Not given	—	4.2	—	7.1	1.4
			women[a]		—	1.6	—	2.3	0.8
Mensch and Kandel (1988)	Young adult men	5,299		Past month	—	5.0	—	8.0	2.0
Newcomb (1988)	Young adults (M age = 22)	221	men	Past 6 months	39.4	28.5	—	22.5	9.5
		518	(women)	Past 6 months	27.2	13.9	—	14.3	9.3
Newcomb (1989)	Adults (M age = 26)	154	men	Past 6 months	27	24	—	13	8
		391	(women)	Past 6 months	13	9	—	6	3
Schneck et al. (1991)	Transportation employees	120,000		Not specified	—	6	3	—	—
White et al. (1988)	Commuting employees	<225[b]	men	Past year	—	7.1[b]	—	31.9[b]	—
			women	Past year	—	1.6[b]	—	23.3[b]	—

[a] These were reported separately for part-time and full-time employees. Although Ns were not reported for these breakdowns, the percentages cited are equal-weighted averages of these two groups.

[b] Precise Ns for men and women workers were not provided. Prevalence rates were based on past year users of each drug.

representing three occupational groups and found that: (1) 8 percent of retail employees reported some drug use on the job; (2) 13 percent of manufacturing employees reported such behavior; as did (3) 3 percent of hospital employees. Lehman and Simpson (1992) found that 10 percent of 1,325 municipal workers admitted using some illicit drug on the job.

Results showed that 8 percent of 1,239 men and 3 percent of 556 women reported using alcohol on the job, while 3 percent of the men and 1 percent of the women reported some illicit drug use in the workplace.

Mensch and Kandel (1988) studied data from large samples of young adults. Among the 5,299 men, 5 percent admitted using alcohol in the workplace, 8 percent had used marijuana, and 2 percent had used cocaine. Of the 4,860 women, 1 percent reported being high on alcohol on the job, 3 percent on marijuana, and 1 percent on cocaine. Martin et al. (in press) also examined national samples of youth, looking separately at part-time and full-time employees. Those who were employed full time reported higher rates of using alcohol, cocaine, and marijuana on the job than those who worked part time. Unfortunately, sample sizes were not provided in this report, although based on the data set used, the numbers should be in the thousands. Estimates of drug use on the job for men (4 percent for alcohol, 7 percent for marijuana, and 1 percent for cocaine) were consistently and substantially higher than those for women (2 percent for alcohol, 3 percent for marijuana, and 1 percent for cocaine). Schneck et al. (1991) examined responses from about 120,000 transportation employees and found that 6 percent had used alcohol at times that would interfere with their job, and 3 percent reported a similar use of illicit drugs.

Newcomb (1988) studied a community sample of 739 young adults and found that among the 221 men, 39 percent reported being "high, drunk, or stoned" on the job at least once during the past 6 months: 29 percent had used alcohol, 23 percent marijuana, 10 percent cocaine, and 6 percent other stimulants. Among the 518 women in the sample, 27 percent reported having been high, drunk, or stoned on the job: 14 percent had used alcohol, 14 percent marijuana, 9 percent cocaine, and 5 percent other stimulants. This same sample was assessed 4 years later with substantially reduced rates of being high, drunk, or stoned on the job (Newcomb, 1989). Of the 154 men whom Newcomb was able to follow, 27 percent had been high on a psychoactive drug in the workplace, with 24 percent reporting alcohol use, 13 percent marijuana use, 8 percent cocaine use, and 3 percent other stimulants. Among the 391 women in the follow-up survey, 13 percent reported using any psychoactive substance on the job, with 5 percent reporting use of alcohol, 6 percent marijuana, 3 percent cocaine, and 1 percent other stimulants.

The different prevalence rates reported by different studies are probably due to the variations in questions asked, samples used, and occupations represented. For instance, long-distance truckers who are paid for the miles they drive may be particularly susceptible to using drugs that will keep them awake, help them drive farther, and earn them more money. Similarly, some of the samples surveyed may consist of people who hold nontraditional attitudes and engage in more atypical behavior than other adults. Newcomb's particularly high prevalence rates may not only reflect the nature of his sample but may also have been due in part to asking participants whether they have been "drunk, high, or stoned," on the job rather than whether they "had used drugs" on the job. This question captures people who while on the job felt the effects of drugs taken before work, during breaks, at lunch, as well as those affected by drugs taken during work hours. If so, this question more adequately assesses the proportion of the work force whose performance might be affected by drugs than does the more commonly asked inquiry into on-the-job drug use.

This is one reason that may explain why White et al. (1988) obtained such high rates of workplace drug use, since their items asked respondents whether they had gone to work "high" on alcohol or marijuana during the past year. Of employed men who used marijuana during the past year, 32 percent reported going to work high on marijuana at least once in the past year, whereas only 7 percent of men who reported drinking reported going to work high on alcohol in the past year. Rates for women were substantially smaller, with 23 percent of current marijuana users admitting to having gone to work high on marijuana and 2 percent of current drinkers reporting showing up at work high on alcohol. Since these figures are based only on users of the particular drug, they do not mean that a large proportion of workers in general show up for work high.

Often data from the HHS and the MWS (discussed earlier in this chapter) also report drug use on the job. Since those studies have been discussed earlier, they are not repeated here. They showed, however, that alcohol use was the most commonly used drug at work and that illicit drug use at work is relatively low. The HSS survey assessed alcohol and other drug use at work by asking respondents in the follow-up surveys if they had used a given drug at work during the past year. Unfortunately, the meaning of the term *at work* was not further specified. Table 3.10 reports data on substance use at work from the 1987 through 1991 follow-up surveys. As depicted in Table 3.10, alcohol is the substance most often used at work. More specifically, in 1991 alcohol had the highest on-the-job prevalence rate, with 8 percent of the men and 5 percent of the women reporting having used alcohol at work in the past 12 months. Illicit drugs have never been used at work by a large proportion of the work force, and the proportion has decreased substantially in recent years. Marijuana was the second most prevalent drug, with use at work reported by 5 percent of the men and 1 percent of the women in 1991. Less than 1 percent of this sample used any

TABLE 3.10 Trends in Alcohol and Other Drug Use at Work, Past 12 Months, Young Adults Aged 19-28 (in percent)

Substance/Sex	Year of Survey				
	1987	1988	1989	1990	1991
Alcohol					
Male	12.2	7.0	9.0	8.8	7.6
Female	7.7	6.3	5.4	6.0	4.6
Marijuana					
Male	8.0	5.6	5.1	4.6	4.5
Female	1.5	1.6	1.5	1.2	0.9
Cocaine					
Male	2.9	2.7	1.5	1.6	0.5
Female	1.0	2.3	0.5	1.1	0.3
Amphetamines					
Male	2.9	2.8	1.5	1.6	0.4
Female	3.0	2.0	2.0	1.3	0.8
Tranquilizers					
Male	0.8	0.3	0.5	0.3	0.2
Female	1.0	0.5	0.1	0.4	0.3

SOURCE: Unpublished data from the High School Senior Surveys (1992).

other illicit drug on the job. Cocaine use at work was reported by 0.5 percent of the men and by 0.3 percent of the women. Corresponding figures for amphetamines were 0.4 and 0.8 percent and for tranquilizers, 0.2 and 0.3 percent. The figures from the HSS follow-ups are likely to underestimate true prevalence of drug use in the work force, since high school dropouts are not in the sample and, like all longitudinal studies, the HSS suffers from attrition; however, the trends nevertheless seem clear: drug use is declining among the broad spectrum of youth, both in general and at work.

The HHS follow-ups show that alcohol and other drug use at work also varies with occupation. In general, protective services workers (police, fire fighters) show very low rates of use at work, and skilled workers show relatively high rates, with little variation across the other categories (Table 3.11). Alcohol use at work (at least once in the previous 12 months) is highest for men in the skilled and managerial categories; professionals and semiskilled workers are also high in their use rates. Controlling for occupation, women are only slightly less likely than men to have used alcohol at work, and among clericals female use rates are slightly higher.

The findings in several studies that more respondents admit to using

TABLE 3.11 Use of Alcohol and Other Drugs at Work in Past 12 Months, Young Adults Aged 19-28 by Occupational Category (in percent)

Sex/Occupation	Alcohol	Marijuana	Cocaine	Amphetamines	Tranquilizer
Males					
Semiskilled[a]	9.6	9.5	2.6	3.4	0.8
Clerical, sales[b]	4.2	3.4	1.8	1.4	0.5
Police, fire[c]	3.6	1.3	0.0	0.9	0.0
Military[d]	5.8	1.1	0.7	1.4	0.0
Skilled[e]	11.3	9.2	3.6	2.4	0.5
Manager, sales rep[f]	10.1	2.8	0.8	1.4	0.4
Professional[g]	8.5	2.8	1.4	0.5	0.3
Females					
Semiskilled[a]	6.8	2.7	1.2	3.0	0.5
Clerical, sales[b]	6.0	1.6	1.6	1.9	0.2
Police, fire[c]	0.0	0.0	0.0	3.2	0.0
Military[d]	5.4	0.0	0.0	3.2	0.0
Skilled[e]	7.0	4.8	1.0	4.0	2.9
Manager, sales rep[f]	7.9	0.5	1.1	0.0	0.9
Professional[g]	5.0	0.2	0.1	0.6	0.4

[a]Semiskilled: laborer (car washer, sanitary worker, farm laborer); service worker (cook, waiter, barber, janitor, gas station attendant, practical nurse, beautician); operative or semi-skilled worker (garage worker, taxicab, bus or truck driver, assembly line worker, welder).

[b]Clerical, sales clerk: sales clerk in a retail store (shoe salesperson, department store, drug store); clerical or office worker (bank teller, bookkeeper, secretary, typist, postal clerk or carrier, ticket agent).

[c]Police, fire; protective service (police officer, fireman, detective).

[d]Military; military service.

[e]Skilled; craftsman or skilled worker (carpenter, electrician, brick layer, mechanic, machinist, tool and die maker, telephone installer).

[f]Manager, sales rep; farm owner, farm manager; owner of a small business (restaurant owner, shop owner); sales representative (insurance agent, real estate broker, bond salesman); manager or administrator (office manager, sales manager, school administrator, government official).

[g]Professional: professional with doctoral degree or equivalent (lawyer, physician, dentist, scientist, college professor).

SOURCE: Unpublished data from the High School Senior Surveys (1992).

marijuana than alcohol in the workplace is surprising, since alcohol is in general the most frequently used drug at the work site. This discrepancy is probably a sample artifact, as in the White et al. (1988) study in which respondents were limited to those who had used the illicit drug.

Summary

Prevalence estimates vary greatly across studies, although alcohol or marijuana are consistently the most prevalent drugs used in the workplace. Nevertheless, three conclusions can be drawn that are also consistent with findings from large-scale survey findings. First, according to employee reports, drug use in the workplace ranges from a modest to a moderate extent (although much of the reported use may be single incidents, perhaps even at events like office parties). Second, men are more likely than women to use drugs in the workplace. And third, the highest rates of workplace drug use seem to be among young adults, with use decreasing substantially with increasing age.

CONCLUSIONS AND RECOMMENDATIONS

Data sources ranging from self-report questionnaires to urinalysis testing to emergency room visits provide important insights about the use of alcohol and other drugs among members of the general population and the work force. Taken together, the data indicate that, since the late 1970s:

(1) The prevalence of illicit drug use among members of the general population and the work force has been decreasing, but continues to affect a sizable proportion of the population, especially young adults.

(2) Illicit drug use may be decreasing among occasional users, but it may be stable or even increasing among hard-core users who are generally not well represented in surveys.

(3) Heavy alcohol use has been relatively stable over the past several years; rates of heavy drinking have been notably high among young adult men, especially those in the military and among workers in such industries as construction, transportation, and wholesale goods.

(4) Cigarette smoking has been declining during the past decade for those 18 and older, but has been relatively stable for youths ages 12 to 17.

(5) Illicit drug use is more common among unemployed than employed persons, and weekly alcohol use is highest among young employed workers.

(6) Illicit drug use is relatively high among male workers in certain industries, such as construction, but relatively low among professionals.

• Given these long-term trends, we must be cautious in attributing short-term changes in alcohol and other drug use in either society or the work force to specific national efforts to stem the use of drugs.

• Few epidemiological studies are targeted directly at the work force, leaving researchers to rely on data sources designed for other uses.

Recommendation: More focused epidemiological studies, including longitudinal studies, are needed to assess the magnitude and severity of alcohol and other drug use among the work force. As a first step, the National Household Surveys on Drug Abuse should be modified to provide specific information about job characteristics, job-related behaviors, and alcohol and other drug use at work. Ultimately a national panel survey devoted to this topic should be instituted. In addition, other studies are needed that provide better information about: (1) employment patterns among persons who use alcohol and other drugs; (2) patterns of alcohol and other drug use among workers; (3) patterns of use in heavily using populations to better understand the employment history and work experience of these individuals; and (4) the impact of illicit drug use and heavy alcohol use on work activity.

Although the workplace offers a unique opportunity to obtain leverage on the alcohol and other drug problems of some users, there are many serious alcohol and other drug abusers who are not regularly employed, if they are employed at all. In 1990 approximately 7 percent of workers reported having used an illicit drug and approximately 6 percent reported having drunk heavily in the past month, compared with 14 percent and 6 percent, respectively, for the unemployed.

• Given the relative low base rate of alcohol and other drug abusers in the employed segment of the work force compared with other selected populations, postemployment workplace alcohol and other drug interventions may help a limited number of abusers, but workplace-oriented interventions cannot solve society's problems with alcohol and other drugs.
• Alcohol and tobacco are the drugs most widely abused by members of the U.S. work force. The adverse health consequences of these drugs are well known. In terms of prevalence rates of work force use and perceived effects of use on performance, alcohol is more likely to have adverse consequences.

Recommendation: Any program that addresses drug use by the work force should include alcohol, the drug most associated with perceived detrimental job performance, as a priority.

Rates of self-reported alcohol and other drug use on the job vary according to occupation, age, gender, and ethnicity. Excluding tobacco and caffeine, most surveys find that fewer than 10 percent of workers report having used alcohol or other drugs while on the job during the prior year. Some studies, however, report significantly higher usage rates. Much of the difference in the rates reported appears attributable to differences in the samples surveyed and the questions asked.

Recommendation: It is important to investigate alcohol and other drug use in different well-specified samples and to develop benchmark measures to allow findings that are comparable across studies.

REFERENCES

Alden, W.F.
  1986   The scope of the drug problem: a national strategy. *Vital Speeches of the Day* 751-
          756.
Backer, T.E.
  1987   *Strategic Planning for Workplace Drug Abuse Problems.* Rockville, Md.: National
          Institute on Drug Abuse.
Blank, D.L., and J.W. Fenton
  1989   Early employment testing for marijuana: demographic and employee retention pat-
          terns. In S.W. Gust and J.M. Walsh, eds., *Drugs in the Workplace: Research and
          Evaluation Data.* NIDA Research Monograph 91. Rockville, Md.: National Insti-
          tute on Drug Abuse.
Bray, R.M., M.E. Marsden, and M.R. Peterson
  1991   Standardized comparisons of the use of alcohol, drugs, and cigarettes among mili-
          tary personnel and civilians. *American Journal of Public Health* 81:865-869.
Bray, R.M., L.A. Kroutil, J.W. Luckey, S.C. Wheeless, V.G. Iannacchione, D.W. Anderson,
          M.E. Marsden, and G.H. Dunteman
  1992   *1992 Worldwide Survey of Substance Abuse and Health Behaviors Among Military
          Personnel.* Research Triangle Park, N.C.: Research Triangle Institute.
Canadian Facts
  1991   *Substance Use and the Work Place Survey of Employees.* Ottawa, Canada: Cana-
          dian Facts.
Cook, R.F., and A.D. Bernstein
  1991   Assessing Drug Abuse in the Workplace: A Comparison of Major Methods. Paper
          presented at the Drug-Free Workplace Conference, Washington, D.C.
Crouch, D.J., D.O. Webb, L.V. Peterson, P.F. Buller, and D.E. Rollins
  1989   A critical evaluation of the Utah Power and Light Company's substance abuse man-
          agement program: absenteeism, accidents, and costs. In S.W. Gust and J.M. Walsh,
          eds., *Drugs in the Workplace: Research and Evaluation Data.* NIDA Research
          Monograph 91. Rockville, Md.: National Institute on Drug Abuse.
Decima
  1990   *Final Report to Transport Canada on the Results for the Substance Use and Trans-
          portation Safety Study.* Toronto, Canada: Decima Research.
Gerstein, D.R., and L.W. Green, eds.
  1993   *Preventing Drug Abuse: What Do We Know?* Committee on Drug Abuse Preven-
          tion Research, Commission on Behavioral and Social Sciences and Education, Na-
          tional Research Council. Washington, D.C.: National Academy Press.
Gleason, P.M., J.R. Veu, and M.R. Pergamit
  1991   Drug and alcohol use at work: a survey of young workers. *Monthly Labor Review*
          August:3-7.

Gordon, J.
1987   Drug testing as a productivity booster? *Training* 24:22-34
Guinn, B.
1983   Job satisfaction, counterproductive behavior and circumstantial drug use among long-distance truckers. *Journal of Psychoactive Drugs* 15:185-188.
Gust, S.W., and J.M. Walsh, eds.
1989   *Drugs in the Workplace: Research and Evaluation Data.* NIDA Research Monograph 91. Rockville, Md.: National Institute on Drug Abuse.
Gust, S.W., J.M. Walsh, L.B. Thomas, and D.J. Crouch, eds.
1990   *Drugs in the Workplace: Research and Evaluation Data,* Vol. II. NIDA Research Monograph 100. Rockville, Md.: National Institute on Drug Abuse.
Holcom, M.L., W.E.K. Lehman, and D.D. Simpson
1991   Employee Accidents: Influences of Personal Characteristics, Job Characteristics, and Substance Use. Unpublished manuscript, Institute of Behavioral Research, Texas Christian University, Fort Worth.
Hollinger, R.C.
1988   Working under the influence (WUI): correlates of employees use of alcohol and other drugs. *Journal of Applied Behavioral Science* 24:439-454.
Johnston, L.D., P.M. O'Malley, and J.G. Bachman
1992   *Smoking, Drinking, and Illicit Drug Use Among American Secondary School Students, College Students, and Young Adults, 1975-1991,* Vol. I and II. Rockville, Md.: National Institute on Drug Abuse.
Kopstein, A., and J. Gfroerer
1990   Drug use patterns and demographics of employed drug users: data from the 1988 Household Survey. Pp. 25-44 in S.W. Gust, J.M. Walsh, L.B. Thomas, and D.J. Crouch, eds., *Drugs in the Workplace: Research and Evaluation Data,* Vol. 2. NIDA Research Monograph 100. Rockville, Md.: National Institute on Drug Abuse.
Lehman, W.E.K., and D.D. Simpson
1992   Employee substance use and on-the-job behaviors. *Journal of Applied Psychology* 77:309-321.
Lehman, W.E.K., M.L. Holcom, and D.D. Simpson
1990a   Employee Health and Performance in the Workplace: A Survey of Municipal Employees of a Large Southwest City. Institute of Behavioral Research, Texas Christian University, Fort Worth.
1990b   Employee Health and Performance in the Workplace: A Survey of Employees of the Housing Authority in a Large Southwest City. Institute of Behavioral Research, Texas Christian University, Fort Worth.
Levy, S.I.
1973   A case study of drug-related criminal behavior in business and industry. In J.M. Sher, ed., *Drug Abuse in Industry.* Springfield, Ill.: Thomas.
Martin, J.K., J.M. Kraft, and P.M. Roman
in press The extent and impact of alcohol and drug problems in the workplace. In S. McDonald and P. Roman, eds., *Drug Screening in the Workplace: Research Perspectives.* Washington, D.C.: Hemisphere.
McDaniel, M.A.
1988   Does pre-employment drug use predict on-the-job suitability? *Personnel Psychology* 41:717-729.
Mensch, B.S., and D.B. Kandel
1988   Do job conditions influence the use of drugs? *Journal of Health and Social Behavior* 29:169-184.

National Institute on Drug Abuse
   1991   *National Household Survey on Drug Abuse: Main Findings 1990.* Rockville, Md.:
            National Institute on Drug Abuse.
Newcomb, M.D.
   1988   *Drug Use in the Workplace: Risk Factors for Disruptive Substance Use Among
            Young Adults.* Dover, Mass.: Auburn House.
   1989   Drug Use and Sensation Seeking: Latent-Variable Comparisons Among Adoles-
            cents. Paper presented at the Western Psychological Association meeting, Reno,
            Nevada.
Normand, J., and S.D. Salyards
   1989   An empirical evaluation of preemployment drug testing in the United States Postal
            Service: interim report of findings. In S.W. Gust and J.M. Walsh, eds., *Drugs in
            the Workplace: Research and Evaluation Data.* NIDA Research Monograph 91.
            Rockville, Md.: National Institute on Drug Abuse.
Normand, J., S.D. Salyards, and J.J. Mahony
   1990   An evaluation of preemployment drug testing. *Journal of Applied Psychology*
            75:629-639.
Osborn, C.E., and J.J. Sokolov
   1989   Drug use trends in a nuclear power company: cumulative data from an ongoing
            testing program. In S.W. Gust and J.M. Walsh, eds., *Drugs in the Workplace:
            Research and Evaluation Data.* NIDA Research Monograph 91. Rockville, Md.:
            National Institute on Drug Abuse.
   1990   Drug use trends in a nuclear power facility: data from a random screening program.
            In S.W. Gust, J.M. Walsh, L.B. Thomas, and D.J. Crouch, eds., *Drugs in the Work-
            place: Research and Evaluation Data*, Vol. II. NIDA Research Monograph 100.
            Rockville, Md.: National Institute on Drug Abuse.
Parish, D.C.
   1989   Relation of the pre-employment drug testing result to employment status: a one-
            year follow-up. *Journal of General Internal Medicine* 4:44-47.
Parker, D.A., and T.C. Harford
   1992   The epidemiology of alcohol consumption and dependence across occupations in the
            United States. *Alcohol Health & Research World* 16(2):97-105.
Rosenbaum, A.L., W.E.K. Lehman, E.K., Olsen, and M.L. Holcom
   1992   Prevalence of Substance Use and its Association with Employee Performance Among
            Municipal Workers in a Southwestern City. Institute of Behavioral Research, Texas
            Christian University, Fort Worth.
Schneck, D., R. Amodei, and R. Kernish
   1991   *Substance Abuse in the Transit Industry.* Washington, D.C.: Office of Technical
            Assistance and Safety.
Sheridan, J.R., and H. Winkler
   1989   An evaluation of drug testing in the workplace. In S.W. Gust and J.M. Walsh, eds.,
            Drugs in the Workplace: Research and Evaluation Data. NIDA Research Mono-
            graph 91. Rockville, Md.: National Institute on Drug Abuse.
Substance Abuse and Mental Health Services Administration
   1993   *National Household Survey on Drug Abuse: Main Findings 1991.* Rockville, Md.:
            Substance Abuse and Mental Health Services Administration.
Taggert, R.W.
   1989   Results of the drug testing program at Southern Pacific Railroad. In S.W. Gust and
            J.M. Walsh, eds., *Drugs in the Workplace: Research and Evaluation Data.* NIDA
            Research Monograph 91. Rockville, Md.: National Institute on Drug Abuse.

Washton, A.M., and M.S. Gold
   1987   Recent trends in cocaine abuse as seen in the cocaine hotline. Pp. 10-22 in A.M. Washton and M.S. Gold, eds., *Cocaine: Clinicians Handbook.* New York: Guilford Press.
White, H.R., A. Aidala, and B. Zablocki
   1988   A longitudinal investigation of drug use and work patterns among middle-class, white adults. *The Journal of Applied Behavioral Science* 4:466-469.
Wish, E.
   1990-   U.S. drug policy in the 1990s: insights from new data from arrestees.
   1992   *International Journal of the Addictions* 25:377-409.
Zwerling, C., J. Ryan, and E.J. Orav
   1990   The efficacy of preemployment drug screening for marijuana and cocaine in predicting employment outcome. *Journal of the American Medical Association* 264:2639-2643.

II
EFFECTS OF USE

4

Impact of Alcohol and Other Drug Use: Laboratory Studies

Despite substantial national efforts, drug abuse remains a serious public health problem for a sizable proportion of the population. Since data presented in Chapter 3 suggest that a sizable portion of the work force uses drugs, reducing use by the active work force would have an impact on drug use overall, reducing the pool of illicit drug users in the United States and moving us closer to the societal goal of eliminating drug abuse. The workplace is thus an obvious site for user-focused interventions.

STRENGTHS AND LIMITATIONS
OF LABORATORY STUDIES

This societal perspective is seldom used to justify programs to reduce or eliminate drug use by the work force, and there may be constitutional problems with workplace drug-testing programs aimed predominantly at this goal. Interventions aimed at securing a drug-free workplace are justified instead largely on safety and productivity grounds. The data obtained in worker population studies, however, do not provide clear evidence of the deleterious effects of drugs other than alcohol on safety and other job performance indicators. This does not mean there are no deleterious effects; it may reflect the paucity of relevant data and the quality of the research done to date.

The extent to which impaired worker performance due to drug use can affect safety and productivity in the workplace is not well understood, although a substantial amount of laboratory research has been carried out evaluating the effects of single doses of various abusable drugs on cognitive and psychomotor performance. The results of such research cannot be extrapolated directly to the workplace because the effects of drugs on workplace performance are a complex function of the interaction between the dynamic workplace environment and the multiplicity of other variables impinging on the worker. For example, the job performance of a worker who has slept little the night before, is anxious about a family member's problem, has not eaten breakfast, must work with a dangerous piece of equipment, and has continually changing job demands is likely to be affected differently by a prior night's use of marijuana or cocaine than a well-rested worker performing a routine task. The challenge of modeling such complex interactions and simplifying the issues so that they can be studied in the laboratory is obvious and may never fully be met. Yet laboratory research can provide a base from which to start understanding such problems. Even if it cannot capture the full richness of the occupational world, it can help us understand how the drugs people take interact with different kinds of ongoing behavior; this is knowledge we must have in order to design and implement effective intervention programs.

A second goal of laboratory research on drug effects is to develop reliable measures of the acute impairment associated with drug use. To date, the most commonly used method for identifying drug use by the work force relies on urinalysis to detect the presence of drugs or their metabolites. Such testing does not address the issue of drug-induced impairment. Although there are data relating dose of alcohol to level of impairment, there are no data relating the level of other drugs (or their metabolites) obtained from urinalysis to levels of impairment. Laboratory-developed measures of impairment that lead to the development of a reliable and easily administered performance battery for the detection of workplace performance impairment could be an enormous improvement over the current technologies (discussed in Chapter 6).

A myriad of laboratory performance studies have been carried out to test the effects, under controlled conditions, of such drugs as stimulants, marijuana, sedatives, benzodiazepines, and alcohol (see Table 4.1).[1] How-

---

[1]This discussion is based on a review, for the National Research Council, of approximately 250 papers by Foltin and Evans (1992). The studies included were published between 1970 and 1991 and involved healthy volunteers tested using laboratory tasks and given single doses of stimulant, sedative-hypnotic, alcohol, or marijuana. A shorter version of that review has recently been published by the *Journal of Human Psychopharmacology* (see Foltin and Evans, 1993). Review of the 250 papers yielded data on 305 tasks, only 118 of which were used in more than one experiment. For simplicity of discussion, tasks were grouped into general categories and only general behavioral effects are discussed.

TABLE 4.1 Examples of Task and Performance Effects of Selected Drugs of Abuse

Drug/Study	Task[a]	Results
Stimulants		
Lane and Williams (1985) (caffeine, 250 mg)	arithmetic	not significant
Klorman et al. (1984) (methylphenidate, 20 mg)	continuous performance	not significant
Hindmarch et al. (1990) (nicotine, 2 mg gum)	complex reaction time	not significant
Heishman and Stitzer (1989) (amphetamines, 20 mg)	circular lights	not significant
Marijuana		
Jones and Stone (1970) (4.5, 9.0 mg)	time estimation	impaired
Pihl and Sigal (1978) (8 mg)	time estimation	impaired
Marks and MacAvoy (1989) (2.6, 5.2 mg)	divided attention	impaired
Heishman et al. (1989) (12, 21 mg)	divided attention	not significant
Hooker and Jones (1987) (12 mg)	arithmetic	not significant
Barnett et al. (1985) (7, 14, 17.5 mg)	tracking	impaired
Evans et al. (1976) (1.75 mg/70 kg)	tracking	impaired
Alcohol		
Strömberg et al. (1988) (1g/kg)	postural stability	impaired
Erwin et al. (1986) (0.8g/kg)	divided attention	impaired
Collins (1980) (3.25 ml)	reaction time	impaired
Wilson et al. (1984) (BAC 100 mg)	tapping	impaired
Taberner et al. (1983) (0.1-0.4 g/kg)	cancellation	impaired
Peterson et al. (1990) (0.132-1.32 ml)	reaction time	impaired
Linnoila et al. (1990) (0.8g/kg)	continuous performance	not significant
Foltin et al. (1993) (19.4-58.1 g)	vigilance	impaired
Linnoila et al. (1990) (0.8g/kg)	complex reaction time	not significant
Peterson et al. (1990) (0.132-1.32 ml)	tracking	impaired

continued on next page

TABLE 4.1 *(Continued)*

Drug/Study	Task[a]	Results
Folton et al. (1993) (19.4-58.1 g)	list recall	not significant
Sedatives		
Mattila et al. (1986) (Buspirone, 15 mg)	divided attention	not significant
Preston et al. (1989) (Lorazepam, 1-4 mg)	circular lights	impaired
Patat et al. (1987) (Diazepam, 10 mg)	tapping	not significant
Mattila et al. (1986) (Diazepam, 10.5, 21 mg)	cancellation	impaired
Curran and Lader (1987) (Lorazepam, 1.2 mg)	arithmetic	impaired
Erwin et al. (1986) (Diazepam, 10 mg)	continuous performance	impaired
Alford et al. (1991) (Clobazam, 10 mg)	complex reaction time	not significant
Patat et al. (1991) (Triazolam, 0.25 mg)	list recall	impaired
Alford et al. (1991) (Lorazepam, 1 mg)	recognition memory	impaired

[a]Definition of tasks:

Arithmetic: subjects required to perform simple mathematical tasks, most often "in their heads" rather than using pencil and paper.

Complex reaction time: subjects required to respond differentially to a change in stimulus conditions.

Time estimation: subjects required to give time estimations.

Divided attention: subjects required to perform two tasks simultaneously.

Tracking: subjects required to track a moving stimulus with their dominant hand.

Postural stability: a range of various tasks to provide measures of gross motor coordination.

Circular lights: measures gross hand/eye coordination.

Tapping: requires subjects to tap a key with one finger for a given number of taps or length of time.

Cancellation: requires subjects to examine a field of information and mark as many target stimuli as possible in a fixed period of time.

Reaction time: requires subjects to respond as rapidly as possible to a visual or auditory stimulus which has only one correct response.

Continuous performance: requires subjects to attend to stimulus presentations and respond when certain patterns of stimuli occur.

Vigilance: reaction time tasks under continuous attention conditions.

List recall: requires subjects to recall previous learned tasks or information.

Recognition memory: requires subjects to recall or list stimuli previously presented to them.

SOURCE: Foltin and Evans (1992).

ever, even apart from the complex interaction effects mentioned above, these studies have numerous shortcomings as guides to understanding the effects of alcohol and other drug use by the work force. Although the doses studied are sometimes (but not always) the same as those being used by drug users in the work force, patterning of drug use comparable to that of many drug users (i.e., multiple doses, periodically repeated doses, etc.) has not been adequately addressed. Moreover, with few exceptions, no attempt has been made to model the specific task used to measure impairment after specific workplace performances, and multiple variations on similar tasks make generalization across studies difficult.

To further complicate the picture, there has been little effort to model the subject population in laboratory studies after the work force population. The most frequently used research subject is a college student, paid to participate in a research project, or expected to participate in order to fulfill a course requirement. In addition, unlike the worker who is experienced in the task being performed, the subjects in most drug use studies are frequently performing the tasks on which impairment is measured for the first time or after only a brief period of training. Behavioral histories are seldom taken into account in laboratory research. Other common weaknesses of experimental design include inattention to doses used, time points for measurements, and contingencies in maintaining behavior. Despite these problems, however, a few generalizations can be drawn about the likely effects of different classes of drugs on performance.

DRUGS AND THEIR EFFECTS

Stimulant Drugs

Stimulant drugs (e.g., caffeine, amphetamine, cocaine) increase general activity, lead to reports of positive subjective effects, and are often used clinically to reduce food intake (Fischman, 1987). Despite users' reports of substantial performance enhancement after stimulant use, this effect has not been systematically replicated in the laboratory (Johanson and Fischman, 1989). When improvement in performance has occurred, the margin of improvement has either been less than 10 percent, or stimulants prevented or reversed a decrement in performance due to fatigue or boredom. Of course in some situations like athletic competitions, a minor improvement in performance could have large positive effects for the performer (Laties and Weiss, 1981), and, when otherwise unavoidable fatigue or boredom are fought off, decrements in performance may be forestalled. In general, however, it is important to point out that significant performance enhancement is not apparent; much of what users report are the subjective effects of stimulants (e.g., increased levels of energy, friendliness), which lead to a belief that behavior is improved without any actual improvement (Fischman, 1987).

Marijuana

The use of marijuana and products containing Δ^9-tetrahydrocannabinol (THC) has a long history, and the literature on the effects of these substances on performance is voluminous. Concentrated efforts to delineate marijuana-related effects on behavior have yielded variable results, with the most consistent effects being decrements in time estimation and divided attention tasks (e.g., Jones and Stone, 1970; Marks and MacAvoy, 1989). Marijuana interfered with performance on a variety of other tasks on approximately 50 percent of the occasions it was studied (e.g., arithmetic, Chesher et al., 1977; tracking, Barnett et al., 1985), suggesting that experimental conditions play a substantial role in determining the effects of this substance. Although there is some evidence that marijuana can affect performance for several hours after it is used (e.g., Miller and Cornett, 1978), there are almost no data on what behaviors are impaired, for how long, and to what extent.

There has been a general belief that smoking marijuana can lead to a cluster of signs and symptoms often referred to as an *amotivational syndrome*. If it does, repeated rather than occasional use of marijuana could have severe implications for behavior and productivity in the workplace. The motivational effects of marijuana have provided a focus for research over the past several decades, with variable results. In general, well-controlled epidemiological studies of marijuana use have failed to confirm the existence of such a syndrome (e.g., Comitas, 1976; Stefanis et al., 1977; Page, 1983), and laboratory research suggests that environmental conditions can influence the amotivational effects of marijuana, determining its presence or absence (Foltin et al., 1989, 1990).

Alcohol and Sedatives

The majority of studies evaluating acute effects of alcohol administration have found that single doses cause decrements in a variety of performance tasks, particularly tracking, visual vigilance, divided attention, postural stability, and cancellation tasks, with less robust effects on memory tasks. Since the problems that alcohol use poses for transportation safety are well recognized, it has received substantial attention from the transportation research community. As with other laboratory studies, the magnitude of impairment in transportation-related tasks has been shown to be dependent on the nature of the task, research subject characteristics (e.g., skill level, tolerance) and environmental factors (e.g., fatigue). Overlearned tasks (e.g., coordination, balance) are relatively resistant to alcohol consumption (Burns, 1992), while divided attention, information processing, and attention processes are highly susceptible to alcohol-induced impairment (Streufert et al., 1992). Performance on these latter tasks are impaired at low blood alcohol levels, implying that relatively small amounts of alcohol can have detrimental consequences for both traffic safety as well as other workplace safety-sensitive positions. Although there is a relationship between blood alcohol level and decrements in performance, there is considerable variability in the alcohol level at which decrements occur. In addition, there is variability in the amount of alcohol required to reach a given blood alcohol level, even when body weight is controlled (O'Neil et al., 1983). This source of variability is largely related to variations in metabolic rate. Furthermore, although the data are not as clear for all the benzodiazepines, data with prototypic benzodiazepines (diazepam, lorazepam, and triazolam) suggest that, as with alcohol, these drugs produce decrements on a full range of performance tasks, from gross motor tasks such as postural stability (Evans et al., 1990) to complex tasks such as divided attention (Erwin et al., 1986).

Residual Drug Effects

Although residual effects can refer to any effects that occur a number of hours after major drug effects have dissipated, this has come to mean *next-day effects* or *hangover effects*. The issue here is whether substances used at home on one day affect job performance the next day. These effects can either be manifested as prolonged drug effects, similar to the initial drug effect, or can differ from the initial drug effect. This latter change in behavior is best characterized by what is commonly called hangover. Thus, alcohol consumed during the evening can produce intoxication, slurred speech, etc. Six or eight hours later, after some sleep and no further alcohol intake, a different set of symptoms (e.g., headache, irritability, inability to concentrate, etc.) might be apparent. Such hangover effects can be disruptive in the workplace, reducing productivity and perhaps interfering with safe and accurate performance and/or social interactions. In addition, it is possible that hangover or drug withdrawal effects are contributing factors in the maintenance of drug-seeking behavior.

In addressing the issue of residual drug effects, we have to differentiate between chronic, regular, daily drug use and acute, or occasional, drug use. Repeated drug use can result in tolerance to some of the effects of the drug. When tolerance develops, it takes a larger dose of the drug to achieve the same effect. The development of tolerance does not by itself affect workplace performance, although it can moderate what would otherwise be the effects of drug-taking behavior or allow greater consumption of a drug than would otherwise occur. The aspect of chronic drug use that can affect workplace performance adversely is the development of dependence. Physical dependence is manifested as a syndrome of effects that appear upon abrupt cessation of a drug after chronic use and can be alleviated by intake of that drug. The most widely described drug dependence is probably for the opiates, as seen with chronic heroin use. Comparable dependence is seen with many if not all classes of psychotropic drugs.

The data on the development of dependence to alcohol, sedatives, and opiates are clear. Repeated and regular intake of these substances has been shown to result in physical dependence, manifested by a replicable withdrawal syndrome that can be alleviated by the administration of the substance that the individual has been taking. The data for marijuana are less clear. A number of laboratory studies have been carried out in which research subjects were given marijuana cigarettes to smoke, or Δ^9-THC to consume, repeatedly for 10-30 days. In general, both tolerance to many of marijuana's effects and dependence are seen (Jones and Benowitz, 1976; Mendelson et al., 1976). Withdrawal is manifested as irritability, restlessness, decreased appetite, tremor, etc., and has been described (Jones, 1978) as a clinical picture similar to that seen after withdrawal of the sedative-hypnotics. It is possible that the maintenance of stable THC blood levels is important for the development of dependence, and that cessation of use could result in a withdrawal syndrome with workplace consequences.

Residual effects of *occasional* marijuana use appear slight if they exist at all. Some researchers searching for hangover effects recount subjective reports of feeling "spacey" or "stoned" or "hung over" the next day (Cousens and DiMascio, 1973). The few objective measures that purport to show decrements attributable to the consumption of marijuana a day earlier are suggestive at best (Yesavage et al., 1985; Leirer et al., 1991). Thus, we cannot at this time conclude that the occasional use of marijuana will have measurable next-day residual effects, nor can we conclude that some subtle effects are not present.

Accuracy in identifying small amounts of cannabis metabolites in urine is excellent. This means that even occasional use of marijuana is often picked up in urine screens taken in relation to an accident or other workplace problems. We cannot, however, on the basis of the available data, assign particular behavioral consequences to the presence of these metabolites in the urine. Thus, when post-accident drug screening reveals that a responsible person tested positive for marijuana, it does not mean that marijuana use played a causal role in the incident.

Alcohol hangover effects can apparently degrade performance. They have been reported to impair drivers' and pilots' performance (Laurell and Tornros, 1983; Yesavage and Leirer, 1986), although the extent of the impairment was in part related to both age and experience with the task. For example, performance of older pilots was more impaired than that of younger pilots, but the older pilots were more aware of their impairment for up to 4 hours after reaching peak blood alcohol levels.

There are no data on the residual effects of occasional stimulant use except for fatigue related to secondary sleep deprivation. When stimulants are used repeatedly in binges, a "crash," marked by irritability, hypersomnolence, and some depression can occur (Fischman, 1987). This constellation of next-day effects, however, has not been linked to specific performance changes, and it may be that the effects do not differ from decrements measured after sleep deprivation in the absence of drug use.

METHODOLOGICAL ISSUES

Where laboratory conditions are different from the conditions that characterize actual drug use, drug users, and job performance, there is a question of how far one can generalize from laboratory results to predict the actual implications of drug use that are of interest (Berkowitz and Donnerstein, 1982; Dipboye and Flanahan, 1979; Locke, 1986; Sears, 1986; Sackett and Larson, 1991). This is the *external validity* problem. Not all differences between the laboratory and the outside world pose serious threats to external validity. This depends on whether there is reason to believe the differences are consequential for the generalizations one would like to make. Unfortunately, in assessing the research done to date on the performance implications of drug use, many of the differences between the currently available laboratory studies and drug use outside the laboratory appear large and potentially important. Often, however, these differences, or at least the size of these differences, are not inherent in the laboratory methodology. Thus identifying important differences not only highlights the limitations of extant research, but it also suggests ways in which future studies can be improved.

The failure to examine combinations of drugs constitutes a major gap in the research on drugs' effects on performance. It is becoming increasingly rare to find a single-drug-class abuser (or even drug user). Polydrug use is generally the norm, and this is particularly the case for alcohol. Many substances, such as marijuana, nicotine, and sedatives, are frequently taken in combination with alcohol, and the effects of these combinations are generally unknown. It has recently been reported that the combined intake of cocaine and alcohol results in formation of a metabolite, cocaethylene, which has a half-life of more than 2 hours, and is considerably more toxic than either drug alone (Hearn et al., 1992; Perez-Reyes and Jeffcoat, 1992). Although not yet studied, it is possible that this active metabolite could result in behavioral changes long after measurable cocaine or alcohol levels are present in the body. Other combinations of drugs may have effects that are different from or longer lasting than the effects of the drugs taken singly.

Research on the performance implications of drug use must also consider carefully the experimental population. There are several research objectives to be met in determining an appropriate research subject population. Initial research studies evaluating a specific substance or a specific task should be carried out in a single well-studied population in which multiple variables can be controlled, motivational variables can be either manipulated or controlled, and basic mechanisms can be addressed. This approach exemplifies much of the research summarized above. Subjects in these studies were generally male college or graduate students. Unfortunately, few studies move on to the next phase of research in which issues of generalizability and predictability are addressed. It is difficult to know how generalizable data from the population of male college or graduate students, tested individually and in isolation, are to the general work force. On one hand, students, who are younger than much of the work force, have commonly learned to perform under less than optimal conditions, often taking tests under conditions of sleep deprivation and substantial stress. On the other hand, student subjects may seldom or never have used the drugs administered, and unlike the occasional or regular user, they may not have learned how to function productively under the influence of the drug. In addition, laboratory performance tests are often novel, with minimal opportunity for practice prior to testing. Members of the work force are generally performing well-learned tasks in familiar, more social environments, with familiar cues designed to enhance performance as the working environment undergoes minor modifications (e.g., illumination changes, personnel changes).

Much of the research being carried out on the effects of psychoactive substances on performance has not been designed with the "at risk" population in mind. For example, at least 20 percent of truck drivers are said to drive under the influence of marijuana, methamphetamine, or cocaine (Beilock, 1988). Yet little research on the effects of these drugs has the specific situations of truck drivers in mind. Prescribed medications (e.g., benzodiazepines) may well impair performance, yet few studies evaluating them in the populations most likely to need them have been carried out. Epidemiologic studies are necessary to help define the populations at risk, the substances most generally used, and the environments in which they are most likely to be used. Data from such statistics can then feed into laboratory research.

As we have already noted, few performance studies model drug use outside the laboratory. With many drugs, it is rare for a user to take a single dose each day. Stimulants such as cocaine, for example, are taken repeatedly, in binges, for several hours or days at a time (Johanson and Fischman, 1989). Under these conditions, it is likely that tolerance will develop to some of the effects of the drug, although dosing can escalate to substantial levels. Thus, the single doses often administered in research settings do not accurately reflect, in either pattern or number, those taken by habitual or even occasional users.

Many of the studies evaluating the effects of single doses of drugs on laboratory performance employ contingencies for correct or efficient performance. Points exchangeable for money, for example, are awarded when tasks are completed according to instructions. In the workplace there may be eventual contingencies (e.g., firing for those whose performance is habitually substandard), but there is rarely a performance monitor providing performance feedback on a minute-by-minute basis. This difference also undercuts the generalizability of the data from laboratory to workplace.

Perhaps the most important effect missed in most laboratory performance studies is the interaction of the drug taken with the behavior of the user and others in the environment (i.e., laboratory studies do not involve a social environment). Although drugs have pharmacological effects that at high doses can be substantial, the effects of using a drug often depend on what else is going on in the environment and the feedback given to the individual performing under the effect of the drug. For this reason, studies that emulate workplace conditions can more accurately assess drug effects than those that do not. In an interesting series of experiments, Kelly and colleagues have examined the behavioral profiles associated with using marijuana (Kelly et al., 1990), amphetamines (Kelly et al., 1991), and diazepam (Kelly et al., 1993). Healthy volunteers resided continuously in a laboratory designed for the long-term unobtrusive measurement of human behavior (Brady et al., 1974). The laboratory day was designed to emulate a normal day, with subjects working in their private rooms from about 9:00 a.m. to 5:00 p.m., followed by a social activities period when subjects had access to other subjects and a common social/exercise space. Data were collected simultaneously on a wide range of behaviors under naturalistic living conditions: performance, social behavior, food intake, cigarette smoking, and subjective effects. By comparing drug effects across multiple dimensions of human behavior, it was possible to ascertain a behavioral profile of each drug's action. In addition, this design addresses the risk factors discussed in the introduction of this section and narrows the gap between laboratory studies and the workplace. By using a social setting, distracting events, extensive training with weeks of practice, and a sample of nonstudents, this study comes closer to simulating the workplace and living conditions associated with ordinary drug use than the studies we have discussed thus far.

Kelly and his colleagues found that smoking marijuana cigarettes decreased accuracy on a digit symbol substitution task (DSST), increased food intake, and decreased verbal interaction and tobacco cigarette smoking (Kelly et al., 1990). When comparing the relative potency of marijuana across these measures, it was clear that DSST performance, food intake, and social behavior were all altered at doses that had no effects on task performance other than the DSST. This suggests that THC doses that affect performance are equal to, if not greater, than doses that affect social and eating behavior.

Oral amphetamine administration decreased food intake, improved accuracy on some work tasks, and increased verbal interaction, cigarette smoking, and verbal ratings of drug effect (Kelly et al., 1991). The relative potency comparisons, in this case, suggested that the doses that were affecting performance also had significant effects on other dimensions of human behavior. Oral diazepam administration, in contrast, increased verbal interaction at low doses and decreased verbal interaction at high doses, disrupted only one measure of task performance, increased food intake at one or both doses, and increased verbal ratings of drug effect (Kelly et al., 1993). The relative potency comparisons in this experiment suggested that diazepam at clinical doses disrupted dimensions of human performance, *other* than task performance.

The Kelly et al. experiments clearly indicate the utility of multiple measures in studying the performance effects of drugs. The unique aspect of these experiments is that measures of normal social and eating behavior were obtained, providing a source of potency comparisons involving normal nonlaboratory-dependent behavior. The findings suggest that, at least for diazepam and marijuana, experiments that measure only task performance may miss the effects that particular drug doses have on other behaviors. Where significant performance effects are found, other significant changes in behavior are also likely. The use of multiple dependent measures in performance experiments will make it easier to put into the context the changes in performance observed in laboratory experiments.

Measures of the subjective effects of test drugs can also provide essential information about the effectiveness of the dose range being studied. For example, in an experiment on the effects of buspirone on performance, Critchfield and Griffiths (1991) did not observe any performance effects of a high buspirone dose (four to five times the therapeutic dose) in sedative users, but did observe significant ratings of "bad drug effect." Without the self-report data, there would have been no verification that an effective dose range was being tested. Visual analog scales, often used in the assessment of momentary changes in affect (Folstein and Luria, 1973), require little effort, represent minimal intrusion on existing protocols, and can be incorporated readily into most laboratory procedures.

LIMITS AND REALITIES OF LABORATORY STUDIES

There are no studies that provide direct estimates of the effects of drug use on job performance or on behavior in organizations. As is often the case with research in the social and behavioral sciences and in medicine, ethical constraints make it impossible to conduct definitive controlled studies of the long-term effects of drug use at work. Rather, it is necessary to infer the impact of drug use at work from a variety of studies conducted in the laboratory and the field. Laboratory studies provide evidence regarding the effects of controlled, short-term exposure to specific drugs on the performance of specific tasks. Field studies provide evidence regarding the links between drug use (either self-reported or detected through other means) and a number of work behaviors, but they lack the controls needed to allow researchers to isolate specific drug effects.

Difficulties in generalizing from behavioral research are by no means unique to research on the impact of drugs in the workplace; these same issues emerge in virtually any area of research that involves human behavior. It is therefore important to keep an appropriate perspective in discussing the methodological limitations of research on drugs and work. Nevertheless, it is important to note at the outset that these difficulties are an important reason why the existing research base does not demonstrate conclusively that the effects of drug use on the work force are either large or small. The challenge is to overcome them.

One way to appraise the generalizability of any specific set of laboratory findings is through a risk factors model, in which each of the potentially important differences between the laboratory and the work setting is treated as a factor that is likely to limit the generalizability of laboratory research. The more risk factors that are present, the greater the likelihood that the effects of the drug examined will be different in the lab than in the field. Table 4.2 lists several risk factors, some of which have already been

TABLE 4.2 Features of Typical Laboratory Studies that Differ from the Workplace

In the Laboratory	In the Workplace
1. Focus on maximal performance	1. Focus on typical performance
2. Controlled processing	2. Automatic processing
3. Novice performers	3. Experienced performers
4. Performance in isolation	4. Performance in social setting
5. Simple task	5. Complex task
6. Clear performance standards	6. Ambiguous standards
7. Homogeneous samples	7. Heterogeneous samples
8. Controlled drug exposure	8. Variable drug exposure
9. Limited time span	9. Long time span
10. Novice drug user	10. Experienced drug user

mentioned, that commonly threaten the external validity of laboratory studies relating drug usage to task performance.

It is common in the workplace to distinguish between tests of maximal performance and tests of typical performance. In laboratory settings, in which subjects are under scrutiny, people are often motivated to perform well and are able to perform with few distractions. Thus, they are likely to demonstrate maximal performance. In work settings, in which people are not under the same level of scrutiny, their typical performance is not likely to be as high or as consistent. The typical-maximal performance distinction is particularly important for studying the effects of drugs that affect attention, fatigue, and vigilance. Subjects may make special efforts to overcome the effects of these drugs in laboratory settings, which they would not make in work settings. The incorporation of distractions (e.g., multiple attention tasks) in laboratory studies is one way to address this issue.

Laboratory studies often present unfamiliar or novel tasks that require constant attention and monitoring. In contrast, many work tasks are over-learned, and individuals may perform those tasks in an automatic processing mode after extensive training and practice. Also, as already pointed out, laboratory studies often employ novice subjects (e.g., college students), whereas in the workplace most workers are relatively experienced with the tasks that need to be performed. Laboratory studies should include over-learned (i.e., highly practiced) tasks as well as novel tasks.

Laboratory studies often require subjects to perform in isolation, whereas job performance is usually carried out in a social setting. The effects of the presence of other workers on performance are themselves complex (e.g., social facilitation effects can enhance performance, whereas distraction can detract from performance); when jobs involve social interactions and interdependencies, the generalizability of studies in which subjects work alone can be especially hazardous. The addition of studies carried out in social settings could address this issue.

Laboratory studies often involve a single, relatively simple task (e.g., a reaction time task), whereas job performance often involves multiple, complex tasks. Furthermore, the evaluation of performance in the laboratory is often considerably simpler than in the field. That is, the standards that define good performance are often clear and well understood in the laboratory, but the same is not always the case in work settings. What is defined as poor performance in a work setting may not be the result of impairment, but rather the effect of disagreement over the definition of adequate performance.

Laboratory studies often employ convenience samples (e.g., college students, military pilots), which tend to be homogeneous. This may cause those studies to underestimate the importance of individual differences, as well as differences in training and experience when generalizing to the workplace. Similarly, the exposure of subjects to drugs in laboratory experiments is usually carefully controlled (e.g., fixed doses of specific drugs taken in specific settings), whereas in the workplace there may be extensive variation in patterns and levels of drug use, including different configurations of polydrug use. Studies using experienced drug users with variations in drug use history as subjects may be useful in this regard; polydrug configurations must be tested.

Finally, laboratory studies are usually limited in scope, and subjects often know the approximate time span of the study. It may be easier to maintain maximal performance levels, or to adopt strategies to mitigate the effects of drugs on performance, in tasks whose duration is known (and is short) than it is over the course of a typical workday. Experimental sessions extending over the course of a workday, or at least for several hours, are more likely to capture drug effects than those of shorter duration.

As in all applications of risk factor approaches, a simple count of the factors that are present or absent in a given study does not necessarily determine its external validity. What is crucial is the plausibility of the threats posed by specific factors in the context of the given research. Indeed, it is possible that a study might exhibit all the potential barriers to generalizability shown in Table 4.2 and still produce generalizable results (e.g., effect of cyanide on performance using animals as subjects). The risk factor approach does provide a rough and probabilistic statement about generalizability; the more factors that are present, the less likely that laboratory results will replicate exactly in the field. It is particularly useful for evaluating the existing body of research on drug effects as a whole; the prevalence of studies that share almost all listed risk factors is disheartening. We reiterate, however, that this is not inherent in the laboratory methodology, as some researchers have shown.

GENERAL FINDINGS

Perhaps the most obvious finding of this survey of the literature on performance effects is the lack of consistent and significant effects. While sufficient amounts of almost any substance will have a deleterious effect on work force behavior, this is not the issue. The question is whether alcohol and other drugs of abuse, taken in the doses and patterns that people are using, either occasionally or regularly have detrimental effects on behavior, particularly workplace performance The literature suggests that, in single doses and under laboratory conditions, stimulant drugs (caffeine, cocaine, methylphenidate, amphetamine and nicotine) either have no effect or they moderately improve performance. Smoking marijuana seems to have variable effects, with inconsistent decrements on performance. Sedative drugs (alcohol, benzodiazepines, barbiturates) generally disrupt performance. There are large differences across experiments and drugs in terms of experimental design, and the proportion of experiments reporting significant drug effects varies widely across tasks and drugs. The extent to which this variation is due to task methodology rather than dose needs investigation. Information gained from such research will also help identify factors that can moderate, as well as accentuate, drug-induced effects on performance.

Given the variability in tasks and procedures, the fact that, at certain doses, drugs affected performance in 40 to 80 percent of the experiments reviewed by the committee indicates that this field, though experimentally mature, requires additional research rooted in more careful attention to methodology. Although an impressive array of tasks has been used in the research to date, experimental protocols have rarely been similar across studies. Suggestions for future protocols include use of control groups, training subjects prior to participation, testing of more than one dose, testing for drug combinations, and testing of performance before and several times after drug administration. A greater range of subject populations beyond the student population should also be sampled. Task standardization, including instructions to subjects, duration of performance, feedback to subjects, motivational conditions, and details of presentation should be maximized across studies at least in some conditions, to provide a common metric for comparison.

The relevance of tasks performed in the laboratory to tasks performed in the workplace is often not clear, and even when there is a plausible link, it has seldom been demonstrated. Clearly it is not possible to model every type of performance by the work force. And yet it should be possible to differentiate several functional categories of tasks to be studied. For example, acquisition of new behavior (i.e., learning) and stable performance of practiced tasks might be differentiated and both aspects modeled in testing. It would be useful for future research designs in which new tasks are being developed to include one or two standardized benchmark tasks for comparison of drug effects across studies. This would provide the systematic replication necessary to generalize across studies. Reliability across tasks could then be evaluated, and importantly, predictive validity could be assessed.

The relationship between drug doses that affect performance and doses that are used clinically, or self-administered for nonmedical purposes, determines the effects of drugs on work force performance. The greater the extent of the overlap between these dose ranges, the greater the potential hazards to both the drug user and society. Therefore, it is important that research in this area incorporate usage information collected in epidemiologic or other laboratory studies so that we can optimize the utility of the data being collected in performance testing for predicting decrements in workplace performance. Future research, using more standardized protocols and tasks with broad subject populations, should address the varied issues relating to public safety and the creation of work and home environments that minimize potential adverse drug effects.

In sum, laboratory research has the potential for providing valuable information about the relationship between alcohol and other drug use, social behavior, and job performance. To date, despite some research designs that are abstractly elegant, that potential has hardly been tapped. Recognizing the important contribution laboratory research can make to improving our understanding of the impact of individual alcohol and other drug use on work performance, and after having carefully reviewed the current scientific knowledge base, the committee offers the following conclusions and recommendations.

CONCLUSIONS AND RECOMMENDATIONS

- Laboratory studies of the effects of alcohol and other drugs on behavior have shown inconsistent results. These differences may be due, in part, to differences in the populations tested, the measurements used, and the range of drug doses administered.

Recommendation: Benchmark measures should be included in laboratory studies to permit generalization across studies. Funding agencies should consider holding conferences to establish such benchmarks.

Laboratory studies show small performance-enhancing effects of commonly used doses of cocaine and other stimulants. Commonly used doses of marijuana produce variable decrements in performance. Alcohol and prescribed sedatives produce decreases in performance depending on the dose, time of consumption, and the time-course of circulating concentrations of the drug's active metabolites, relative to the work schedule. All drug effects are influenced by dose and prior experience. The age of individuals and the presence of other drugs may also mediate the influence of particular drugs.

- The use of alcohol and other drugs away from the work site, including prescription drugs and over-the-counter medication, may have detrimental effects during work, especially for those in safety-sensitive positions. Thus, a long-acting drug taken the night before work or alcohol taken at lunch away from the job may have on-the-job effects like those of drugs taken at the work site. In addition, cessation of drug use may produce either withdrawal or hangover effects that affect work site performance. To date there has been little research directed toward any of these issues.

Recommendation: Researchers and funding agencies should devote more attention to the ways in which prescription and over-the-counter medications affect job performance, especially for safety-sensitive positions.

Recommendation: Studies of work site alcohol and other drug use should encompass off-site use that may have on-the-job effects. Hangover and withdrawal effects should also be considered in assessing the workplace implications of alcohol and other drug use.

REFERENCES

Alford, C., J.Z. Bhatti, S. Curran, G. McKay, and I. Hindmarch
  1991   Pharmacodynamic effects of buspirone and clobazam. *British Journal of Clinical Pharmacology* 32:91-97.

Barnett, G., V. Licko, and T. Thompson
  1985   Behavioral pharmacokinetics of marijuana. *Psychopharmacology* 85:51-56.

Beilock, R.
  1988   RCCC Motor Carrier Safety Survey. Regular Common Carrier Conference, Alexandria, Va.

Berkowitz, L., and E. Donnerstein
  1982   External validity is more than skin deep. *American Psychologist* 37:245-257.

Brady, J.V., G. Bigelow, H. Emurian, and D.M. Williams
  1974   Design of a programmed environment for the experimental analysis of social behavior. Pp. 187-208 in D.H. Carlson, ed., *Man-Environment Interactions: Evaluations and Applications. 7: Social Ecology*. Milwaukee, Wis.: Environmental Design Research Associates.

Burns, M.
  1992   Alcohol and drug effects on performance. Pp. 49-59 in *Alcohol and Other Drugs in Transportation: Research Needs for the Next Decade*. Transportation Research Board, National Research Council. Washington, D.C.: National Academy Press.

Chesher, G.B., H.M. Franks, D.M. Jackson, G.A. Starmer, and R.K.C. Teo
  1977   Ethanol and Δ^9-tetrahydrocannabinol: interactive effects on human perceptual, cognitive and motor functions. *Medical Journal of Australia* 1:478-481.

Collins, W.E.
  1980   Performance effects of alcohol intoxication and hangover at ground level and at simulated altitude. *Aviation, Space, and Environmental Medicine* 51:327-335.

Comitas, L.
  1976   Cannabis and work in Jamaica: a refutation of the amotivational syndrome. *Annals of the New York Academy of Sciences* 282:24-32.

Cousens, K., and A. DiMascio
  1973   (-)A9THC as an hypnotic: an experimental study of three dose levels. *Psychopharmacologia* 33:355-364.

Critchfield, T.S., and R.R. Griffiths
  1991   Behavioral and subjective effects of buspirone and lorazepam in sedative abusers: supra-therapeutic doses. In L. Harris, ed., *Problems of Drug Dependence*. NIDA Research Monograph 105. Rockville, Md.: National Institute on Drug Abuse.

Curran, H.V., and M. Lader
  1987   Differential amnesic properties of benzodiazepines: a dose-response comparison of two drugs with similar elimination half-lives. *Psychopharmacology* 92:358-364.
Dipboye, R.L., and M.F. Flanahan
  1979   Research settings in industrial and organizational psychology: are findings in the field more generalizable than in the laboratory? *American Psychologist* 34:141-150.
Erwin, C.W., M. Linnoila, J. Hartwell, A. Erwin, and S. Gutherie
  1986   Effects of buspirone and diazepam, alone, and in combination with alcohol, on skilled performance and evoked potentials. *Journal of Clinical Psychopharmacology* 6:199-209.
Evans, M.A., R. Martz, B.E. Rodda, L. Lemberger, and R.B. Forney
  1976   Effects of marihuana-dextroamphetamine combination. *Clinical Pharmacology and Therapeutics* 20:350-358.
Evans, S.M., F.R. Funderburk, and R.R. Griffiths
  1990   Zolpidem and triazolam in humans: behavioral and subjective effects and abuse liability. *Journal of Pharmacology and Experimental Therapeutics* 255:1246-1255.
Fischman, M.W.
  1987   Cocaine and the amphetamines. Pp. 1543-1543 in H.Y. Meltzer, ed., *Psychopharmacology: A Third Generation of Progress*. New York: Raven Press.
Folstein, M.F., and R. Luria
  1973   Reliability, validity, and clinical application of the visual analogue mood scale. *Psychosomatic Medicine* 3:479-486.
Foltin, R.W., and S.M. Evans
  1992   Performance Effects of Drugs of Abuse: A Methodological Survey. Manuscript prepared for the Committee on Drug Use in the Workplace, Commission on Behavioral and Social Sciences and Education, National Research Council, Washington, D.C.
  1993   Performance effects of drugs of abuse: a methodological survey. *Journal of Human Psychopharmacology* 8:9-19.
Foltin, R.W., M.W. Fischman, J.V. Brady, T.H. Kelly, D.J. Bernstein, and M.N. Nellis
  1989   Motivational effects of smoked marijuana: behavioral contingencies and high-probability recreational activities. *Pharmacology, Biochemistry, and Behavior* 34:871-877.
Foltin, R.W., M.W. Fischman, J.V. Brady, D.J. Bernstein, R.M. Capriotti, M.N. Nellis, and T.H. Kelly
  1990   Motivational effects of smoked marijuana: behavioral contingencies and low-probability activities. *Journal of the Experimental Analysis of Behavior* 53:5-19.
Foltin, R.W., M.W. Fischman, P. Pippen, and T.H. Kelly
  1993   Behavioral effects of ethanol and marijuana, alone and in combination with cocaine in humans. *Drug and Alcohol Dependence* 32:93-106.
Hearn, W.L., S. Rose, J. Wagner, A. Ciarleglio, and D.C. Mash
  1992   Cocaethylene is more potent than cocaine in mediating lethality. *Pharmacology, Biochemistry and Behavior* 39:531-533.
Heishman, S.J., and M.L. Stitzer
  1989   Effect of d-amphetamine, secobarbital, and marijuana on choice behavior: social versus nonsocial options. *Psychopharmacology* 99:156-162.
Heishman, S.J., M.L. Stitzer, and J.E. Yingling
  1989   Effects of tetrahydrocannabinol content on marijuana smoking behavior, subjective reports, and performance. *Pharmacology, Biochemistry, and Behavior* 34:173-179.

Hindmarch, I., J.S. Kerr, and N. Sherwood
  1990   Effects of nicotine gum on psychomotor performance in smokers and non-smokers. *Psychopharmacology* 100:535-541.
Hooker, W.D., and R.T. Jones
  1987   Increased susceptibility to memory intrusions and the Stroop interference effect during acute marijuana intoxication. *Psychopharmacology* 91:20-24.
Johanson, C.E., and M.W. Fischman
  1989   The pharmacology of cocaine related to its abuse. *Pharmacological Reviews* 41:3-52.
Jones, R.T.
  1978   Marijuana: human effects. Pp. 378-412 in L.L. Iversen et al., eds., *Handbook of Psychopharmacology*, Vol. 12. New York: Plenum Press.
Jones, R.T., and N. Benowitz
  1976   The 30-day trip—clinical studies of cannabis tolerance and dependence. Pp. 627-642 in M.C. Braude and S. Szara, eds., *The Pharmacology of Marijuana*. New York: Raven Press.
Jones, R.T., and G.C. Stone
  1970   Psychological studies of marijuana and alcohol in man. *Psychopharmacologia* 18:108-117.
Kelly, T.H., R.W. Foltin, C.S. Emurian, and M.W. Fischman
  1990   Multidimensional behavioral effects of marijuana. *Progress in Neuro-Psychopharmacology* 14:885-902.
Kelly, T.H., M.W. Fischman, R.W. Foltin, and J.V. Brady
  1991   Response patterns and cardiovascular effects during response sequence acquisition by humans. *Journal of the Experimental Analysis of Behavior* 56:557-574.
Kelly, T.H., R.W. Foltin, L. King, and M.W. Fischman
  1993   The effects of repeated diazepam exposure on multiple measures of human behavior. *Biological Psychiatry*. (In press.)
Klorman, R., L.O. Bauer, H.W. Coons, J.L. Lewis, L.J. Peloquin, R.A. Perlmutter, R.M. Ryan, L.F. Salzman, and J. Strauss
  1984   Enhancing effects of methylphenidate on normal young adults' cognitive processes. *Psychopharmacological Bulletin* 20:3-9.
Lane, J.D., and R.B. Williams, Jr.
  1985   Caffeine affects cardiovascular response to stress. *Psychophysiology* 22:648-655.
Laties, V.G., and B. Weiss
  1981   The amphetamine margin in sports. *Federation Proceedings* 40:2689-2692.
Laurell, H., and J. Tornros
  1983   Investigation of alcoholic hang-over effects on driving performance. *Blutalkohol* 20:489-499.
Leirer, V.O., J.A. Yesavage, and D.G. Morrow
  1991   Marijuana carry-over effects on aircraft pilot performance. *Aviation, Space, and Environmental Medicine* 62:221-227.
Linnoila, M., J.M. Stapleton, R. Lister, H. Moss, E. Lane, A. Granger, D.J. Greenblatt, and M.J. Eckardt
  1990   Effects of adinazolam and diazepam, alone and in combination with ethanol, on psychomotor and cognitive performance on autonomic nervous system reactivity in healthy volunteers. *European Journal of Clinical Pharmacology* 38:371-377.
Locke, E.A.
  1986   *Generalizing from Laboratory to Field Settings*. Lexington, Mass.: Heath.
Marks, D.F., and M.G. MacAvoy
  1989   Divided attention performance in cannabis users and non-users following alcohol and cannabis separately and in combination. *Psychopharmacology* 99:397-401.

Mattila, M., T. Seppala, and M.J. Mattila
1986   Combined effects of buspirone and diazepam on objective and subjective tests of performance in healthy volunteers. *Clinical Pharmacology and Therapeutics* 40:620-626.

Mendelson, J.H., J.C. Kuehnle, I. Greenberg, and N.K. Mello
1976   Operant acquisition of marijuana in man. *Journal of Pharmacology and Experimental Therapeutics* 198:42-53.

Miller, L.L., and T.L. Cornett
1978   Marijuana: dose effects on pulse rate, subjective estimates of intoxication, free recall and recognition memory. *Pharmacology, Biochemistry and Behavior* 9:573-577.

O'Neil, B., A. Williams, and K. Dubowski
1983   Variability in blood alcohol concentrations. *Journal of Studies in Alcohol* 44:222-230.

Page, J.B.
1983   The amotivational syndrome hypothesis and the Costa Rica study: relationship between methods and results. *Journal of Psychoactive Drugs* 15:261-267.

Patat, A., M.J. Klein, and M. Hucher
1987   Effects of single oral doses of clobazam, diazepam and lorazepam on performance tasks and memory. *European Journal of Clinical Pharmacology* 32:461-466.

Patat, A., M.J. Klein, M. Hucher, and J. Grainer
1991   Study of the potential reversal of trizolam memory and cognitive deficits by RU 41 656 in healthy subjects. *Psychopharmacology* 104:75-80.

Perez-Reyes, M., and A.R. Jeffcoat
1992   Ethanol-cocaine interaction: cocaine and cocaethylene plasma concentrations and their relationship to subjective and cardiovascular effects. *Life Sciences* 51:553-563.

Peterson, J.B., J. Rothfleisch, P.D. Zelazo, and R.O. Pihl
1990   Acute alcohol intoxication and cognitive functioning. *Journal of Studies on Alcohol* 51:114-122.

Pihl, R.O., and H. Sigal
1978   Motivational levels and the marijuana high. *Journal of Abnormal Psychology* 87:280-285.

Preston, K.L., J.J. Guarino, W.T. Kirk, and R.R. Griffiths
1989   Evaluation of the abuse potential of methocarbamol. *Journal of Pharmacology and Experimental Therapeutics* 248:1146-1157.

Sackett, P.R., and J.R. Larson
1991   Research strategies and tactics in industrial and organizational psychology. In M. Dunnette and L. Hough, eds., *Handbook of Industrial and Organizational Psychology*, 2nd ed., Vol. 1. Palo Alto, Calif.: Consulting Psychologists Press.

Sears, D.O.
1986   College sophomores in the laboratory: influence of a narrow data base on social psychology's view of human nature. *Journal of Personality and Social Psychology* 51:515-530.

Stefanis, C., R. Dornbush, and M. Fink
1977   *Hashish: Studies of Long-Term Use.* New York: Raven Press.

Streufert, S., R.M. Pogash, J. Roach, D. Gingrich, R. Landis, W. Severs, L. Lonardi, and A. Kantner
1992   Effects of alcohol on risk taking, strategy, and error rate in visuomotor performance. *Journal of Applied Psychology* 77:515-524.

Strömberg, C., T. Seppälä, and M.J. Mattila
    1988   Acute effects of maprotiline, doxepin and zimeldine with alcohol in healthy volun-
            teers. *Archives of International Pharmacodynamics* 291:217-228.
Taberner, P.V., C.J.C. Roberts, E. Shrosbree, C.J. Pycock, and L. English
    1983   An investigation into the interaction between ethanol at low doses and the benzodi-
            azepines nitrazepam and temazepam on psychomotor performance in normal sub-
            jects. *Psychopharmacology* 81:321-326.
Wilson, J.R., V.G. Erwin, G.E. McClearn, R. Plomin, R.C. Johnson, F.M. Ahern, and R.E.
Cole
    1984   Effects of ethanol: II. Behavioral sensitivity and acute behavioral tolerance. *Alco-
            holism: Clinical and Experimental Research* 366-374.
Yesavage, J.A., and V.O. Leirer
    1986   Hangover effects on aircraft pilots 14 hours after alcohol ingestion: a preliminary
            report. *American Journal of Psychiatry* 1546-1550.
Yesavage, J.A., V.O. Leirer, M. Denari, and L.E. Hollister
    1985   Carry-over effects of marijuana intoxication on aircraft pilot performance: a pre-
            liminary report. *American Journal of Psychiatry* 142:1325-1329.

5

Impact of Alcohol and Other Drug Use: Observational/Field Studies

Use of alcohol or illicit drugs by employees at work or even away from work has long been associated with harmful consequences. In fact, much of the impetus behind the movement for a drug-free workplace has been due to widely publicized accidents that have been tied to the use of drugs. Marijuana use was implicated in the U.S.S. Nimitz accident in 1981, in which a Navy pilot crashed into the aircraft carrier's deck and destroyed several planes, resulting in damage estimates in excess of $100 million. Marijuana use was also implicated in several fatal train accidents, most notably the Conrail-Amtrak collision in 1987, in which 16 people died. Alcohol use is seen as an important cause of the Exxon Valdez catastrophe, one of the worst and most publicized oil spills in U.S. history.

These isolated catastrophic incidents are, however, of little scientific value in assessing the magnitude of the effects of alcohol and other drugs on job-related outcome measures. Studies that have attempted to assess such effects with worker populations have been observational in nature, since, as noted in the previous chapter, ethical constraints prevent definitive studies of the effects of drug use at work (e.g., it would be unacceptable to design a longitudinal double-blind study in which a large number of workers were randomly assigned to various drug use conditions to allow researchers to observe the impact of drug use). But observational field studies, like controlled laboratory studies, have potentially serious limitations as a means of obtaining true estimates of the effects of alcohol and other drugs on job-related outcomes.

COMMON PROBLEMS WITH FIELD STUDIES

One problem with field studies is that their measures of alcohol and other drug use are often flawed. Self-reports are frequently suspect, although there are conditions under which they can be relatively trustworthy (Rouse et al., 1985; Reinisch et al., 1991; Freier et al., 1991). Bioassays (e.g., urine tests) indicate the recent use of drugs, but they provide little information about the frequency of use or the impairment (if any) associated with drug use.

A second problem is conceptual. The phrase *alcohol and other drug use* refers to a broad array of patterns of use of different drugs or combinations of drugs. Thus the findings of different studies are often not strictly comparable, and it is difficult to make sensible generalizations about the effects of alcohol and other drug use without numerous qualifications. Finally, while many field studies indicate a statistical relationship between indicators of alcohol and other drug use and work behaviors (e.g., absenteeism), most do not provide a basis for determining the causal role (if any) of alcohol and other drug use in determining these behaviors. Reported correlations between use and job performance could be due to the effects of some third, unmeasured variable rather than to the direct effects of alcohol and other drugs themselves. Job stresses, for example, might lead people both to take alcohol and other drugs and to absent themselves from work. If so, eliminating alcohol and other drug use without decreasing job stress might actually increase absenteeism, because one coping mechanism would be gone. Alternatively, alcohol and other drug use, absenteeism, and carelessness on the job might all result from a rejection of conventional social standards, in which case, attitude change rather then the coerced abstinence from alcohol and other drugs might be the key to better job performance.

Links Between Deviance, Alcohol and
Other Drug Use, and Work Behavior

Researchers have found that measures of alcohol and other drug use (both bioassay and self-report measures) are related to a number of problematic work behaviors, notably absenteeism, and perhaps accident rates and performance levels. It is plausible to assume that these work problems result from alcohol- and other drug-induced impairment but, as we have just pointed out, this is not the only possibility, and it may not be the most plausible one. Even if alcohol and other drug use has little or no direct effect on these workplace behaviors, it is still possible to find substantial correlations between such use and absenteeism, poor performance, and the like because these behaviors are all part of a general pattern or syndrome of behavior often referred to as deviance. Knowing whether alcohol and other drug use makes an independent contribution to undesirable behaviors in the workplace is an important issue, since it bears substantially on how best to treat use by the work force. If alcohol and other drug use is strongly associated with other types of deviant attitudes and behaviors, confronting only the inappropriate use may not correct a worker's problems. In what follows, we first briefly review research on the construct of deviance; we then present a simplified model of the role deviance might play in explaining the relationship of reported associations between alcohol and other drug use and workplace behaviors; finally, we discuss the empirical evidence relating the effects of alcohol and other drugs to job-related outcomes.

Alcohol and Other Drug Use and Deviance

Alcohol and other drug use and abuse do not occur as isolated events, but rather seem to be components of a cluster of behaviors and attitudes that form a syndrome or lifestyle referred to as problem behavior or deviance. Problem behavior theory, developed by Jessor and Jessor (1977, 1978), sees alcohol and other drug use as only one aspect of a deviance-prone lifestyle, particularly in adolescents and young adults (who represent the majority of those likely to use illicit drugs in or in connection with the workplace). For adolescents, aspects of the deviance-prone lifestyle include alcohol abuse, illicit drug use, precocious sexual involvement, frequent sexual activity, academic problems, deviant attitudes, and delinquent behavior. This theory has been tested in several studies, which, consistent with the theory, have shown high correlations among these deviant behaviors (Donovan and Jessor, 1985; Gillmore et al., 1991; Newcomb and Bentler, 1988).

Newcomb (1988) found that the use of alcohol and other drugs in the workplace was most highly correlated with low law abidance and selling drugs, followed by thefts and confrontational acts, and then sexual involvement. Alcohol use on the job (which is typically considered less deviant than other drug use) was less tightly bound to other types of deviance. Deviance variables accounted for 6 percent of the variance in self-reported alcohol use on the job, whereas they accounted for 20 percent of the variance in cocaine use at work and for 36 percent of the variance in the use of other hard drugs at work.

Several of the workplace correlates of alcohol and other drug use appear to be part of the general pattern of behavior associated with deviance, including work avoidance, abuse of benefits, irresponsibility, and low workplace rule abidance. Although some of these behaviors may be directly caused by alcohol and other drug use, many of them appear to be aspects of general deviance rather than the consequences of specific alcohol- or other drug-induced impairment.

Role of Deviance in the Correlation of Alcohol and Other Drug Use and Work Behavior

The research reviewed above suggests that deviance is a potentially critical variable in explaining why measures of problem drinking and illicit drug use are related to workplace behaviors such as absenteeism and poor performance. If they are, the simplified model depicted in Figure 5.1 may assist in understanding the complex processes involved in the deviance in alcohol and other drug use/workplace behavior relationship.

This figure includes four critical links. First, general deviance (A) is related to and is probably a causal factor in alcohol and other drug use. In fact, such use is often used as a marker variable or a measure of deviance. Although a reciprocal link is possible (i.e., alcohol and other drug use may increase deviance, which leads to greater exposure to alcohol and other drugs), research on deviance suggests that use is originally and primarily an aspect of or a result of a generally deviant pattern of behavior rather than a cause of that behavior. The magnitude of the reciprocal causal relation probably increases with the individual level of alcohol and other drug involvement.

Second, alcohol and other drug use can lead to impairment (B), which may depend on the dosage and purity of the drug, the time and setting in which drugs were consumed, the individual's prior experience with the drug, the nature of the task, and a host of other factors. Laboratory research suggests that various drugs can either enhance, impair, or have no effect on performance (see Chapter 4). Similarly, the direct effects of alcohol and other drugs on other workplace behaviors (e.g., absenteeism) may be highly uncertain or variable. Nevertheless, it is possible that some of the observed alcohol and other drug use/work behavior correlations are due to the direct effects of these drugs on judgment, coordination, vigilance, overall health, and other variables.

Third, impairment may lead to changes in work behavior (C), although the strength of this effect will depend on the degree of impairment, the subject's experience with performing under impairment, the nature of the task, and the like. Finally, deviance may directly affect behaviors (D) such as absenteeism, performance, counterproductive behavior, etc., independent of any of the pharmacological effects of the drugs taken. For example,

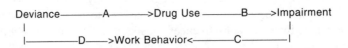

FIGURE 5.1 Relating deviance, drug use, and work behavior.

individuals who engage in deviant behavior patterns may be absent or care-
less, even on days when no drug or drug withdrawal effects are present.

There is research evidence to justify all four of the linkages shown in
Figure 5.1. It is difficult, however, to make well-supported statements
about the relative strength or importance of the various links, since, among
other things, they may vary in both magnitude and direction, depending on
the characteristics of an individual's alcohol and other drug use involvement. However, it is useful to note that the links between use, impairment,
and work behavior appear to be more context-dependent than the links between deviance, use, and work behavior. That is, the probable effects of
drugs on impairment and work behavior appear to depend on a large number of variables (e.g., dosage, experience, nature of the task), whereas the
links between deviance, alcohol and other drug use, and work behavior
appear to be more resilient to context, as they would if use and undesirable
work behavior are simple manifestations of a broader underlying deviance.
This suggests that deviance may be a better explanation than impairment of
the links between alcohol and other drug use and undesirable work behavior. If so, confronting deviant behaviors and attitudes may be a more effective strategy than narrow antidrug programs for both preventing workplace
decrements and treating poorly performing workers.

Because there are no studies that directly examine the impacts of alcohol and other drug use on work force performance, we must examine the
cumulative evidence from laboratory and field studies, each of which examines some facets of the possible connections between alcohol and other
drugs and work, to make inferences about the overall impact of their use.
For example, to the extent that laboratory studies demonstrate alcohol- and
other drug-induced impairment on tasks that are essentially similar to those
encountered on the job, it is reasonable to infer the possibility of workplace
impairment from the consumption of the studied drugs. The interpretability
of field studies on the effects of alcohol and other drugs is enhanced to the
extent that multiple studies employing different methods consistently estimate the correlates of alcohol and other drug use in the work environment,
and as the probable confounds in reported alcohol and other drug use/work
behavior correlations are identified and controlled for. While the individual
studies reviewed below are all subject to methodological criticism, the cumulative body of research may nevertheless provide a basis for making
reliable, empirically grounded statements about the impact of alcohol and
other drug use on work-related behaviors.

FIELD STUDIES

In general, alcohol and other drug use by the work force have been
associated with absenteeism, accidents, turnover, and other negative work

behaviors. Research support is most consistent for their association with absenteeism. For other types of outcomes, there is mixed or weak support, with very little support from better-designed studies. The research literature for different outcomes is reviewed below and is summarized in Table 5.1.

Absenteeism

The relationship of illicit drug use and absenteeism is perhaps the most robust of any of the outcomes that have been linked with employee drug use. A prospective study of preemployment drug testing in the U.S. Postal Service (Normand and Salyards, 1989; Normand et al., 1990) showed after 1.3 years of employment that employees who had tested positive for illicit drug use at the time they were hired had a mean absence rate of 6.6 percent of hours worked, which was 60 percent higher then the mean absence rate of 4.1 percent for employees who tested negative for drugs at the time of hire. When examining positive tests by type of drug, it was found that employees who tested positive for marijuana use were 1.5 times more likely to use leave time heavily, and employees who tested positive for cocaine were more than 4 times as likely as employees who tested negative to be heavy leave users.

Zwerling et al. (1990) examined preemployment drug test results for postal hires in the Boston area and found similar results for absenteeism. Employees testing positive for marijuana had a mean absence rate of 7.1 percent of scheduled hours worked, those testing positive for cocaine had a mean absence rate of 9.8, and those testing positive for other drugs a rate of 7.9, compared with a rate of 4.0 for employees who tested negative.

In surveys of municipal employees in the southwestern United States (Lehman et al., 1990a,b; Rosenbaum et al., 1992), there were strong relationships between self-reported alcohol and other drug use and unscheduled absenteeism. In one municipal sample (Lehman et al., 1990a), employees who reported having unscheduled absences during the last year were more likely than employees without unscheduled absences to get drunk frequently (18 compared with 13 percent), to drink at work (9 compared with 6 percent), and to report alcohol-related problems (26 compared with 15 percent). In terms of illicit drug use, employees with unscheduled absences were more likely to have used marijuana (30 compared with 20 percent) or other illicit drugs (17 compared with 10 percent) in their lifetime and to have used marijuana in the last year (11 compared with 6 percent). They also were more likely to have used illicit drugs in the last month (7 compared with 4 percent) and to have worked under the influence of illicit drugs in the last year (4 compared with 2 percent).

Results in a sample of municipal employees from a different city (Rosenbaum et al., 1992) also showed strong relationships between alcohol and other drug use and absenteeism. Employees were classified into three groups based on use in the last year: (1) nonusers who did not report use of any illicit drugs and did not drink frequently or experience negative consequences due to drinking; (2) heavy alcohol users who either drank frequently or experienced negative outcomes due to drinking but did not use illicit drugs; and (3) illicit drug users who reported at least some use of any illicit drug in the last year. Illicit drug users were much more likely than others to report having at least three unscheduled absences in the last year (79 percent), and heavy alcohol users (59 percent) were more likely than nonusers (52 percent) to have excessive absences.

Alcohol and other drug use was also more likely among employees with unscheduled absences in a sample of employees from the local housing authority from the same city as the first municipal sample above. Employees with unscheduled absences were more likely than others to drink at work (27 compared with 9 percent) and to report alcohol-related problems (24 compared with 12 percent). They were more likely to report lifetime use of marijuana (30 compared with 11 percent) and cocaine (12 compared with 3 percent), and last year use of marijuana (15 compared with 3 percent) and cocaine (9 compared with 1 percent).

It should be noted that, in the three samples above, alcohol and other drug use and absenteeism were based on self-reports and thus are subject to common methods variance. In addition, the relationships reported are based on two-way cross-tabulations and may possibly be explained by other variables. For example, younger employees are more likely to drink heavily and use illicit drugs, and they are also more likely than older employees to have higher absenteeism rates. It is possible that age or other variables can account fully or in part for the observed relationships.

A drug abuse management program at the Utah Power and Light Company was evaluated by Crouch et al. (1989). In this study, employees who tested positive for alcohol and other drugs in mandatory drug screens (usually for cause) and employees who self-referred to the employee assistance program (EAP) were compared with frequency-matched control groups. Employees in the drug-positive group had significantly higher absenteeism rates than did the matched control groups (75.3 accumulated sick hours versus 55.8 hours). The drug-positive group had a mean of 63.8 hours of unexcused absences compared with 18.7 hours for the control group. For the self-referred EAP group, the mean number of accumulated sick hours was 81.7 compared with 56.3 for the control group; the EAP group had 32.2 hours of unexcused absences on average compared with 10.1 for the control group.

This study is limited in several ways. There were only 12 employees in the drug-positive group and 27 in the EAP group, numbers too small to

TABLE 5.1 Alcohol and Drug Use and Job Outcomes

Outcome	Study	Sample
Absenteeism	Normand and Salyards (1989)	Postal service hires
	Zwerling et al. (1990)	Postal service hires in Boston
	Lehman et al. (1990a,b); Rosenbaum et al. (1992)	Municipal employees
	Crouch et al. (1989)	Utah Power and Light employees
	Sheridan and Winkler (1989)	Georgia Power Company employee testing positive and negative on drug tests
Accidents — transportation	Fell (1982); Fell and Klein (1986); Klein (1986)	Traffic fatalities in 15 states
	Transportation Research Board (1987)	Commercial vehicle fatalities
	National Transportation Safety Board (1990)	182 fatally injured truck drivers
	Moody et al. (1990)	Mandatory postaccident testing for railroad accidents

Data	Result
Preemployment urines; absenteeism records	Applicants testing positive for drug use had higher subsequent absenteeism; cocaine positives had more absenteeism than marijuana positives.
Preemployment urines and absenteeism records	Cocaine positives had highest rate of absenteeism followed by marijuana and other drug positives, and then negatives.
Self-report drug use and absenteeism	Employees reporting unscheduled absences more likely to get drunk, have alcohol problems, and recent illicit drug use.
Urine tests (usually for cause) and employee assistance program (EAP) referrals; absenteeism records	Drug positive group had more absences than matched control group; self-referred EAP group had more absences than matched control group.
Urine test for cause and random; absenteeism records	Positives not more absent in general than negatives; positives more absent than negatives for unpaid sickness, personal time, and suspensions in 1986 but not 1987.
Analysis of body fluids	More than half of fatal accidents involved alcohol, with about 75% of those with BAC above 0.10%; 16% of injury crashes and 8% of accidents with property damage only involve alcohol.
Analysis of body fluids	15% of commercial drivers involved in fatal accidents had detectable alcohol levels; in accidents in which truck driver is killed, 22% had been drinking, and 16% had BAC above 0.10%.
Analysis of body fluids	One-third of drivers tested positive for drugs of abuse; marijuana and alcohol 13%, cocaine 9%, other stimulants 8%, amphetamines 7%; drug impairment judged a factor in 87% of cases in which driver tested positive.
Analysis of body fluids, primarily urinalysis	In 26.8% of fatal accidents and 16.3% of nonfatal accidents, at least one employee involved in accident tested positive for illicit drug; marijuana 62% of positives, cocaine 20%, alcohol 9%, in one-third of positive events, drugs or alcohol were factors in accident.

continued

TABLE 5.1 *(Continued)*

Outcome	Study	Sample
	Taggart (1989)	Southern Pacific Railroad
	Kuhlman et al. (1991)	377 aviation fatalities
Accidents — other industries	Alleyne et al. (1991)	459 deaths at work in Alberta, Canada
	Lewis and Cooper (1989)	207 fatal work-related accidents in Harris County, Texas
	Hingson et al. (1985)	1,740 randomly sampled, employed adults in New England
	Holcom et al. (in press)	1,325 municipal workers
	Crouch et al. (1989)	Utah Power and Light Company
	Zwerling et al. (1990)	Postal service applicants in Boston

Data	Result
Urine tests; company accident records	Positive drug tests decreased from 23 to 6% in 3 years; personal injuries declined from 15.5 per 200,000 person hours to 5.8 during same time period; 22.2 human factor train accidents per 1 million train miles dropped to 2.2 in time period.
Analysis of body fluids	Alcohol found in less than 5%, marijuana in 1.3%, and cocaine metabolites in 1.3%.
Analysis of body fluids	11% had detectable alcohol with 4% over 0.08%; marijuana found in 8.5%, prescription drugs found in 8.5%, when alcohol present, 65% of deaths result of motor vehicle accident or getting caught in or under an object compared with 47% when alcohol not present.
Analysis of body fluids	Alcohol found in 13.3% with BACs over 0.10% for 9.2%; only one illicit drug found; 7% tested positive for prescription drugs that could have altered key functions such as reaction time or coordination.
Self-report alcohol and drug use and accidents	17% reported accidental injuries, 41 of which occurred at work; logistic regression indicated drinking at work not associated with accidents, but 5 or more drinks per day or use of psychoactive drugs elevated accident risk.
Self-report alcohol and drug use and accidents	Employees in high-risk jobs more likely to use drugs and drink frequently; alcohol and drug use not related to accidents in low-risk jobs; drug use best predictor of accidents for high-risk jobs.
Company drug-testing program and company accident records	Accidents increased from 1983 to 1985 when drug testing began; accidents decreased in 1986 and 1987; drug positive employees 5 times more likely to be in accident than control group although included tests for cause.
Preemployment drug tests and company accident records	Marijuana positive showed increased risk for accidents and injuries during first year of employment; cocaine positives showed slight risk increase for injuries.

continued

TABLE 5.1 *(Continued)*

Outcome	Study	Sample
	Normand et al. (1990)	Postal service applicants
Turnover	Blank and Fenton (1989)	1,052 naval recruits
	McDaniel (1988)	10,000 military recruits
	Normand et al. (1990)	Postal service applicants
	Zwerling et al. (1990)	Postal service applicants in Boston
	Kandel and Yamaguchi (1987)	1,325 young adults in New England
	Newcomb (1988)	Young adults followed up in Los Angeles
	White et al. (1988)	376 middle-class, white adults in longitudinal study
Job satisfaction	Mangione and Quinn (1975)	1,327 wage and salaried workers
	Perone et al. (1979)	Industrial workers with extreme scores on drug use

Data	Result
Preemployment drug tests and company accident records	No significant relationship found between preemployment drug test and subsequent accidents.
Preemployment drug tests and military retention records	2.5 years after entering service, 81% of THC-negative and 57% of THC-positive recruits still in service; 14% of THC-positive left because of drug/alcohol problems, 21% for behavioral problems compared to 1% and 8% of THC-negative group.
Self-report drug use and military discharge records	Preservice drug use correlated 0.08 with unsuitability discharge.
Preemployment drug tests and company retention records	No significant relationship between preemployment drug use and turnover; drug positive 1.5 times more likely to be fired, although firing usually related to excessive absenteeism.
Preemployment drug tests and company retention records	Marijuana positive 1.6 times higher turnover than drug negatives and 2 times as high involuntary turnover.
Self-report drug use and job mobility	Concurrent use of marijuana, other illicit drugs, and daily drinking associated with reduction of job tenure; drug effects more likely to lead to job loss rather than job change.
Self-report drug use and job status	Frequently losing jobs significant predictor of disruptive alcohol, marijuana, and other drug use.
Self-report drug use and occupational status	No relationship found between chronic or current use of marijuana or alcohol and occupational status.
Self-report drug use and job satisfaction	Small correlation (-0.12) between job satisfaction and drug use at work only for men 30 years or older.
Self-report drug use and job satisfaction	No differences between drug users and nonusers in either real or simulated jobs.

continued

TABLE 5.1   *(Continued)*

Outcome	Study	Sample
	Hollinger (1988)	9,175 employees from 47 organizations
	Lehman et al. (1990a, 1991)	1,325 municipal employees
Other outcomes	Mangione and Quinn (1975)	1,327 wage and salaried workers
	Newcomb (1988)	Young adults followed-up in Los Angeles
	Lehman and Simpson (1992)	1,325 municipal employees
	Rosenbaum et al. (1992)	1,081 municipal employees
	Blum et al. (1993)	136 employed men
	Salyards (1993)	Postal service applicants
	Lehman et al. (1992)	1,325 municipal employees

Data	Result
Self-report drug use and job satisfaction	Employees dissatisfied with jobs 75% more likely to drink at work.
Self-report drug use and job satisfaction	Dissatisfied employees more likely than satisfied employees to drink heavily, use illicit drugs.
Self-report drug use and job behaviors	Drug-using males over the age of 30 more likely than nonusing counterparts to engage in counterproductive behaviors.
Self-report drug use and job behaviors	Engaging in vandalism at work significant predictor of disruptive alcohol use, marijuana use, and hard drug use.
Self-report drug use and job behaviors	Drug use significant predictor of physical withdrawal behaviors, and antagonistic psychological and behaviors.
Self-report drug use and job behaviors	Illicit drug users more likely than alcohol users who were more likely than nonusers to engage in variety of negative work behaviors.
Self-report alcohol and drug use; collateral ratings of conflict avoidance and performance	Heavy drinkers rated as significantly lower on technical performance, self-direction, interpersonal relations, and higher on conflict avoidance.
Preemployment drug tests and company EAP utilization, disciplinary action, and medical claims	Employees testing positive for drugs at hire used EAP more for substance abuse problems, had higher utilization of medical benefits, and more likely to be disciplined for conduct offenses.
Self-report drug use, attitudes, and perceptions of co-workers	Employees exposed to co-worker drug or alcohol use more likely to report problems in work group, more likely to have negative attitudes toward management efforts to combat drug use, and have lower job satisfaction and faith in management.

make stable estimates. It is not known how the samples were selected, and the time period being evaluated in the study is not stated. Furthermore, members of both the drug-tested group and the EAP group may have been in those groups precisely because of problems like absenteeism. Most importantly, the use of frequency-matched control groups is problematic when attempting to produce equivalent groups for comparison purposes (Salyards and Normand, 1991).

Sheridan and Winkler (1989) report on an evaluation of drug testing at the Georgia Power Company. Their data on absenteeism were less consistent than in other studies. Employees who tested positive on company drug tests were compared with employees testing negative. However, results of for-cause and random tests were mixed, and tests for cause are given for employees who have already been identified as having work-related problems. Results showed that positives were not significantly more absent than negatives, but for absenteeism based on unpaid sick leave, personal time, and disciplinary suspensions, negatives were significantly more absent than the company norm, and positives were significantly more absent than negatives in 1986 but not in 1987. These results are, no doubt, influenced by the presence of for-cause tested individuals in both the positive and negative groups. For-cause negatives probably had the kinds of problems associated with alcohol and other drug use or else they would not have been tested.

Accidents

The relationship between employee alcohol and other drug use and accidents is mixed, despite the heavy media attention given to accidents by employees working under the influence and the seemingly obvious association between working while impaired and having accidents. Perhaps the most well-known findings linking alcohol and other drug use and accidents are found in the transportation industry. Accidents involving public carriers are often highly publicized in the media. A single accident can have catastrophic consequences, by resulting in significant loss of life or injury to the public, extensive environmental damage, and huge damage costs. A few well-publicized accidents can both seriously damage the public's confidence in the safety of the transportation system and give rise to lawsuits for substantial damages, thus greatly affecting the economic health of transportation companies. For these reasons, the relationship between alcohol and other drug use and transportation accidents has long been a well-funded focus of research attention.

Evidence on the relationship between alcohol and drug use and accidents in industries other than transportation is mixed. There are many possible reasons for the failure to find consistent associations, one being that on-the-job accidents are relatively rare events and thus difficult to predict. Moreover, there is little evidence that working under the influence is widespread; many employees who do work under the influence may be able to compensate for their impairment, and there is a substantial amount of variation across individuals as to how a specific drug at a given dose affects performance. Given the evidence of higher rates of absenteeism among alcohol and other drug abusers, it is possible that many workers who are too impaired to work and thus more susceptible to accidents stay home from work. Some workers who may be impaired on the job work in positions in which they are not at risk for accidents, such as office settings. Other workers impaired on the job who work in positions in which they are at risk for accidents may be able to avoid dangerous tasks, thus reducing the likelihood of an accident.

In the transportation industry, in contrast, workers who operate vehicles cannot avoid jobs in which they are at risk for accidents. Thus, impairment may become a more important issue for vehicle operators than for some other jobs. Even minimizing risky tasks may be different for vehicle operators. For example, truck or bus drivers need to complete their routes and do not often have alternative activities they can be involved in if they are impaired. Moreover, the stigma that attaches to alcohol and other drug use by transportation workers may lead them to work for fear that excessive absences would call attention to their use, whereas workers in other industries would see absence from work as the best solution. Finally, certain stimulant drugs like caffeine and methamphetamines may in certain circumstances slightly improve performance. Transportation workers may feel that such boosts are necessary to meet job demands, even if in the long run dependence has adverse safety consequences.

Because of the special significance of alcohol and other drug use and accidents in the transportation industry, we review the literature on accidents in transportation first, followed by a discussion on the evidence of alcohol and other drug use and accidents in other industries. (For a more detailed treatment of the transportation literature, the reader is referred to *Alcohol and Other Drugs in Transportation: Research Needs for the Next Decade* (Transportation Research Board, 1993).

Accidents in the Transportation Industry

Much of the public concern regarding alcohol and other drugs in the work force has been precipitated by highly publicized accidents in the transportation industry. Table 5.2 recalls some examples that helped sensitize public perceptions to problems associated with drugs on the job. Although a few accidents involving alcohol or other drug use do not establish a significant relationship for an industry as a whole, the effect of such accidents on public confidence and perceptions and the significant damage even

TABLE 5-2 Transportation Accidents and Incidents Involving Alcohol or Drug Abuse

Industry	Incident	Date	Drugs	Description
Aviation	Northwest Airline pilot and crew	1990	Alcohol	The night before flying, pilot drank 20 mixed drinks and first officer and flight engineer shared six pitchers of beer; after the flight, BAC was found of 0.13 percent, 0.06 percent, and 0.08 percent for the pilot, first officer, and flight engineer, respectively. Three officers convicted of flying under the influence, received jail terms, and lost their licenses.
	Trans-Colorado Airline commuter plane crash	1988	Cocaine	Degradation of captain's performance resulting from cocaine use night before crash: 2 crew members and 7 passengers killed.
	K-Airlines air cargo plane crash	1986	Alcohol	Pilot had BAC of 0.158 percent and 7 DWI convictions: pilot, only person on board, killed.
Military aviation	Navy pilot crashes while landing on aircraft carrier U.S.S. Nimitz	1981	Marijuana	Use of marijuana implicated in crash: several expensive military fighterplanes destroyed, totaling over $100 million.
Railroad	Southern Pacific Transportation Company collision of two trains	1972	Alcohol alcohol	Engineer of one train failed to control his train because of impairment.
	Derailment at Livingston, Louisiana	1982	Alcohol	Alcohol-impaired engineer relinquished controls to unqualified employee: 36 tank cars derailed, 20 punctured or breached; 3,000 people evacuated; 200,000 gallons of toxic chemicals spilled; $16 million damage.

	Year	Drug	Details
Collision of two Missouri Pacific Railroad Company trains near Possum Grape, Arkansas	1982	Alcohol	Alcohol-impaired engineer relinquished controls to unqualified employee: 2 railroad employees killed, 1 seriously injured; $1,047,000 damage.
Rear-end collision between two Seaboard System Railroad trains at Sullivan, Indiana	1984	Alcohol	Alcohol-impaired engineer and brakeman of striking train fell asleep: 2 railroad employees killed.
Conrail freight train improperly passed stop signal at Chase, Maryland and entered main track, where it was hit by an Amtrak passenger train at 120 miles per hour.	1987	Marijuana	Freight train engineer and brakeman were heavy marijuana users and impaired by marijuana at time of accident: engineer and 15 passengers were killed; 174 persons suffered injuries.
Commercial trucking			
Tractor-trailer driving through Colorado mountains lost control on horseshoe turn and slid 350 feet down mountain		Marijuana, cocaine	Inexperienced driver tested positive for cocaine and marijuana; syringe with cocaine residue found in suitcase: driver killed.
Speeding tractor-trailer crashed into properly marked truck on the side of road in California		Amphetamine, methamphetamine, marijuana, cocaine	Driver tested positive for multiple drugs of abuse: driver killed in fire.
Maritime			
Exxon Valdez oil tanker runs aground in Prince William Sound, Alaska	1989	Alcohol	Captain impaired by alcohol, relinquished control to inexperienced third mate: 8 cargo tanks ruptured, spilling 258,000 barrels of crude oil; catastrophic environmental and economic damage.

a single accident can cause mean that such reports are important in their own right.

Alcohol has long been heavily implicated in fatal automobile accidents. In a study of data from 15 states with relatively complete reporting statistics, Fell (1982) estimated that 59 percent of drivers killed in accidents had alcohol in their blood, and 49 percent had blood alcohol content (BAC) at 0.10 percent or higher. A discriminant analysis approach to estimating alcohol-involved fatal crashes developed by Klein (Klein, 1986; Fell and Klein, 1986) estimated alcohol involvement in about one-half of fatal crashes, with 75 percent of those involving BACs at 0.10 percent or higher. Sixteen percent of injury crashes and 8 percent of property damage accidents were estimated to involve alcohol. Although the presence of alcohol in a fatal accident does not necessarily imply that alcohol was a cause of the accident, the data are so overwhelming that a general causal link cannot be denied.

A report by the Transportation Research Board (TRB) (1987) estimated that 750 fatal crashes occur annually in which a commercial vehicle driver has been drinking. Although this is a substantial number of accidents, only 15 percent of commercial vehicle drivers in fatal crashes had detectable levels of alcohol, compared with 45 percent of all drivers in fatal crashes. However, in 75 percent of fatal crashes involving trucks, someone other than the truck driver is killed. In accidents in which the truck driver is killed, 22 percent of drivers are found to have been drinking and 16 percent to have BACs above 0.10 percent. The TRB, we should note, was forced to estimate the number of alcohol-related crashes because the BACs of commercial vehicle drivers involved in fatal crashes are not well reported. Its report states that BACs are reported for only 11 percent of surviving drivers, and 14 percent of those have alcohol in their bloodstreams, 8 percent above 0.10 percent.

The National Transportation Safety Board (1990) reported on a study of truck drivers from 182 heavy-truck crashes in which the driver was fatally injured. One-third of drivers tested positive for illicit drugs. Marijuana and alcohol were found most frequently (13 percent each) followed by cocaine (9 percent), other stimulants (8 percent), and amphetamines (7 percent). Forty-one percent of the alcohol and other drug-positive drivers tested positive for multiple drugs. Impairment from alcohol and other drugs was determined to be a factor in the accident for 87 percent of cases in which the drivers tested positive for drugs.

Mandatory post-accident drug and alcohol testing for railroad accidents was examined by Moody et al. (1990). Overall, 351 events involving 1,398 persons were included in the study. Of these, 6 percent tested positive for illicit drugs or alcohol. However, results showed that, in 27 percent of fatal accidents and 16 percent of nonfatal accidents, at least one employee involved in the accident tested positive for an illicit drug. Marijuana was the most common illicit drug found (62 percent of positives) followed by cocaine (20 percent). In approximately one-third of the events that involved drug positives, alcohol or other drugs were found to be causally related to the accident. The raw figures suggest that marijuana plays a greater role compared with alcohol than it probably does, possibly because marijuana metabolites are present in urine for days or weeks (for chronic users) after consumption, yet alcohol is rapidly metabolized. Moreover, as Chapter 4 makes clear, while performance decrements attributable to alcohol emerge clearly in laboratory studies, decrements attributable to marijuana are harder to find.

An analysis of the drug testing program of the Southern Pacific Railroad (Taggart, 1989) describes accident rates before and after widespread drug testing was begun. Urinalysis testing was begun in August 1984 and included for-cause and preemployment testing. Alcohol was also included in the testing protocol. Positive tests decreased from a high of 23 percent at the beginning of the program, to 12 percent in the first full year, to 6 percent in 1987. Personal injuries showed similar declines during the same time period, decreasing from 15.5 per 200,000 person hours worked in the last full year before testing began to 5.8 in the first 6 months of 1988. Train accidents attributable to human failure also dropped from pretest levels. In 1983 there were 22.2 human factor train accidents per 1 million train miles, and in the first 7 months of 1988 there were 2.2 human factor train accidents per 1 million train miles. Although these appear to be impressive changes in accident rates, there were no comparison groups and so it is not possible to determine whether the change in accident rates was due to the testing program. For example, new company policies or programs or changes to the old ones may have been implemented or improvements in track beds or other conditions could have been made during that period, resulting in lower accident rates.

Alcohol and other drug use does not appear to be an important factor in aviation fatalities, according to a study by Kuhlman et al. (1991). Blood, urine, and tissue samples from 377 aviation fatalities in 1989 were analyzed. Alcohol was found in 5 percent of cases, marijuana in 1 percent, and cocaine metabolites in 2 percent. There was minimal use of therapeutic depressants or stimulants. The authors concluded that the data showed no consistent pattern of alcohol or other drug use among aviation fatalities.

Accidents in Other Industries

The incidence of alcohol and other drug use among workers fatally injured on the job in Alberta, Canada, was examined by Alleyne et al.

(1991), and among workers killed on the job in Harris County, Texas, by Lewis and Cooper (1989).

Alleyne et al. (1991) studied 459 deaths occurring at work in Alberta between 1979 and 1986. Of these deaths, 373 were tested for alcohol, 82 for marijuana, and 329 for other drugs. Eleven percent of fatalities tested for alcohol had detectable alcohol levels, with 4.3 percent over 0.10 percent. The only illicit drug identified was marijuana, which was found in 9 percent of cases tested. Prescription drugs were found in 9 percent of cases, and nonprescription drugs in 7 percent. When alcohol was present in a fatally injured worker, 65 percent of deaths were the result of a motor vehicle accident or getting caught in or under an object. When alcohol was not present, 47 percent of fatalities were due to these types of accidents.

A study of 207 fatal work-related injuries occurring in 1984 and 1985 in Harris County, Texas (including the city of Houston), examined the incidence of alcohol and licit and illicit drugs (Lewis and Cooper, 1989). Detectable levels of alcohol were found in 13 percent of fatalities and 9 percent had BACs over 0.10 percent. Only one case of illicit drug use was detected, and one person tested positive for both alcohol and other drugs. Seven percent of the workers tested positive for prescription drugs that could have altered key functions, such as reaction time or the coordination needed to prevent injury. In neither study of fatal injuries do the authors show that the presence of alcohol or drugs was causally related to the fatal accidents, nor did either study seek to determine whether the deceased workers who tested negative were killed in accidents caused by impaired coworkers.

A telephone survey of 1,740 randomly sampled employed adults in the New England region was conducted by Hingson et al. (1985). Respondents were asked about their levels of alcohol consumption, whether they consumed alcohol at work, and general patterns of drug use. They were also asked about any injuries that required medical attention in the previous year, whether these injuries resulted in an overnight hospitalization, whether they occurred on the job, and the nature of the injuries. If respondents reported injuries, they were asked whether they had consumed any alcohol or other drugs in the 6 hours before the accident.

Overall, 17 percent of respondents reported accidental injuries in the last year, and of these 41 percent occurred at work. More than three-fourths of respondents drank alcoholic beverages, but only 7 percent averaged 3 or more drinks per day. Four percent had been drunk on the job in the month before the interview, and 13 percent reported coming to work hung over or high. A total of 8 percent had taken illicit drugs in the previous month that might have affected their functioning at work.

Results of logistic regression analyses indicated that alcohol consumption at work was not associated with job accidents, but averaging 5 or more drinks per day elevated the relative risk of accidents compared with abstainers. Heavy drinkers were 1.7 times as likely as abstainers to report an accidental injury, 3.8 times as likely to report injuries requiring hospitalization, and 2 times as likely to report a job-based injury. Respondents reporting use of psychoactive drugs were 1.7 times as likely as abstainers to report work accidents and 2.4 times as likely to report having been hospitalized as the result of an accident.

Holcom et al. (in press) examined the relationship between alcohol and other drug use and accidents in a sample of municipal employees. Information on alcohol and other drug use, accidents, personal background, and job characteristics and background was collected via self-report survey of 1,325 randomly selected employees. Measures of use included lifetime use of any illicit substance, alcohol consumption away from work, illicit drug use in the last year, and use of alcohol or illicit drugs at work in the last year. The accident outcome was a composite measure that included three types of accidents in which the respondent was the source of the accident, not just an accident victim: minor personal injury accidents, major personal injury accidents, and equipment damage accidents. Employees were categorized into high-risk (safety-sensitive) and low-risk job groups for analysis.

Discriminant function analyses were used to classify employees within each risk sample into accident and no-accident groups. Variable domains from personal background, including demographic variables and measures of deviance/social maladjustment, job background, including job characteristics and job attitudes, and alcohol and other drug use were used as discriminators. Employees in the high-risk job category were more likely than employees in low-risk jobs to use alcohol frequently (39 compared with 29 percent) and to use alcohol or other drugs at work (13 compared with 8 percent). In the low-risk job category, there were no differences between employees in the accident and no-accident groups on any of the alcohol and other drug use measures. In the high-risk category, employees who had reported an accident in the last year were more than four times as likely as accident-free employees to report illicit drug use in the last year (17 compared with 4 percent). In the discriminant function analyses, drug use at work and illicit drug use in the last year were the best discriminators of accidents for the high-risk jobs; for low-risk jobs, illicit drug use did not contribute to the discrimination of accident groups. As we have noted when discussing other studies, the significant association of alcohol and other drug use with accidents does not necessarily mean that the relationship is causal.

In the evaluation of the Utah Power and Light Company's substance abuse program (Crouch et al., 1989), accident rates increased between 1983 and 1985, but the trend upward stopped in 1985 when the drug-testing program was initiated, and there were statistically fewer accidents in 1986 and 1987. Drug-positive employees were five times more likely to be in an accident than their control group. However, the drug-positive group was small and included employees tested for cause. It is unknown how many were tested because of an accident. The evidence does not allow one to conclude that the decrease in the accident rate after initiating the drug-testing program was due to the drug-testing program.

The two postal service studies showed mixed results for accidents and injuries. In the Boston area sample reported by Zwerling et al. (1990), marijuana positives showed an increased risk for accidents and injuries during the first year of employment, and cocaine positives showed a slight increased risk for injuries. Marijuana positives were 1.55 times as likely as drug negatives to have an accident and 1.85 times as likely to be injured; cocaine positives were 1.85 times as likely as drug negatives to be injured. The national study of postal service employees (Normand et al., 1990) did not find a significant relationship between testing positive and having an accident at work. This lack of a relationship may, however, be due to the low rate of accidents.

Turnover

A number of studies have addressed the issue of turnover or job mobility in relation to alcohol and other drug use. One approach involves the measuring of preemployment illicit drug use, using self-report or urinalysis data, and then following employees after employment to evaluate turnover (e.g., Blank and Fenton, 1989; McDaniel, 1988; Normand et al., 1990; Parish, 1989; Zwerling et al., 1990). Other studies have used population studies of several different populations and analyzed job mobility in relation to alcohol and other drug use (e.g., Kandel and Yamaguchi, 1987; Newcomb, 1988; White et al., 1988).

Several studies examining the relationship between preemployment illicit drug use and turnover were conducted with military recruits. Blank and Fenton (1989) collected data on 1,052 naval recruits who were tested for marijuana and other illicit drugs before entering the Navy. A positive marijuana test did not disqualify potential recruits. Half of the studied sample were marijuana-positive; an equal number of marijuana-negative subjects was selected from the same applicant pool as a comparison group. Approximately 2.5 years after entering the service, 81 percent of the marijuana-negative group and 57 percent of the marijuana-positive group were still in the Navy. Fourteen percent of the marijuana-positive group had left the service due to alcohol or other drug problems and 21 percent because of behavioral or performance problems, compared with 1 percent and 8 percent, respectively, for the marijuana-negative group. However, the increased attrition in the marijuana-positive group may be due to the increased surveillance these positive new recruits were subjected to as a result of the positive preenlistment test.

McDaniel (1988) used self-reports of illicit drug use among over 10,000 military recruits and compared preservice illicit drug use to unsuitability discharges. Preservice illicit drug use correlated .08 with discharge, although discharge was also correlated with cognitive ability (r = –.06). Thus, even though the prevalence rate of previous illicit drug use was relatively high (49 percent), the validity for predicting job suitability was rather low. McDaniel concludes that other selection factors would probably do a better job of selecting employees who are likely to do well on the job.

In the studies of postal employees, Normand et al. (1990) reported that there was not a significant relationship between drug test results and overall turnover or voluntary turnover. However, drug positives were 1.55 times as likely as drug negatives to be fired. Zwerling et al. (1990) found similar results for turnover, with marijuana positives having 1.56 times higher total turnover than did drug negatives and 2.07 times as high involuntary turnover.

Kandel and Yamaguchi (1987) examined job mobility in relation to alcohol and other drug use in a sample of 1,325 young adults aged 24 to 25 in New York state. Three patterns of drug use were investigated, including daily alcohol use, monthly use of marijuana, and monthly use of other illicit drugs. Job mobility was examined as job separations, job changes, and job losses. Other illicit drug use among men and women and daily alcohol use among women were found to have strong associations with job separation, but these were attributed to selection rather than to impairment because the effects of former and current use of these drugs were equally strong. In other words, these data suggest that those who chose to use alcohol and other drugs are people who would probably experience employment instability even if they did not use them. Current daily use of alcohol among men and marijuana use among women were also associated with higher job separation rates; there were differences between those who continued and those who stopped using these drugs, suggesting that alcohol and other drug use may have played a causal role. When other factors were controlled, concurrent use of marijuana, other illicit drugs, and daily alcohol drinking was associated with a reduction of job tenure of 1.3 years for women and just under 1 year for men. Alcohol and other drug effects were more likely to lead to job losses rather than to job changes.

A study of alcohol and other drug use and work patterns for a sample of middle-class, white "baby boomers" did not find a relationship between alcohol and other drug use and employment status (White et al., 1988). A longitudinal analysis of 376 respondents available in a follow-up found that neither chronic nor current use of marijuana or alcohol had any adverse effect on the respondent's employment status. However, the sample used in the study was unique, and the authors warn against extrapolating these results to the larger population.

Newcomb's (1988) follow-up study of young adults in the Los Angeles area reversed the hypothesized causal relationship and used work-related factors to predict measures of problem drinking, marijuana, cocaine, and any drug use. Frequently losing jobs in the last 4 years was a significant predictor of any disruptive drug use, disruptive hard drug use, and disruptive cannabis use. Losing a job in the last 6 months was a significant predictor of disruptive alcohol use, disruptive cannabis use, and any disruptive drug use. Although job instability was one of the most consistent predictors of disruptive alcohol or other drug use among the work-related factors, correlations tended to be small.

Job Satisfaction

A number of studies have found significant associations of alcohol and other drug use with employees' job satisfaction. Depending on the theoretical perspective, job satisfaction can be considered a precursor or an outcome of use. However, the same can be true of many of the other work-related outcomes associated with use. No studies have been able to adequately assess causal direction. However, job satisfaction is an important work-related variable that has been associated with a variety of other work outcomes, such as intentions to quit, turnover, and job performance.

Mangione and Quinn (1975) studied responses from a sample of 1,327 wage and salary workers in the Quality of Employment Survey. Men and women were analyzed separately, and within gender, employees younger than 30 were analyzed separately from employees age 30 and older. There was a significant but small ($r = -.12$) correlation between job satisfaction and illicit drug use at work, but only for men age 30 and older.

In a laboratory simulation task, Perone et al. (1979) first surveyed industrial workers about drug use, and then, to enhance the likelihood of finding a relationship, placed only those subjects with extreme scores on illicit drug use into their user and nonuser groups. The subjects in these groups were given a laboratory simulation involving a repetitive task. Job satisfaction was measured for both the subject's real jobs and their simulated jobs. There were no major differences between illicit drug users and nonusers with regard to either real or simulated jobs.

Hollinger (1988) examined 9,175 responses to a mailed survey of employees in 47 organizations representing 3 industries. Working while intoxicated was predicted in a logistic model by variables representing age, gender, social interaction with coworkers, and job satisfaction. Dissatisfied employees reported that they worked while intoxicated at a rate 75 percent higher than satisfied employees.

The Lehman et al. (1990a) study of municipal employees also showed significant relationships between job satisfaction and alcohol and other drug use. Employees with low satisfaction were more likely than employees with high satisfaction to report using alcohol (79 compared with 72 percent), getting drunk (52 compared with 44 percent), and having alcohol problems (23 compared with 13 percent). Dissatisfied employees also reported more often that the use of prescription or over-the-counter drugs adversely affected their ability to work (11 compared with 5 percent for over-the-counter; 12 compared with 3 percent for prescription drugs). Finally, dissatisfied employees were more likely than satisfied employees to report lifetime use of marijuana (28 compared with 16 percent) and other illicit drugs (18 compared with 7 percent), marijuana use in the last year (10 compared with 3 percent), last year use of other illicit drugs (7 compared with 2 percent), use of illicit drugs within the last month (7 compared with 2 percent), and use of illicit drugs at work in the last year (3 compared with 0 percent). In a multivariate analysis, including other work and personal background variables, job satisfaction was not found to be a significant predictor of use, suggesting that bivariate relationships may not be causal in nature (Lehman et al., 1991).

Other Outcomes

Employees' alcohol and other drug use has also been associated with a variety of other job outcome measures. These include counterproductive behaviors such as theft, vandalism, and purposely doing work wrong (Mangione and Quinn, 1975; Newcomb, 1988); job withdrawal behaviors (Lehman and Simpson, 1992; Rosenbaum et al., 1992); low job productivity and difficult interpersonal relations at work (Blum et al., 1993); higher medical claims, EAP referrals, and disciplinary infractions (Salyards, 1993); and negative coworker attitudes (Lehman et al., 1992).

Mangione and Quinn (1975) and Newcomb (1988) found that alcohol and other drug users were more likely than nonusers to engage in counterproductive behaviors. In Mangione and Quinn's study, men over age 30 who reported using illicit drugs at work were more likely than their nonusing counterparts to engage in such deviant behaviors as spreading rumors or gossip, intentionally doing poor work, stealing merchandise or equipment, not reporting accidentally damaged equipment or merchandise, and damaging equipment or merchandise on purpose. There was no significant relationship between these behaviors and use at work for women or for men under age 30. Newcomb found that engaging in vandalism at work was a significant predictor of problem drinking, marijuana use, hard drug use, and any drug use.

Several different measures of on-the-job behaviors were analyzed in

Lehman and Simpson's (1992) study of municipal employees. Job behaviors included positive work behaviors (doing more work than was required, volunteering to work overtime, trying to improve working conditions), psychological withdrawal behaviors (thinking of being absent, daydreaming, chatting with coworkers, spending work time on personal matters), physical withdrawal behaviors (leaving work early, falling asleep at work, taking long lunch breaks), and antagonistic behaviors (arguing with coworkers, filing formal complaints, insubordination). A measure of counterproductive behaviors was examined but not used because of restricted variance.

Examination of bivariate relationships between the work behavior factors and alcohol and other drug use indicated that employees reporting alcohol or other drug use at work, illicit drug use in the last year, lifetime illicit drug use, or heavy alcohol use tended to engage in more frequent psychological and physical withdrawal and antagonistic behaviors. There were no differences between user groups on positive work behaviors, except that employees who reported lifetime illicit drug use reported slightly higher levels of positive work behaviors than did employees who never used illicit drugs.

Each of the four job behavior factors was then regressed on domains of predictor variables, including personal background, job background, job climate, and alcohol and other drug use. The unique contribution of use to the prediction of job behaviors was assessed by adding the block of variables on alcohol or other drug use to the regression equation after the other variable blocks had been entered. These results indicated that use uniquely accounted for significant although small amounts of variance in each of the four job behavior factors, with the amount of uniquely explained variance ranging from 4 percent in the case of physical withdrawal behaviors to 1 percent for positive work behaviors.

An examination by Rosenbaum et al. (1992) of bivariate relationships between a variety of job behaviors and alcohol and other drug use in a sample of municipal workers showed that illicit drug users were more likely than heavy alcohol users, who in turn were more likely than nonusers, to engage in negative work behaviors. For example, 73 percent of illicit drug users argued with coworkers compared with 63 percent of heavy alcohol users and 52 percent of nonusers. Forty percent of illicit drug users disobeyed supervisors' instructions, 32 percent stole work supplies, and 22 percent intentionally did their job wrong compared with 29 percent, 12 percent, and 10 percent of heavy alcohol users and 19 percent, 11 percent, and 6 percent of nonusers, respectively. Likewise, illicit drug users were more likely than others to let coworkers do their work (57 compared with 44 percent of heavy alcohol users and 36 percent of nonusers), complain of illness at work (69 compared with 54 and 48 percent), daydream about nonwork activities (40 compared with 17 and 15 percent), and fall asleep at work (42 compared with 21 and 17 percent). It should be noted, however, that these measures are based on self-reports and thus are subject both to the biases this method entails and to common methods variance.

Alcohol use and job performance measures were examined by Blum et al. (1993), in their study of 136 employed men. Measures of alcohol consumption and job performance, including assessments of conflict avoidance, technical performance, self-direction, and interpersonal relations, were obtained from the workers and the collateral sources they had named for referrals. Although light and heavy drinkers did not generally differ on their self-assessments of job performance, heavy drinkers were rated as significantly lower on all four scales by their references. Thus heavy drinkers were seen by others as having lower technical performance, self-direction, interpersonal relations, and higher conflict avoidance than light drinkers. More consistent differences were found, however, for the two social aspects of job performance (conflict avoidance and interpersonal relations) than for the technical aspects (technical performance and self-direction).

An expanded analysis of the postal service data examined use of medical benefits, EAP referrals, and disciplinary infractions an average of 3.3 years after hire (Salyards, 1993). Results indicated that employees who tested positive at the time of hire were more than 2.7 times as likely as employees who tested negative to subsequently experience problems requiring EAP intervention, with marijuana positives being twice as likely and cocaine positives being 6.27 times as likely to do so. Positives were 3.5 times as likely as negatives to use the EAP because of alcohol problems and 5.7 times as likely to do so because of illicit drug problems. Although drug positives were more likely than negatives to be disciplined, much of the difference was due to attendance-related offenses. However, positives were 1.6 times as likely as negatives to be disciplined for conduct offenses.

Those who tested positively for illicit drugs at the time they were hired also showed significantly higher utilization of medical benefits than those who tested negative. Comparisons between positives and negatives indicated that, compared with negatives, positives were 1.7 times as likely to be above the median on the total number of claims filed, 1.9 times as likely to be above the median on the total dollar amount of their claims, and 3.4 times as likely to file claims involving alcohol or other drug-related diagnoses (Salyards, 1993).

Alcohol and other drug use has also been linked to employees' job attitudes and perceptions of coworkers. Lehman et al. (1992) asked municipal employees about their awareness of use among their coworkers, whether use in their work group affected their ability to get the work done, and their attitudes toward company policies regarding employee use of alcohol and other drugs. More than 40 percent of respondents reported that coworker use sometimes caused poor-quality work in their work group; more than 30 percent blamed coworker use for poor communication, more chances for injuries, and damaged equipment. Employees exposed to higher levels of alcohol and other drug use by coworkers also were much more likely to attribute work-related problems to coworker use.

Employees exposed to alcohol and other drug use in their work group viewed management efforts to deal with the problem much more negatively than did employees who were not exposed. Employees not aware of coworker use were much more likely not to have an opinion about company efforts to deal with the matter. Employees exposed to coworker use were also more likely to favor preemployment and random urine testing programs. A discriminant analysis used attitudes such as job satisfaction, job involvement, faith in management, and organizational commitment to discriminate between employees not exposed to coworker use, and those exposed to low or high levels of coworker use. Job attitudes significantly discriminated between coworker use groups. Employees with a high exposure to coworker use had lower job satisfaction and less faith in management than did employees not aware of coworker use.

Summary

A wide variety of job outcomes and behaviors has been associated with employees' use of alcohol and other drugs. These include absenteeism, accidents, turnover, job satisfaction, counterproductive behaviors, psychological and physical withdrawal behaviors, and coworker attitudes. Despite the wide variety of research in the studies reviewed above, few definitive statements can be made about the impact of using alcohol and other drugs on job performance. The abundance of evidence presented here indicates that the relationship between use and job behaviors and outcomes is clearly negative. However, the magnitude of the relationships found is generally small, and causal spuriousness and direction are problems that have not been adequately addressed in the literature.

Part of the problem is that the research designs and methods are not amenable to establishing causality. Even when reliable relationships can be reported, the current research does not allow unequivocal causal assertions about those relationships. Perhaps the most reliable relationship involves use and absenteeism. However, the evidence does not necessarily show that use causes higher absenteeism. It is possible that other variables can account for the relationship, for example, general deviance or subjective job stress that induces both use and absenteeism.

The other job outcome that has shown consistent results involves accidents in the transportation industry. Although the presence of alcohol and other drugs in transportation accidents is considerable, it is much lower than that found generally in motor vehicle accidents. However, accidents in the transportation industry, perhaps to a greater extent than most other industries (except possibly the nuclear industry), have the potential to cause great harm to the public and thus are more likely to result in public concerns regarding employees' use of alcohol and other drugs and lack of confidence in public carriers. Alcohol is by far the most implicated drug in transportation industry accidents. Laboratory studies on the effects of alcohol as well as predicted differences in the role alcohol plays in single versus multiple car fatalities allow cause to be ascribed with more confidence in transportation accidents.

When attempting to understand the complex relationships between alcohol and other drug use and job performance across diverse industries, the issues of deviance and impairment are often pertinent. Untangling the magnitude and direction of causal links—which may include deviance and impairment and which may go from behavior to alcohol and other drug use or vice versa or both—poses difficult but critically important issues that must be attended to when attempting to attribute negative work outcomes to use. And yet, as we point out in Chapter 7, it is less critical if the goal is simply to decide whether a drug-testing program will have an impact on an organization's overall productivity level.

To date, most of the research efforts that have sought to shed some light on the potential causal relationship between alcohol and other drug use and job performance have used designs and research methods that do not allow these relationships to be satisfactorily untangled. Relationships that are reported are often mixed and generally not very strong. For example, some studies have found positive relationships of use to turnover; others have not. Some of the inconsistency can be attributed to different or flawed research designs. Inconsistencies can also be attributed to the highly skewed distributions of most variables of interest. Most employees do not abuse illicit drugs or alcohol, most employees do not have accidents at work, and most employees do not abuse absence policies. Thus, finding consistent relationships between relatively rare events such as alcohol and other drug abuse and accidents requires a carefully designed study with a large sample size and reliable measures—a difficult task indeed. It is not enough, however, to show consistency or even causality. From a policy standpoint, attention must be paid to the magnitude of these effects as well.

The use of flawed research designs is also an important issue to be considered when interpreting these studies. Unreliable variables and common method variance plague studies based on self-report data; specification errors abound in models attempting to find the most relevant predictors of job-related behaviors; urine test results are erroneously used to classify employees as users or nonusers (i.e., high rate of false negatives); and evaluation studies use inadequate comparison or control groups, or no comparison groups at all, to name some of the problems that a reader encounters. Each of the studies reviewed here contains serious limitations. However, consistent results across even seriously flawed designs can help increase our understanding of this difficult area. This is fortunate because, even though we can and should do much better than we have done, flaws are often unavoidable in studies of complex human behaviors.

It is thought that alcohol and other drug use by the work force has a significant impact on society. This perception appears corroborated by the extant research, for virtually all of it, including the best-designed studies, report some associations between alcohol or other drug use and distressing, dangerous, or other dysfunctional behaviors. However, it is difficult, given the current research base, to make definitive statements regarding the magnitude of the impact of alcohol and other drug use at work. Many of the effects found, though significant statistically, are small to moderate. Indeed, the available research, taken as a whole, should soften the concern about employee alcohol and other drug use often found in the popular media. But the picture that science presents of alcohol and other drug problems in the workplace may change in either direction. Our current understanding of the area is limited, and much more research needs to be done.

PRODUCTIVITY COSTS OF ALCOHOL AND OTHER DRUG USE

The field studies reviewed above have attempted to assess the causal link between alcohol and other drug use and work-related behavior. Other researchers, primarily economists, have tried to go further and estimate the costs that such use imposes on society. This research has received substantial attention both in the scientific community and among the public. This section describes the nature of such studies and critically evaluates their methods and conclusions. We begin by briefly summarizing one of the best and most widely cited such studies. We then explain why this study and related studies are by themselves inadequate to guide public policies. Finally, we examine in detail how such studies attempt to evaluate the effect of alcohol and other drug use on worker productivity.

Overview of a Typical Cost-of-Drug-Use Study

Rather than summarize the cost-of-drug-use studies done to date, we focus on one recent, widely cited study that subsumes the results of most previous studies and represents perhaps the best example of such studies. This study (Rice et al., 1990) determines the costs of alcohol and other drug use to society by totaling estimates of treatment, morbidity, mortality, and crime costs. We discuss each of these cost estimates in turn. For brevity, our discussion of those cost estimates focuses most strongly on results related to illicit drugs, and we only briefly discuss the results related to the use of alcohol. We note, however, that Rice et al. estimate costs of alcohol use at $70 billion compared with $44 billion for illicit drug use.

Treatment and support costs are those health care expenditures that result from illicit drug use. They include expenditures for short-term hospitalization, outpatient care, medicine, research and training, program administration, and the net cost of private insurance related to illicit drug treatment. For the year 1985, Rice et al. estimate illicit drug treatment and support costs of approximately $2.1 billion. The vast majority of this total stems from visits to hospitals and other institutions devoted specifically to the treatment of illicit drug-abuse-related conditions.

Morbidity costs reflect the "lowered" productivity that results from illicit drug use. Cost-of-drug-use studies equate productivity with income. They compare the income of illicit drug users and nonusers to determine the reduction in income due to illicit drug use. Personal characteristics such as age, sex, and education are commonly controlled in making these comparisons. Rice et al. estimate morbidity costs for 1985 of just under $6 billion.

Mortality costs equal the income that would have been earned by individuals who die from illicit drug use had they not died prematurely. To estimate mortality costs, it is assumed that a person of a given age and sex who dies of illicit drug use would have had a future income stream consistent with the current cross-sectional age-sex distribution of income. The estimated mortality costs for 1985 are $2.6 billion.

Crime-related costs have two main components. The first consists of public and private expenditures on the portion of the criminal justice system that deals with illicit drug-related offenses, including federal efforts at drug traffic control. This component of crime-related costs is estimated at $13.2 billion for 1985. The second component is the losses imposed on the victims of illicit drug-related crimes and the forgone earnings of individuals who are incarcerated for their illicit drug use or who engage in criminal activity, rather than legal employment, because of their illicit drug use. This component of crime-related costs is estimated at $19.3 billion for 1985, of which almost $14 billion represents forgone earnings of individuals who engage in criminal activity because of illicit drug use.

Interpreting Cost-of-Drug-Use Studies

Although their conclusions are widely cited by the media, politicians, and others in the public policy arena, cost-of-drug-use studies do not by themselves provide an economic justification for any particular public policy toward alcohol and other drugs. The reason they do not is that, as emphasized by Harwood et al. (1984), Harwood (1991) and Sindelar (1991), economically based policy recommendations should reflect an evaluation of the costs and benefits of particular policies, not an evaluation of the total costs of the activity the policy seeks to change. This point is fundamental and well recognized by the authors of many cost-of-drug-use studies (e.g., Harwood et al., 1984), but it is often overlooked by those who cite these studies to justify government actions.

Measuring the costs associated with alcohol and other drug use does not, in other words, determine the extent to which these costs might be increased or decreased by specific public policies. For example, consider the policy proposal that funding for alcohol and other drug abuse treatment centers be increased. If those who would receive treatment as a result of additional funding are likely to be program dropouts, additional funding might be ineffective in reducing alcohol and other drug use and its associated costs. If, however, the new clientele consists of people who are strongly desirous of reducing their alcohol and other drug use but are unable to afford existing treatment programs, such expenditures might be highly cost-effective. Estimating the total amount of money currently spent on treatment, which is essentially what occurs in studies like those by Rice et al. (1990), tells us nothing about the likely effects of increased funding for treatment.

Costs of Alcohol and Other Drug Use: Worker Productivity

The component of cost-of-drug-use studies that is most relevant to understanding the interactions between alcohol and other drugs and the workplace is the "diminished" worker productivity attributable to alcohol and other drug use. Existing studies estimate this cost component by comparing the wage rates (or income) of individuals (or households) who use illicit drugs or alcohol with the wage rates (or income) of those who do not, controlling in the better studies for other observable characteristics such as age, sex, race, education, health status, marital status, and family background. A finding that illicit drug or alcohol use is correlated with wage rates or income, possibly controlling for other factors, is usually interpreted as showing that illicit drug or alcohol use affects worker productivity. It should be noted, however, that, for the purpose of this report, productivity effects and earning effects are used interchangeably. Ideally, one would like to be able to obtain a direct measure of productivity; however, because such measures are not easily obtained, researchers must settle for using less than perfect indices or proxies of the construct of interest (i.e., productivity). That is, earning differentials are typically evaluated in attempts to estimate the impact of alcohol and other drug use on productivity.

Despite important differences in data sets, productivity measures, control variables, sample periods, and estimation procedures, a consistent set of

empirical regularities emerges from this literature.   These are described in
the sections that follow.

Alcohol Use and Productivity

Problem or heavy drinking is negatively related to household income,
although the strength and statistical significance of the relation depends on
the measure of problem drinking considered.   Berry and Boland (1977),
using a 1968 National Household Survey, show that the mean income of
households with a male problem drinker (defined as having a large number
of alcohol-related consequences) is 18 percent lower than the mean income
of households without a problem drinker.   Harwood et al. (1984), extending
work by Cruze et al. (1981), use 1979 National Household Survey data from
NIAAA to show that most available indicators of problem drinking are
negatively correlated with household income (controlling for other characteristics) and that a few of these indicators display large and significantly
negative correlations with household income.   Rice et al. (1990), using
1980-1984 Epidemiological Catchment Area (ECA) data, find that a measure of lifetime alcohol abuse or dependence is significantly negatively
correlated with household income.   These results do not, however, exclude
the possibility that low income either contributes to or proxies for variables
that contribute to problem drinking.

Mullahy and Sindelar (1989) also examine the relation between alcohol
abuse and income using ECA survey data.   They find that alcoholism has no
direct relation with earnings but does have an indirect relation: alcohol
abuse is associated with lower educational attainment and marital stability,
which in turn are associated with lower earnings.   In a follow-up study,
Mullahy and Sindelar (1991) examine gender differences in labor market
responses to alcoholism.   Using multiple-site data from the ECA survey,
they find that alcoholism is typically negatively related to both labor force
participation and income for the full sample.   However, the relation varies
by stage of the life cycle and by gender.   They demonstrate that their results
depend on the variables controlled for and whether the dependent variable
is labor force participation or income.

Low to moderate drinking is associated with higher wages.   Berger and
Leigh (1988) use the Quality of Employment Survey to estimate separate
wage equations for drinkers and nondrinkers among both men and women.
They find that drinkers earn higher wages than nondrinkers, after controlling for differences in observable characteristics.   Their result is robust to
changes in model specification, identification assumptions, and definition
of drinker status.   Harwood et al. (1984) find that over a range of alcohol
consumption of up to two ounces per day, the amount of alcohol consumed

is positively correlated with household income. This might occur because higher income leads to increased discretionary consumption of alcohol.

Marijuana Use and Productivity

Heavy or long-term marijuana use is negatively related to both household income and wages for men but appears to be positively related to wages and household income for women. Harwood et al. (1984), considering a population that aggregates men and women, find that daily marijuana use for a period of at least a month at some point in the past is negatively related to household income. Register and Williams (1992), considering men only, report that in the 1984 National Longitudinal Survey of Youth (NLSY), marijuana use for longer than 8 years is negatively related to current wages. Kaestner (1991), who also examines the 1984 NLSY, finds that heavy lifetime or past-30-day marijuana use is insignificantly negatively related to wages for men and significantly positively related for women.

Current or moderate lifetime marijuana use is either essentially uncorrelated with wages or income or is modestly positively correlated. Harwood et al. (1984) report that all measures of current marijuana use or lifetime marijuana use other than having smoked marijuana daily for at least a month display insignificant correlations with household income, with some point estimates positive and some negative. Rice et al. (1990) state that results based on use of particular drugs are ill defined and therefore do not report any details. Register and Williams (1992) find that, averaged over the whole sample, marijuana users had slightly lower wages than nonusers. Controlling for a range of observed characteristics, however, reveals a positive and significant correlation between marijuana use and current wages. Kaestner (1991) reports negative, insignificant correlations for men and positive, generally significant correlations for women with all measures of marijuana use.

Cocaine and Other Drug Use and Productivity

The relation between any level of cocaine or other nonmarijuana drug use and wage rates or income is either insignificant or positive. Harwood et al. (1984) state that they could find no significant results relating illicit drug use to household income for any illicit drug other than marijuana. Again, Rice et al. (1990) state that results based on the use of particular illicit drugs were ill defined and therefore do not report any details. Gill and Michaels (1992), using 1980 and 1984 NLSY data, find that a wage differential that favors illicit drug users over nonusers increases when the comparison is made between hard drug users (cocaine, heroin, etc.) and all other illicit drugs. Register and Williams (1992) document a higher average wage for cocaine users than nonusers, and they show that cocaine use is positively although insignificantly correlated with wages after accounting for observable characteristics. Kaestner (1991) finds that virtually all measures of cocaine use are positively correlated with wage rates, and these correlations are substantially larger and more significant for women than men.

Demographic Differential Effects

In studies for which comparisons are available, the relation between alcohol and other drug use and productivity is usually more negative (less positive) for men than for women. Rice et al. (1990) show that alcohol abuse is more negatively correlated with household income for men than women up through age 34, after which the relation reverses, and that illicit drug abuse is negatively correlated with household income for men of all ages but positively correlated for women of all ages. Kaestner (1991) documents a negative and usually insignificant correlation between various measures of marijuana use and wages for young men and a positive and usually significant correlation for young women. He documents a positive but small and usually insignificant correlation between various measures of cocaine use and wages for men and a positive, larger, and usually significant correlation for women.

Variations in Results Across Outcome Measures

The comparisons that employ household income as a measure of productivity suggest, on average, associations that are more negative between alcohol and other drug use than comparisons based on wages. However, no study uses data on both measures of productivity, so it is difficult to isolate the effects of using a particular productivity measure. In comparing studies with one measure or the other, one also faces differences in data sets, drug variables, control variables, sample periods, and population characteristics (e.g., only young people in the wage regressions whereas all ages in household income regressions). Nevertheless, when similar alcohol and other drug variables are employed, household and individual measures of productivity display similar correlations with alcohol and other drug use. In large part, earlier studies appear to have obtained substantially more negative relations than more recent studies because they emphasized those results that used measures of heavy use or abuse. Even in the early studies, most measures of use for alcohol and other drugs show small negative to small positive correlations with productivity.

The failure of alcohol and other drug use to display the "expected" negative correlation with productivity does not appear to result mainly from an effect of alcohol and other drug use on productivity via the labor supply. Register and Williams (1992), using the NLSY data, find that marijuana use is associated with a decreased probability of being employed but that cocaine use has no significant relation to the probability of employment. Zarkin et al. (1992), using the 1990 National Household Survey on Drug Abuse, examine the prevalence of illicit drug use by work status and the relation between illicit drug use and measures of labor supply: weeks worked during the past year, number of sick days taken during the past month, and number of days of work skipped for nonmedical reasons during the past month. Their prevalence estimates indicate that the working population has a slightly higher rate of alcohol and other drug use than the total household population. Their regression results indicate that illicit drug use is associated with fewer weeks worked, whereas alcohol use is associated with more weeks worked. Illicit drug use is not related to the number of sick days taken, but past-month illicit drug use is related to an increased number of work days skipped. Kaestner (1992) finds a negative relation between illicit drug use and labor supply in cross-sectional estimates but little significant relation in longitudinal estimates.

INTERPRETING THE EMPIRICAL RESULTS

Despite the substantial differences in results across studies, careful reading suggests some consistencies in the empirical results. Heavy or problem use of marijuana or alcohol is generally associated with lower productivity (with the possible exception of women in the case of marijuana) and low to moderate use of any illicit drug or alcohol is either positively associated with productivity or simply not significantly related.

Despite the consistency of the empirical evidence, however, interpretation of this evidence must proceed cautiously. The key problem of interpretation may be called the heterogeneity effect. Put simply, individuals differ along several dimensions, some observable and some not. Observable characteristics include sociodemographics such as education, age, race, and gender. These variables are likely to influence job compensation and are usually included in wage equations. However, several unobservable characteristics may be equally or even more likely to influence wages. These unmeasured variables include motivation, aggression, intelligence, ambition, discipline, and the like. If characteristics such as these influence wages, and if alcohol or other drug use is correlated with one or more of these variables, then the estimated relation between such use and wages will tend to pick up these latent effects. Thus, an estimated negative relation between use and wages or income may simply indicate that less ambitious people are likely to both use alcohol or other drugs and have low wages; the inference that such use causes low wages would not be justified. Similarly, an estimated positive relation could indicate that creative or gregarious individuals are likely to both use alcohol or other drugs and have high wages without suggesting any causal effect.

Another problematic aspect of some of these studies and others (Mills and Noyes, 1984; Newcomb and Bentler, 1986, 1988; Kandel 1984; White et al., 1988) that have examined the association between alcohol and other drug use and income level is that most results are based on cross-sectional data largely among youthful samples. Potential problems associated with cross-sectional designs and the use of restricted age range samples is illustrated by the results of recent analyses of longitudinal data. In analyzing income and alcohol and other drug use data, Newcomb and Bentler (1988) found that greater polydrug use by teenagers was associated with increased income 4 years later. They explained this finding by noting that adolescent polydrug users were more likely than those who used few or no drugs to begin working right out of high school and not attend college. Those who used few or no drugs as teenagers were more likely to go to college and delay entry into the work force. Therefore, adolescent heavy alcohol or other drug users may be expected to earn higher incomes than less heavy users as young adults, since they will have been in the work force for 4 years while those less involved in drugs continued their education.

In a follow-up of this same sample, Newcomb and Bentler (1992) found that 4 years later the relationship between income and teenage polydrug involvement had reversed. Both adolescent alcohol and other drug use and increased use of alcohol and other drugs into adulthood was associated with reduced income by the time people reached their mid-to-late twenties. The researchers explain this reversal by assuming that the greater education of the low alcohol and other drug users eventually resulted in higher income (an elevated earning potential ceiling) than that enjoyed by those who were involved with alcohol and other drugs as teenagers and maintained or continued such involvement. The latter had a short-term income benefit but suffered over the long run from a low ceiling to their earning potential.

Clearly, more prospective data must be analyzed to characterize more adequately and precisely the dynamic relationship between alcohol and other drug use and income. Reliance on cross-sectional data is inappropriate and possibly gravely misleading. Furthermore, a much wider age range must be studied than the primarily young groups represented in these studies.

In addition to these general problems, there are some more technical but nonetheless fundamental problems with most cost-of-drug use research. Wage rates as a measure of productivity are biased because they are observed only for employed individuals and do not reflect the productivity costs that would be incurred by individuals out of the labor force. While researchers today commonly recognize and attempt to address this problem (Gill and Michaels, 1992; Register and Williams, 1992; Kaestner, 1991), the methods used, so-called Heckman corrections (Heckman, 1976, 1979), do not seem adequate to the task. Not only are they sensitive to model misspecification, but at best they can only estimate how alcohol and other drug use would have affected the wages of the unemployed if they were employed. What matters, however, is the extent to which alcohol and other drug use leads individuals to become unemployed. But even these criticisms are less important than the fact that Kaestner (1991) demonstrates that the corrections appear to make no difference to the results in any event.

Some of the studies that use wages as the productivity measure attempt to control for the fact that the relationship between wages and alcohol and other drug use is potentially bidirectional; each may affect the other (e.g., Kaestner, 1991). Such similarity, if it exists, will inflate the estimated correlation between alcohol and other drug use and wages. Correcting for the simultaneity problem requires the availability of "instrumental" variables that affect alcohol and other drug use and not wages. Spousal income is commonly treated as such a variable, but Gill and Michaels (1992) demonstrate that the spouses of alcohol and other drug users typically have low income. If, holding other demographic characteristics constant, users of alcohol and other drugs tend to marry people with low incomes, then simultaneous equation estimation techniques will incorrectly adjust for the effect of income on alcohol and other drug use and could lead to overestimates of the negative relation between such use and wages. Simultaneous equations estimates may thus be worse than the estimates that make no correction for simultaneity bias.

In sum, there are serious difficulties with estimating the causal relations between alcohol and other drug use and productivity and with attempts to estimate the costs of use in general. Current estimates can be taken only as ballpark figures. They are probably correct in suggesting that there are great costs, even if the most concretely measured costs are those incurred in the attempt to control alcohol and other drug use because of the assumed magnitude of nonenforcement costs. Work to refine cost-of-drug-use measures should proceed, but even if substantial progress is made, we should not confuse measures of the cost of drug use with the expected net benefits of policies aimed at limiting those costs.

The committee's conclusions and recommendations that follow are based on a critical review of the literature on the impact of alcohol and other drug use on employees' work-related behavior as well as studies that have explored the relationship between use and productivity/cost estimates. They are intended to highlight the need to expand scientific knowledge of how alcohol and other drug use affects work-related behavior and to improve the quality of research aimed toward this end.

CONCLUSIONS AND RECOMMENDATIONS

• Field studies have consistently linked alcohol and other drug use to higher rates of absenteeism; they also provide evidence of an association between alcohol and perhaps other drug use and increased rates of accidents, particularly in the transportation industry. Less consistent evidence exists linking alcohol and other drug use to other negative work behaviors, although the current research base is insufficient to support firm conclusions. When associations between alcohol and other drug use and counterproductive workplace behavior are found, relationships are most often of moderate or low strength even when they are statistically significant.

• The empirical relationships found between alcohol and other drug use and job performance are complex and need not imply causation. Relationships may exist for some job performance outcomes like absenteeism but not for others. Alcohol and other drug use may be just one among many characteristics of a more deviant lifestyle, and associations between use and degraded job performance may be due not to drug-related impairment but to general deviance or other factors.

Recommendation: To intervene more effectively in improving job performance, we must develop a better research base from which to assess how alcohol and other drug use and other factors act alone and in combination to degrade job performance.

• Widely cited cost estimates of the effects of alcohol and other drug use on U.S. productivity are based on questionable assumptions and weak measures. Moreover, these cost-of-drug-use studies do not provide estimates of potential savings associated with implementing particular public policies toward alcohol and other drugs.

Recommendation: Further research is needed to develop refined, defensible estimates of how much alcohol and other drug use costs specific organizations and society at large. Business decision makers and policy makers should be cautious in making decisions on the basis of evidence currently available.

REFERENCES

Alleyne, B.C., P. Stuart, and R. Copes
   1991   Alcohol and other drug use in occupational fatalities. *Journal of Occupational Medicine* 33:496-500.
Berger, M.C., and J.P. Leigh
   1988   The effect of alcohol use on wages. *Applied Economics* 20:1343-1351.

Berry, R.E., Jr., and J.P. Boland
  1977   The work-related costs of alcohol abuse. In C.J. Schram, ed., *Alcoholism and Its Treatment in Industry*. Baltimore, Md.: The Johns Hopkins University Press.
Blank, D.L., and J.W. Fenton
  1989   Early employment testing for marijuana: demographic and employee retention patterns. In S.W. Gust and J.M. Walsh, eds., *Drugs in the Workplace: Research and Evaluation Data*. NIDA Research Monograph No. 91. Rockville, Md.: National Institute on Drug Abuse.
Blum, T.C., P.M. Roman, and J.K. Martin
  1993   Alcohol consumption and work performance. *Journal of Studies on Alcohol* 54:61-70.
Crouch, D.J., D.O. Webb, L.V. Peterson, P.F. Buller, and D.E. Rollins
  1989   A critical evaluation of the Utah Power and Light Company's substance abuse management program: absenteeism, accidents, and costs. In S.W. Gust and J.M. Walsh, eds., *Drugs in the Workplace: Research and Evaluation Data*. NIDA Research Monograph No. 91. Rockville, Md.: National Institute on Drug Abuse.
Cruze, A., H. Harwood, P. Kristiansen, J. Collins, and D. Jones
  1981   Economic Costs of Alcohol and Drug Abuse and Mental Illness-1977. Research Triangle Institute, Research Triangle Park, N.C.
Donovan, J.E., and R. Jessor
  1985   Structure of problem behavior in adolescence and young adulthood. *Journal of Consulting and Clinical Psychology* 53:890-904.
Fell, J.C.
  1982   Alcohol involvement in traffic accidents. In *Alcohol and Highway Safety: A Review of the State of the Knowledge*. Report DOT-HS-806-269. Washington, D.C.: U.S. Department of Transportation.
Fell, J.C., and T. Klein
  1986   The Nature of the Reduction in Alcohol in U.S. Fatal Crashes. SAE Technical Paper 860038, Society of Automotive Engineers, Warrensdale, Pa.
Freier, M.C., R.M. Bell, and P.L. Ellickson
  1991   *Do Teens Tell the Truth? The Validity of Self-Reported Tobacco Use by Adolescents*. Santa Monica, Calif.: The RAND Corporation.
Gill, A.M., and R.J. Michaels
  1992   Does drug use lower wages? *Industrial Labor Relations Review* 45:419-434.
Gillmore, M.R., J.D. Hawkins, R.F. Catalano, Jr., L.E. Day, M. Moore, and R. Abbott
  1991   Structure of problem behaviors in preadolescence. *Journal of Consulting Clinical Psychology* 59(4):499-506.
Harwood, H.J.
  1991   Economics and drugs: promises, problems, and prospects. In W.S. Cartwright and J.M. Kaple, eds., *Economic Costs, Cost-Effectiveness, Financing, and Community-Based Drug Treatment*. Rockville, Md.: National Institute on Drug Abuse.
Harwood, H.J., D.M. Napolitano, P.L. Kristiansen, and J.J. Collins
  1984   Economic Costs to Society of Alcohol and Drug Abuse and Mental Illness: 1980. Report to Alcohol, Drug Abuse, and Mental Health Administration. Research Triangle Institute, Research Triangle Park, N.C.
Heckman, J.J.
  1976   The common structure of statistical models of truncation, sample selection, and limited dependent variables and a single estimator for such models. *Annals of Economic and Social Measurement*. 5:475-492.
  1979   Sample selection bias as a specification error. *Econometrica* 47:153-161.

Hingson, R.W., R.I. Lederman, and D.C. Walsh
  1985   Employee drinking patterns and accidental injury: a study of four New England States. *Journal of Studies on Alcohol* 46:298-303.
Holcom, M.L., W.E.K. Lehman, and D.D. Simpson
  in press Employee accidents: Influences of personal characteristics, job characteristics, and substance use. *Journal of Safety Research.*
Hollinger, R.C.
  1988   Working under the influence (WUI): correlates of employees' use of alcohol and other drugs. *Journal of Applied Behavioral Science* 24:439-454.
Jessor, R., and S.L. Jessor
  1977   *Problem Behavior and Psychosocial Development: A Longitudinal Study of Youth.* New York: Academic Press.
  1978   Theory testing in longitudinal research on marijuana use. In D. Kandel, ed., *Longitudinal Research on Drug Use.* Washington, D.C.: Hemisphere.
Kaestner, R.
  1991   The effect of illicit drug use on the wages of young adults. *Journal of Labor Economics* 9:381-412.
  1992   The Effect of Illicit Drug Use on the Labor Supply of Young Adults. Unpublished manuscript, Rider College, Trenton, N.J.
Kandel, D.B.
  1984   Marijuana users in young adulthood. *Archives of General Psychiatry* 1:200-209.
Kandel, D.B., and K. Yamaguchi
  1987   Job mobility and drug use: an event history analysis. *American Journal of Sociology* 92:836-878.
Klein, T.
  1986   *A Method for Estimating Posterior BAC Distributions for Persons Involved in Fatal Traffic Accidents.* Washington, D.C.: Sigmastat.
Kuhlman, J.J., B. Levine, M.L. Smith, and J.R. Hordinsky
  1991   Toxicological findings in Federal Aviation Administration general aviation accidents. *Journal of Forensic Sciences* 36:1121-1128.
Lehman, W.E.K., and D.D. Simpson
  1992   Employee substance use and on-the-job behaviors. *Journal of Applied Psychology* 77:309-321.
Lehman, W.E.K., M.L. Holcom, and D.D. Simpson
  1990a   Employee Health and Performance in the Workplace: A Survey of Municipal Employees of a Large Southwest City. Unpublished manuscript, Institute of Behavioral Research. Texas Christian University, Fort Worth.
  1990b   Employee Health and Performance in the Workplace: A Survey of Employees of the Housing Authority in a Large Southwest City. Unpublished manuscript, Institute of Behavioral Research. Texas Christian University, Fort Worth.
Lehman, W.E.K., D.J. Farabee, M.L. Holcom, and D.D. Simpson
  1991   Prediction of Substance Use in the Workplace: Unique Contributions of Demographic and Work Environment Variables. Unpublished manuscript, Institute of Behavioral Research. Texas Christian University, Fort Worth.
Lehman, W.E.K., D.J. Farabee, and D.D. Simpson
  1992   Co-Worker Substance Use and Its Relationship with Employee Attitudes and Morale. Unpublished manuscript, Institute of Behavioral Research. Texas Christian University, Fort Worth.
Lewis, R.J., and S.P. Cooper
  1989   Alcohol, other drugs, and fatal work-related injuries. *Journal of Occupational Medicine* 31:23-28.

Mangione, T.W., and R.P. Quinn
    1975   Job satisfaction, counterproductive behavior, and drug use at work. *Journal of Applied Psychology* 60:114-116.
McDaniel, M.A.
    1988   Does pre-employment drug use predict on-the-job suitability? *Personnel Psychology* 41:717-729.
Mills, C.J., and H.L. Noyes
    1984   Patterns and correlates of initial and subsequent drug use among adolescents. *Journal of Consulting and Clinical Psychology* 52:231-243.
Moody, D.E., D.J. Crouch, D.M. Andrenyak, R.P. Smith, D.G. Wilkins, A.M. Hoffman, and D.E. Rollins
    1990   Mandatory post accident drug and alcohol testing for the Federal Railroad Administration (FRA). In S.W. Gust, J.M. Walsh, L.B. Thomas, and D.J. Crouch, eds., *Drugs in the Workplace: Research and Evaluation Data*, Vol. II. NIDA Research Monograph No. 100. Rockville, Md.: National Institute on Drug Abuse.
Mullahy, J., and J.L. Sindelar
    1989   Alcoholism and Human Capital. Discussion paper QE89-06, Quality of the Environment Division, Resources for the Future, Washington, D.C.
    1991   Gender differences in labor market effects of alcoholism. *AEA Papers and Proceedings* May:161-165.
National Transportation Safety Board
    1990   *Safety Study: Fatigue, Alcohol, Other Drugs, and Medical Factors in Fatal-to-the-Driver Heavy Truck Crashes*, Vol 1. NTSB/SS-90/01. Washington, D.C.: National Transportation Safety Board.
Newcomb, M.D.
    1988   *Drug Use in the Workplace: Risk Factors for Disruptive Substance Use Among Young Adults*. Dover, Md.: Auburn House.
Newcomb, M.D., and P.M. Bentler
    1986   Cocaine use among adolescents: longitudinal associations with social context, psychopathology, and use of other substances. *Addictive Behaviors* 11:263-273.
    1988   *Consequences of Adolescent Drug Use: Impact on the Lives of Young Adults*. Newbury Park, Calif.: Sage Publications.
    1992   Adolescent and Subsequent Changes in Young Adult Drug Use: Effects on Psychosocial Functioning in Adulthood. Unpublished manuscript, University of Southern California.
Normand, J., and S.D. Salyards
    1989   An empirical evaluation of preemployment drug testing in the United States Postal Service: interim report of findings. In S.W. Gust and J.M. Walsh, eds., *Drugs in the Workplace: Research and Evaluation Data*. NIDA Research Monograph No. 91. Rockville, Md.: National Institute on Drug Abuse.
Normand, J., S.D. Salyards, and J.J. Mahony
    1990   An evaluation of preemployment drug testing. *Journal of Applied Psychology* 75:629-639.
Parish, D.C.
    1989   Relation of the pre-employment drug testing result to employment status: a one-year follow-up. *Journal of General Internal Medicine* 4:44-47.
Perone, M., R.J. DeWaard, and A. Baron
    1979   Satisfaction with real and simulated jobs in relation to personality variables and drug use. *Journal of Applied Psychology* 64:660-668.
Register, C.A., and D.R. Williams
    1992   Labor market effects of marijuana and cocaine use among young men. *Industrial Labor Relations Review* 45:435-448.

Reinisch, E.J., R.M. Bell, and P.L. Ellickson
  1991   *How Accurate are Adolescent Reports of Drug Use?* Santa Monica, Calif.: The RAND Corporation.
Rice, D.P., S. Kelman, L.S. Miller, and S. Dunmeyer
  1990   The Economic Costs of Alcohol and Drug Abuse and Mental Illness: 1985. Institute for Health and Aging, University of California, San Francisco.
Rosenbaum, A.L., W.E.K. Lehman, K.E. Olson, and M.L. Holcom
  1992   Prevalence of Substance Use and Its Association with Performance Among Municipal Workers in a Southwestern City. Unpublished manuscript, Institute of Behavioral Research. Texas Christian University, Fort Worth.
Rouse, B.A., N.J. Kozel, and L.G. Richards, eds.
  1985   *Self-Report Methods of Estimating Drug Use: Meeting Current Challenges to Validity.* NIDA Research Monograph No. 57. Rockville, Md.: National Institute on Drug Abuse.
Salyards, S.D.
  1993   Preemployment drug testing: associations with EAP, disciplinary, and medical claims information. *PharmChem Newsletter* 21(1):1-4.
Salyards, S.D., and J. Normand
  1991   Methodological issues in the evaluation of employee drug-testing programs. In M.J. Burke, chair, *Drugs in the Workforce.* Symposium conducted at the 15th Annual Convention of the International Personnel Management Association Assessment Council, Chicago.
Sheridan, J.R., and H. Winkler
  1989   An evaluation of drug testing in the workplace. In S.W. Gust and J.M. Walsh, eds., *Drugs in the Workplace: Research and Evaluation Data.* NIDA Research Monograph No. 91. Rockville, Md.: National Institute on Drug Abuse.
Sindelar, J.
  1991   Economic cost of illicit drug studies: critique and research agenda. In W.S. Cartwright and J.M. Kaple, eds., *Economic Costs, Cost-Effectiveness, Financing, and Community-Based Drug Treatment.* Rockville, Md.: National Institute on Drug Abuse.
Taggart, R.W.
  1989   Results of the drug testing program at Southern Pacific Railroad. In S.W. Gust and J.M. Walsh, eds., *Drugs in the Workplace: Research and Evaluation Data.* NIDA Research Monograph No. 91. Rockville, Md.: National Institute on Drug Abuse.
Transportation Research Board
  1987   *Zero Alcohol and Other Options: Limits for Truck and Bus Drivers.* Special report 216. Washington, D.C.: Transportation Research Board, National Research Council.
  1993   *Alcohol and Other Drugs in Transportation: Research Needs for the Next Decade.* National Research Council. Washington, D.C.: National Academy Press.
White, H.R., A. Aidala, and B. Zablocki
  1988   A longitudinal investigation of drug use and work patterns among middle-class, white adults. *Journal of Applied Behavioral Science* 4:455-469.
Zarkin, G.A., M.T. French, and J.V. Rachal
  1992   The Relationship Between Illicit Drug Use and Labor Supply. Research Triangle Institute, Research Triangle Park, N.C.
Zwerling, C., J. Ryan, and E.J. Orav
  1990   The efficacy of preemployment drug screening for marijuana and cocaine in predicting employment outcome. *Journal of the American Medical Association* 264:2639-2643.

III
EFFECTIVENESS OF
WORKPLACE INTERVENTIONS

6

Detecting and Assessing Alcohol and Other Drug Use

The response of many employers to the perceived problem of alcohol and other drug use has been to establish drug-testing programs, either voluntarily or in compliance with federal regulations. Drug-testing programs typically have two main purposes: (1) to determine drug use among a firm's employees or prospective employees and (2) to deter such use for reasons of safety, productivity, and health. Given the preponderance of drug-testing programs among the drug intervention programs of U.S. corporations, a substantial portion of this chapter is devoted to describing what these programs entail; committee members thought it was critical to provide the reader with a thorough description of the technological issues associated with commonly used analytical methods of urinalysis drug testing. The extent to which these programs have been shown to be effective in achieving these goals is the subject of Chapter 7.

Both direct and indirect methods are used to detect alcohol and other drug use among the work force. Biochemical analysis and self-reports are the two most commonly used direct methods for assessing substance use. Each has limitations. Biochemical methods, primarily urinalysis, usually detect only recent use and generally cannot measure patterns or frequency of use. Although hair analysis can potentially trace longer-term patterns of use, data on the measurement properties of this analytical technique are still limited. Self-report methods can measure patterns and frequency of alcohol and other drug use but are limited by validity problems, primarily involving the failure of some respondents to disclose use.

To avoid the limitations of the direct methods, the use of indirect methods for assessing drug use and identifying drug users has been rapidly growing. Indirect approaches typically involve measuring or observing behaviors or responses that are frequently associated with alcohol and other drug use and inferring use from what is observed. They too have significant limitations, but they can complement the information gleaned from biochemical analysis and self-reports.

This chapter first provides a brief historical perspective on the evolution of what is currently the most common biochemical method for detecting applicant and employee alcohol and other drug use in corporate America. It then reviews the main procedural components of forensic drug-testing programs. That is followed by a description of the most widely used indirect methods for assessing alcohol and other drug use: personal profiles, and behavioral indicators. The chapter ends with the committee's conclusions and recommendations.

EVOLUTION OF BIOCHEMICAL DRUG TESTING

The analysis of urine specimens and other body fluids to determine if particular individuals have used various drugs is not new. Drug testing in forensic toxicology and some clinical hospital laboratories predates President Reagan's executive order of September 1986 by at least 15 years (Finkle, 1972; Hawks and Chiang, 1986). The results of urine testing and their use as evidence in legal contexts has been tacitly accepted in the United States for many years. Large-scale drug testing was originally stimulated by the Department of Defense's (DoD) need to monitor its armed forces during the Vietnam War era, and by the heroin "epidemic" in the 1970s, which resulted in thousands of patients being treated with methadone (*Federal Register*, 1972) and were required to be drug free and monitored to confirm that they were not taking additional drugs. In late 1980 the testing industry further expanded as the Navy, following a series of incidents that highlighted the pervasive use of marijuana among their personnel, announced a policy of "zero tolerance" for illicit drugs (Cangianelli, 1989). Over a period of 2 years they designed and implemented a testing program that required contracted laboratories to analyze more than 2 million urine specimens each year in order to monitor and control illegal drug use in the Navy. By the time the naval program was in place, the other branches of the services had followed suit (Willette, 1986). Private industry then followed. By 1985, several major U.S. corporations included drug testing in applicant screening programs, and some selected employees with the stated motive of promoting occupational safety and employee assistance (Frings, 1986; Hanson, 1986).

The technical, logistical, and laboratory operations requirements to support these massive testing programs were wholly inadequate in the beginning. They rested primarily on cumbersome, inefficient, and nonspecific techniques, such as thin layer chromatography (TLC) and gas chromatography (GC). Many of the laboratories doing drug testing had little notion of what constituted legally adequate work, and experienced forensic analytical toxicologists were few. Performance testing surveys revealed serious inaccuracies in some laboratory results. These survey reports still haunt toxicologists and are quoted repeatedly by antagonists to today's employee drug-testing programs, although the data are now obsolete (Hansen et al., 1985; McBay, 1986; Boone, 1987). Throughout the 1970s the National Institute on Drug Abuse (NIDA), mainly through their Research Technology Branch, and the DoD sponsored projects to develop new techniques and analytical methods for the detection of illicit drugs and their metabolites in urine and other body fluids (Foltz et al., 1980). Immunoassays such as EMIT, an enzyme-based assay, and Abusescreen, a radio-labeled assay, came to fruition in 1981, and improved gas chromatography, and eventually mass spectrometry (GC/MS) became available. Variants of these techniques now form the core of almost all urine analysis methods for detecting evidence of illicit drug use.

Against this long background and the example provided by the DoD, President Reagan issued an executive order in 1986 directing federal agencies to achieve a drug-free federal workplace, an action that was catalyzed by the report of the President's Commission on Organized Crime (1986). In July 1987 Congress expanded on the executive order by enacting a law that required urine testing for federal employees, including employees of federal contractors, and also required that technical and scientific guidelines and standards of practice be met by all laboratories testing urine specimens covered by the law. Scientists from NIDA and forensic toxicologists worked intensively to define a practical laboratory program that would permit testing human urine for five commonly used illicit drugs and their metabolites, with a minimum of error and a maximum of protection for employees. The results of their work were published as "Mandatory Guidelines for Federal Workplace Drug Testing Programs" in April 1988 (*Federal Register*, 1988). Just 3 months later, a National Laboratory Certification Program was implemented by NIDA, which required strict adherence to the guidelines and certification standards. Today there are almost 100 laboratories certified by HHS[1] as competent to conduct forensic urine drug testing for, at a minimum, marijuana, cocaine, opiates, amphetamines, and phencyclidine and

---

[1]Note that the 1992 ADAMHA Reorganization Act (P.L. 102-321) resulted in NIDA's National Laboratory Certification Program and related activities being transferred to the Substance Abuse and Mental Health Services Administration of the U.S. Department of Health and Human Services.

their metabolites. The HHS-NIDA guidelines have since been revised and updated (*Federal Register*, 1993). In 1989 the Nuclear Regulatory Commission (NRC) established its own regulations, and following the Omnibus Transportation Act of 1991 the Department of Transportation (DOT) issued regulations that included testing for alcohol and permitted individual urine specimens to be split into two before submission to the laboratory. The DOT issued proposed rule making for their program in January 1993 (*Federal Register*, 1993).

Professional organizations have shown an interest in certifying laboratories in which their members are employed. Most notably, the College of American Pathologists, which has a long history of monitoring, improving, educating, and regulating clinical laboratories, has established a program to which many laboratories subscribe. Their guidelines compare well with those of NIDA and differ only in detail (College of American Pathologists, 1990). Similarly, some states have enacted statutes and regulations specifically to control laboratories doing employee drug testing. These regulations vary greatly. Although the laboratory aspects of federal testing programs have become a model, and proposed new federal legislation may set minimum standards for all drug testing (The 1993 Drug Testing Quality Act—HR33), for the moment, a vast amount of testing is not done in NIDA-certified laboratories. These unregulated programs often include preemployment, random, for-cause, and penal testing.

In a period of about 20 years, urine testing has moved from identifying a few individuals with major criminal or health problems to generalized programs that touch the lives of millions of citizens. It has given rise to a distinct and lucrative industry, with activities ranging from specimen collection to medical treatment, that was unimagined just 10 years ago. Tens of millions of urine specimens are analyzed every year in laboratories that vary from NIDA-certified operations to uncertified testing at workplaces, in amateur and professional sports, in doctor's offices, and in jails. One idea that motivates such widespread testing is the well-intentioned and generally popular goal of deterring the abuse of drugs among employed people and in other selected populations. There are, however, serious differences between the deterrence-oriented *identify, catch, and punish* philosophy and the less punitive *identify, treat, and rehabilitate* approach. These orientations often conflict and can seriously confound forensic toxicologists and medical review officers who are responsible for interpreting drug test results.

At the end of 1989 NIDA's Division of Applied Research sponsored a consensus conference to assess technical, scientific, and procedural issues of employee drug testing after about 18 months of operations following the President's executive order. A report was published early in 1990 (Finkle et al., 1990) that expressed the views and recommendations of the conference participants, that included politicians, government officials, representatives of business, industry and labor, as well as laboratory scientists and physicians. Their recommendations for improvements in the guidelines for testing as well as concerns related to laboratory certification and other important aspects have not been implemented nearly 4 years later, although few minor recommendations have been included in the revised HHS-NIDA guidelines (*Federal Register*, 1993). This type of inaction is particularly unfortunate and has recently been paralleled with another important report (Rollins, 1992), which evaluated the efficacy of on-site testing (still not released by NIDA).

BIOCHEMICAL METHODS FOR DETECTING DRUG USE

Forensic urine drug testing begins with specimen collection from the donor, proceeds to laboratory analysis, and then, in properly run programs, culminates in the interpretation of reported results by a medical review officer. These three components of the test are interdependent and essential to the integrity of the process and the validity of the laboratory results. The laboratory, however, is the only actor in this sequence that is subject to certification and regulation under the federal guidelines. Since actions based on drug tests may often be contested legally, the testing process must have sufficient integrity to establish the validity of test results. Showing such integrity requires detailed attention to prescribed procedures, quality control, and documentation.

Specimen Collection

When a specimen is collected for clinical purposes, there is no suspicion that the donor altered the specimen or attempted to subvert the analysis. It is generally part of a medical evaluation, the donor has health incentives to cooperate, and there is no legal attention to the test results. The same is not true for employee testing, which may involve use of illegal drugs and possible loss of employment. Thus, special procedures must be used to ensure that a specimen reaching the laboratory can be clearly identified as coming from a particular donor's urinary bladder, at a particular time and place, and that the specimen is unadulterated and has not been tampered with between collection and submission to the laboratory.

These procedures have been described by Caplan and Dubey (1992). They begin with specimen collection under either direct or indirect observation. Direct observation means that the collector observes the urination and can attest to the fact that the specimen came directly from the donor into the collection container. This is not a common practice in typical employee-testing programs. In the indirect collection process, the actual voiding of urine is not witnessed, but safeguards are taken to ensure specimen integrity. Common measures include ensuring no access to water taps, placing a bluing agent in the toilet bowl, and measuring of the urine specimen temperature immediately after collection to detect any dilution or specimen substitution. In collections by either procedure after the urine is voided, a tamperproof seal is placed over the collection bottle for transportation by courier to the laboratory. In addition, security seals are generally preprinted with unique identification numbers, and the specimen donor is required to date and initial the seal after it is placed on the collection container. The specimen is accompanied to the laboratory by a completed chain-of-custody form. This form not only requests the particular analysis but it also documents the date, time, and process of collection and provides the link between the specimen and the donor. A new government-approved form designed by DOT with the advice of scientists in the field and based on the past 5 years experience is likely to become the standard by the end of 1993 (D. Smith, personal communication, 1992).

A minor industry has developed to provide specimen collection services. Managing urine collection systems is not a trivial task. Simply keeping track of specimens poses difficulties when, as is frequently the case, collection sites send samples to several different laboratories and serve several different employers. While there is some uniformity in the federal system, in the private sector employers use different chain-of-custody forms, collection kits, seals, and courier services. Neither the companies who provide collection services, urine collectors, nor the sites at which they work are in any way regulated. It is generally the responsibility of employers and laboratories to select experienced and trustworthy collectors.

Tactics often used in attempts to confound urine analyses include dilution of the urine, substitution of drug-free urine, and the addition of substances that may render the urine unsuitable for analysis. Typical adulterants are salt, bleach, detergents, vinegar, bicarbonate, hand soap, vitamin C, ammonia, peroxide, and phosphate (Warner, 1989; Pearson et al., 1989). Recording specimen temperature at the time of collection is a useful check against possible urine substitution or dilution with cold water. Specific gravity and concentration of creatinine (a component of urine) may also indicate dilution, but recent studies strongly suggest they are of limited value for this purpose (Needleman et al., 1992; Peat, personal communication, 1992). The likely use of acidic or alkaline adulterants is suggested by massively altered urine pH.

Temperature, specific gravity, and pH are easily measured. When the urine collection procedure is indirect (not observed), then determination of creatinine at the laboratory may be a useful determinant that the submitted specimen is actually human urine. None of these tests is specific for adulteration or particular diseases, however, and the general health status of the donor may also affect the values.

At present the specimen submitted to the laboratory for analysis is invariably urine. Although more difficult to analyze, blood or plasma can be more informative and useful for forensic and clinical interpretations; however, the routine use of venopuncture to obtain blood specimens is not likely to be acceptable by either donors or the law. In special circumstances, such as testing for drug-induced impairment following a vehicular or industrial accident, blood testing is commonly seen as appropriate and often occurs. Deep lung air exhaled into a breath-testing device to assess blood alcohol concentration is now the specimen of choice in drinking-driving law enforcement programs (Dubowski, 1992). The National Highway and Transportation Safety Administration has approved a variety of portable and larger instruments for breath testing, which will undoubtedly be used as a convenient way to test for alcohol under the new DOT regulations. Saliva is another possible specimen. Saliva has been used to test for some therapeutic drugs and their metabolites, and there is evidence that certain illicit drugs are also detectable through saliva tests (Schramm et al., 1992). Practical difficulties, which include collecting an adequate volume of defined saliva, problems posed by the mixing of parotid saliva with common mixed mouth secretions, and the analytical sensitivity required have limited, perhaps unduly, research on saliva tests, and so little is known about the pharmacokinetics or biodispositional properties of those markers of illicit drugs that can be found in saliva.

In contrast, the use of head hair as a specimen to determine illegal drug use is under intensive study. Since Baumgartner (Baumgartner, 1984, 1989) used an immunoassay technique to detect the most commonly used illicit drugs and their metabolites in hair, the analytical toxicology of hair has been the subject of symposia, position papers, and extensive research in both the United States and Europe (Sunshine, 1992; Moeller, 1992). Hair can be and is analyzed in specific forensic cases but has not yet found favor in employee drug-testing programs. Although the question of whether hair analysis reliably and accurately detects drug use is being extensively studied, there is at present no body of reference data like that which exists for urine that would allow hair to become a routinely examined specimen. A consensus conference held under the auspices of the Society of Forensic Toxicologists with NIDA support concluded that the use of hair analysis for employee and preemployment drug testing is premature given current information on hair analysis for illicit drugs (National Institute on Drug Abuse, 1990; Keegan, 1991; U.S. Food and Drug Administration, 1990).

Technical issues relating to analytical accuracy, precision, sensitivity, and specificity are as yet unresolved and the threshold concentrations that are needed to define potentially false-positive or false-negative results for either screening or confirmation procedures have not been established. One important point to note is that no reference material is available with which to standardize analytical methods. In addition, the quantities of drugs and metabolites incorporated into hair, especially cannabinoids, may be below the detection limits of routine confirmatory (GC/MS) procedures. Issues relating to the external contamination of hair, washing or other aspects of sample preparation, and minimum sample sizes for analysis are all unresolved. The pharmacology and toxicology of drugs in hair is also poorly understood at present.

Among the matters we should know more about are the relationship between the dose of the drug and the concentration of the drug or its metabolites in hair over time, the minimum dose required to produce a positive analytical result, the time interval between drug use and the appearance or detection of the drug in the hair shaft, and the implications of individual variation by race, age, sex, and hair characteristics. There is however, research under way on all of these topics, and much has been published in the last 2 years, suggesting that answers to questions that must be resolved may soon be available, and that head hair will in fact be a useful specimen for the detection of illegal drug use (Sunshine, 1992). Perhaps in 1994 a follow-up consensus conference to the Society of Forensic Toxicologists Symposium would be in order to reassess current knowledge. However, even if current questions regarding hair analysis are clearly answered, the results could not address the issue of intoxication at the time of collection nor could they determine whether the individual's use of the drug resulted in intoxication at the time of consumption. Furthermore, hair analysis results may provide accurate information concerning whether past drug use occurred, but not in relation to where it occurred (e.g., on the job or off the job).

Laboratory Methods

As already stated, NIDA requires urine analysis for only five drug classes: marijuana (cannabinoids), cocaine (benzoylecgonine), opiates (morphine and codeine), amphetamine and methamphetamine, and phencyclidine. A complete analysis for these substances (analytes) is a multistep procedure that is carried out serially, from specimen receipt and verification to authenticated final report. Two of the three steps are analytical methods. The initial or screening test is designed to efficiently identify those urine specimens that are negative—that is, no drugs or metabolites are detected at concentrations above established cutoff values. Those specimens that test positive initially are subject to a confirmatory test which specifically identifies the drug, metabolite, or both, and assays the concentration. In all laboratories that are part of government-regulated programs, this two-stage procedure must be followed. The screening method, under NIDA guidelines, must be based on an immunoassay, and the confirmation method must be an acceptable form of gas chromatography-mass spectrometry (GC/MS).

Although there are many immunoassay techniques, the demands of high volume (often thousands of specimens each day), efficiency, quality control, and laboratory management limit the techniques in practice to enzyme immunoassay (EMIT), fluorescence polarization immunoassay (FPIA), and radio immunoassay (RIA). For reasons of cost, efficiency, and adaptability to automated chemistry analyzers, most NIDA-certified laboratories use EMIT as the initial screening method. The only large-scale forensic drug-testing laboratories using RIA are those supporting DoD programs. FPIA is an excellent method, but largely because of cost it has found favor principally as a second-stage screening method for specimens that test positive for amphetamines by EMIT. FPIA reagents are more specific for amphetamines than the EMIT reagents and therefore screen out specimens that otherwise might needlessly go to the confirmation stage.

These screening tests are necessarily designed to be highly sensitive to the analytes but not specific in their response, which means that at the screening stage some false-positive results can be expected. Thus, positive screening results alone do not necessarily imply the presence of a tested-for drug or its metabolite, and positive screening results cannot support a final report, nor can different immunoassays be used as screening and confirmation in tandem. The confirmation test must be based on a different chemical principle. This approach to forensic, analytical toxicology accords with the recommended guidelines and standards of the best-informed professional societies (American Academy of Forensic Sciences, Society of Forensic Toxicologists, 1991).

Despite what careful science demands, there are unregulated drug-testing programs that do not employ confirmation testing, including testing within the penal system for compliance with parole conditions and probation and for prisoner evaluation; testing for compliance in methadone maintenance programs; and some workplace programs that use on-site "laboratories." Relying on screening test results is an unacceptable practice that is particularly serious in contexts in which personal liberty is at stake. The FDA requires manufacturers of immunoassay test kits to include a statement in the kit: "The assay provides only a preliminary test result. A specific alternative method must be used to obtain a confirmed analytical result. Gas chromatography/mass spectrometry (GC/MS) is the preferred confirmatory method." This clear and carefully worded statement is ignored in some programs (Rollins, 1992; Finkle et al., 1990).

When used by an appropriately trained and skilled laboratory technician, GC/MS is the best method for confirming positive screening tests results (Hoyt et al., 1987; Foltz et al., 1980). Although the types of GC/MS instruments and techniques for GC/MS analysis vary, the techniques in use can provide very sensitive, specific identification either by analyzing a full mass spectrum or, more usually, by monitoring at least three selected ions and quantitation using deuterated internal standards of the drug or metabolite sought. In most GC/MS assays, the analyses are derivatized to provide for improved chromatographic characteristics and greater sensitivity.

This two-stage analytical procedure can achieve reliable results within defined limits of sensitivity and precise quantitation at concentrations significantly less than the HHS-NIDA established cutoff threshold values. Not all programs use the NIDA cutoff concentrations; even government agencies differ (see Table 6.1). The Nuclear Regulatory Commission allows licensees to use cutoffs more stringent than NIDA requirements, and they often do so. DoD has cutoffs for drugs not in the NIDA panel, such as barbiturates and LSD. The variation in private-sector programs is even greater. There is nothing intrinsically wrong with going beyond what NIDA requires, but there should be a rationale for such choices that are supported by laboratory quality assurance data and external blind performance testing that demonstrates laboratory capability at and below the cutoffs chosen.

Although the two-stage method approved by NIDA appears well suited to its task, there is a cost associated with rigidly setting the analytical methods to be used in drug testing. Innovation may be stifled, and the drug testing industry may fail to take advantage of new advancements in analytical chemistry or, indeed, of existing methods that might find limited application in some workplace programs. For example, thin layer chromatography (TLC) and high performance liquid chromatography (HPLC) may not enjoy all the attributes of sensitivity and specificity and efficiency required by very large programs and high-volume laboratories, but these techniques have advanced far in the last several years. The Toxi Lab system of thin layer chromatography has been carried to a remarkable degree of sophisti-

TABLE 6.1 Example of Administrative Threshold (cutoff) Concentrations (nanograms/milliliter, January 1992)

| Drug | NIDA | | DoD | |
	Immunoassay	GC/MS	Immunoassay	GC/MS
Marijuana	100[a]	15	50	15
Cocaine	300	150	150	100
Opiates	300	300	300	300
Amphetamine(s)	1,000	500	500	500
Phencyclidine	25	25	25	25

[a]The 1993 revised HHS guidelines recommend 50 ng/ml.

cation (DeZeeuw, 1992), and the same may be said of HPLC with diode array ultraviolet detection systems (Logan et al., 1990). These techniques may well be appropriate as qualitative confirmatory methods in small-volume, carefully defined workplace programs. NIDA should be encouraged to support applied research efforts to improve existing methods and develop new ones, even though ultimately changing existing government regulations can be very laborious and time-consuming.

No matter which analytical methods are used, their reliability depends on laboratory quality control and assurance and demonstrated proficiency in the processes employed. In government-regulated programs, the NIDA-certified laboratory is the only component of the urine-testing process that is tightly controlled and regulated with regard to quality. Quality control requirements include review of documentation from specimen receipt to final report and of the complete data package for every urine specimen analyzed. In addition, analyses must take place in secure laboratories with limited access to specimens by necessary personnel, and the integrity of the specimens must be documented by internal chain-of-custody, quality control and analytical data review. All records documenting tests results and quality control procedures must be available for examination if the analysis is subject to legal challenge. These documents are often referred to as litigation packages and provide a reviewable history of the specimen in question. A litigation package should contain the following documents (Crouch and Jennison, 1990; Crouch et al., 1988):

- Collection site information (external chain of custody, temperature, identification)
- Courier receipt
- Internal chain of custody form (note abnormal circumstances)
- Specimen identification confirmation
- Integrity check (pH, SG, etc.)
- Accessioning chain of custody
- Screening data (controls, calibrators, quality control, and certifying scientist signatures)
- Accessioning chain of custody for confirmation(s)
- GC/MS data (controls, calibrators, quality control, and certifying scientist signatures)
- Positive identification validation report (signatures, numbers, cut offs)
- Specimen long-term storage

Every NIDA-approved laboratory must have a quality assurance program. Quality assurance programs involve documented procedures that the laboratory follows to minimize human and technical error and to ensure the reliability of the analysis and final report by controlling the way specimens are extracted and handled and the way analytical instruments are checked for correct function. A typical flow of specimens in which checks and control points are incorporated is shown in Figure 6.1 (Crouch and Jennison, 1990). Quality assurance programs should at a minimum include: auditing specimen collection and protocols; quality control of laboratory assays; participation in open and external blind proficiency testing programs; and continuous training of laboratory staff. The most complex of these components is the control of laboratory assays. Quality assurance and control is described in detail in the NIDA Standards for Certification of Laboratories; it must include the analysis of instrument calibrators, open specimen controls, blind specimen controls and establishment of specificity and sensitivity limits for all assays. For confirming quantitative data, statistical linearity and precision must be defined. The following should be regarded as the fundamental components of a laboratory quality control program (Peat and Finkle, 1992):

1. Limits of detection and quantitation should be known for each analyte and may be determined by one of the following procedures:

    (a) mean value of the blank plus three standard deviations;
    (b) extension of the calibration curve to zero;
    (c) a designated signal-to-noise ratio;
    (d) a limit of at least 40 percent of the administrative cutoff value.

2. For studies involving quantitation of an analyte, the following should also be known:

    (a) linearity over the appropriate concentration range, which should include a blank, and concentrations less than the cutoff value.
    (b) precision at designated concentrations over the linear range;
    (c) if available, deuterated internal standards should be used for GC/MS assays. If not, then analogs of the analyte are preferred; and
    (d) each assay batch should include matrix-matched controls, both blanks and positives.

3. For qualitative identification, controls should also be matched with the biological specimen-urine and include a negative. At least one positive and one negative should be included with each set of specimens for analysis.

NIDA-certified laboratories are challenged with proficiency specimens

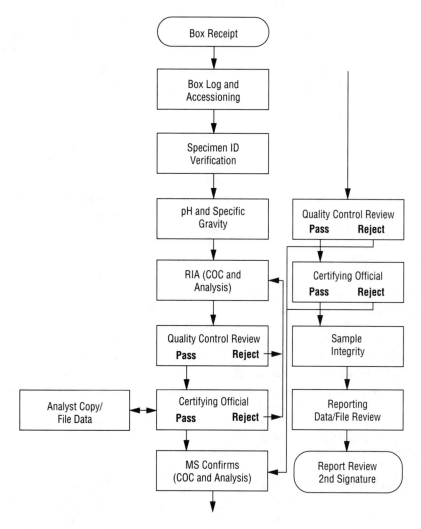

FIGURE 6.1   Typical flow of NIDA HHS samples at the laboratory.   SOURCE:
Crouch and Jennison (1990).

every 2 months and are also inspected on site by three NIDA inspectors
every 6 months.   At the inspection the laboratory director and certifying
scientists must be able to demonstrate that their urine-testing methods follow the HHS-NIDA guidelines and NIDA Standard Operating Procedures.
This is an exacting, costly, and often stressful aspect of the NIDA Certification Program, but it is absolutely essential to the integrity and credibility of
certified forensic laboratories.   There are, however, growing complaints

that NIDA inspections are becoming too expensive, detailed, intrusive, punitive, and bureaucratic. NIDA should review with their Drug Testing Advisory Board and representatives of the laboratories ways of reducing the financial burden and complexity of obtaining and maintaining certification. The fine balance between tight control and professional freedom needs guarding; respecting this balance was the intent of the toxicologists who prepared the original guidelines.

On-Site Testing Facilities

Although millions of tests are performed annually in NIDA-certified urine drug-testing laboratories, there are perhaps hundreds of other facilities, usually small and often on site at industrial plants or near a major work force, that do urine testing for drugs but do not generally meet the exacting standards required by government-regulated HHS-NIDA laboratories. The reliability and performance of on-site testing was discussed briefly at the NIDA Employee Drug Testing Consensus Conference (Finkle et al., 1990). The delegates at that conference recommended that facilities performing screening tests only should be subject to basic forensic standards for specimen collection, chain-of-custody documentation, and security. In addition, their test results should be subject to inspection and review and, most important, all presumptive positive specimens should be submitted to a certified laboratory for confirmation. It was also recommended that these facilities should participate in open and blind performance-testing surveys. Since that time NIDA has sponsored a survey of selected on-site facilities to assess the scope of their work, their purposes, and the apparent quality of their programs (Rollins, 1992). Although this report has not yet been released to the public, it is clear that there is substantial variability in program quality and that some level of control is necessary.

NIDA-certified laboratories are exempt from the 1988 Amendments (published February 1992) to the Clinical Laboratory Improvement Act (CLIA) but facilities conducting on-site drug screening are not exempt (*Federal Register*, 1992b, 1993). Companies with on-site laboratories conducting drug screening will have to obtain CLIA laboratory certification—an exacting process that will include inspections at least every 2 years by officials from the Health Care Financing Administration (HCFA). They will also be required to have a quality assurance program and to analyze quality control samples through their methods and instruments each day. The staff at the facility or laboratory will also have to meet certain standards, particularly the designated laboratory director. Implementation of standards for on-site drug testing is a high priority, and attention should be given to establishing some consistency across standards, regardless of whether the employment drug testing is performed on site or by an external NIDA-certified laboratory—especially with regard to the need for confirming initial screening test results. Standards similar to those recommended by delegates who attended the NIDA employee drug-testing consensus conference should be given serious consideration.

Adding to the List of Drugs to be Tested

As we have noted, laboratories that run NIDA-certified programs test urine for one or more of a panel of five drugs. Private-sector programs and laboratories that engage in drug testing and are not certified by NIDA are free to test for whatever panel of drugs they are able to identify and may choose cutoff concentrations at any level. By far the most common of the drugs that can affect work performance is ethanol (alcoholic beverages). Other legal drugs that may be used or abused and that can harm work performance can be bought over the counter in drug stores or supermarkets or are prescribed by physicians. Examples include the benzodiazepine sedative and antianxiety drugs, barbiturates, and some antihistamines that have sedative properties. In addition, other illegal drugs such as LSD and a variety of amphetamine derivatives are not part of the NIDA panel.

Alcohol testing, using NHTSA-approved breath testing devices, will soon be included in drug-testing programs conducted under the auspices of the Department of Transportation. The result will indicate blood alcohol concentration. Urine testing to identify alcohol use also presents no particular difficulties for most laboratories. Urine test results do not, however, show whether there is alcohol-induced impairment, whether alcohol has been used in the workplace, or whether there is alcohol in the blood while at work. Establishing impairment due to alcohol is important because the Americans With Disabilities Act (ADA) does not protect current users of illicit drugs, but it does protect those who are diagnosed as alcoholics. Thus under the ADA, any test result that is to be the basis of negative action has to establish impairment. This requirement inevitably leads to the need to establish threshold blood alcohol concentrations (BAC) above which the employee may be presumed to be under the influence of alcohol with attendant physiological and behavioral impairments. For drivers in the regulated commercial transportation industry, a BAC of 0.04 percent has been proposed (*Federal Register*, 1992a), which is substantially lower than the 0.1 or 0.08 percent level for drivers as defined by most states.

The example of alcohol, about which there is more scientific knowledge than any other legal drug, illustrates some of the technical difficulties and procedural complexities consequent to adding other groups of drugs to testing panels. Additional difficulties arise in testing for legal prescription and nonprescription drugs, since this poses ethical issues of confidentiality, employer and employee rights, and the involvement of physicians who treat employees as patients. Undaunted, many employers have added drug classes that contain dozens of individual drugs and metabolites to their requests for laboratory analysis. Testing for some of these drugs and their metabolites poses difficult analytical problems, although reliable immunoassays exist for other drug classes.

The NIDA consensus conference, which considered the proliferation of tested drugs, recommended that testing should not extend to additional drugs unless the criteria regarding analytical methods and procedures in the present NIDA guidelines with respect to an initial screening test and an independent confirmatory test could be met. This means that, for each candidate drug, screening and confirmation cutoff concentrations must be determined, and these cutoffs should be applied nationally. Also, proficiency testing and open and blind quality control programs should be in place for each additional drug before any testing of employee urine samples is undertaken, and the laboratory performance in testing for these drugs should be subject to the same NIDA inspection requirements.

Since the addition of other drugs to the present NIDA-5 opens a Pandora's box of procedural and technical issues, it seems prudent to prohibit their inclusion unless there is evidence that their misuse has serious detrimental consequences in the workplace. With the exception of alcohol, evidence of significant detriments associated with non-NIDA-5 drugs does not exist at the present time. Some employers may expand their definition of a drug-free workplace, but they do so at the risk of inadequate technical and forensic support.

Accuracy and Interpretation

Given that the current NIDA-specified cutoff concentrations are generous and sensitivity and specificity requirements are high, when a urine specimen is analyzed for the five illicit drugs and their metabolites in strict accordance with NIDA guidelines, including a report to the medical review officer, the likelihood that an individual employee will be falsely accused of illicit drug use in this situation is remote. Almost all known problems with false-positive reports in the past 5 years have been caused by procedural, documentation, and administrative errors or have been recorded by unregulated, uncertified laboratories (D. Bush, personal communication, 1992). This is a strong argument in support of the tight regulation and certification of laboratories, whether by NIDA or by professional organizations in the private sector. In this connection, it cannot be overemphasized that without confirmatory testing and careful medical review, treating the results of urine drug screening as evidence of drug use is unacceptable and scientifically indefensible.

Unexpected technical difficulties do occur, but they can be detected by the quality control and assurance procedures in place in the NIDA-certified laboratories. For example, it was learned that massive concentrations of ephedrine or pseudo-ephedrine, especially in the presence of low concentrations of methamphetamine, could lead to false identification and quantitation of methamphetamine but, as soon as this became apparent, procedural changes were made and technical improvements implemented through the NIDA laboratory network (National Institute on Drug Abuse, 1991). This type of experience is nonetheless sobering and argues for the intelligent and continuous examination of quality assurance data. NIDA and DoD have huge amounts of data resulting from blind performance testing, which confirm the extraordinary reliability of regulated laboratories. These data should be critically reviewed, analyzed, and published.

Despite their accuracy and precision, analytical results seldom allow clear answers to the questions that most concern medical review officers, employers, and lawyers. These questions include: (a) was the individual impaired at the time the specimen was taken, (b) when was the drug taken, (c) route of consumption, (d) what was the dose of the drug taken, and (e) is the individual a chronic abuser of the drug? The establishment of cause-and-effect relationships and retrospective calculations of drug dose and time of consumption generally cannot be made from single urine drug and metabolite concentrations alone. Most of the metabolites detected in urine are not pharmacologically active and, although clinical studies provide pharmacokinetic, time-course reference data, without blood or plasma concentrations and supporting circumstantial evidence, urine assay data lend themselves to only general interpretation. There is no reliable evidence that urine drug and metabolite concentrations correlate with behavior. The blood alcohol concentration model that is so valuable in the highway safety context is unique and not useful as a basis from which to evaluate the role of other drugs. Clinical studies and data banks of case experiences are being published in increasing numbers and are a useful reference for interpretation, but they must be used conservatively by knowledgeable forensic toxicologists.

A positive analytical result indicates only exposure to the identified drug. In unusual or extreme circumstances, it is possible that the exposure did not result from an individual's conscious or intentional action. This does not render positive test results false, but it does highlight the importance of accurate interpretation. Two of the most commonly claimed sources of unintentional exposure are the passive inhalation of cannabinoids from marijuana smoke and the unintentional consumption of morphine and codeine from poppy seeds. Research has shown, however, that the passive inhalation of marijuana smoke is very unlikely to result in a positive urine analysis at the present NIDA confirmation (GC/MS) cutoff concentration of 15 ng/mL (Cone and Johnson, 1986; Cone et al., 1987). Although the passive inhalation of marijuana smoke can lead to detectable levels of cannabinoids in urine, it is extremely improbable that a person not intending to inhale marijuana smoke would be able to tolerate the noxious environment of heavy marijuana smoke for the time needed to absorb a sufficient dose of cannabinoids to test positive.

Poppy seeds, which are commonly used on bagels and other baked foods, often do contain sufficient amounts of morphine to cause detectable concentrations of morphine, codeine, or both in urine. Published data on urine concentrations of these opiates following measured doses of poppy seeds (Elsohly and Elsohly, 1990; Selavka, 1991) permit cautious interpretations when this reason is offered for the positive urine results. Moreover, if the heroin metabolite 6-monoacetylmorphine is identified despite alleged poppy seed consumption, then the sole cause of the positive test is heroin use. Unfortunately, because of urinary excretion time and the inability of some laboratories to detect the low concentrations, the absence of this metabolite has no interpretive significance (Cone et al., 1991). Because of the poppy seed effect, every urine reported to the medical review officer as containing morphine must be investigated to determine, if possible, whether it resulted from intentional drug use.

The possible confounding of ephedrine and methamphetamine has already been noted. It should be recognized, however, that the concentrations of ephedrine and pseudo-ephedrine or of the decongestant drug phenylpropanolamine that must exist for positive tests means that these drugs have been consumed in far greater amounts than anything required for reasonable medical therapy. The widely used Vicks inhaler is also sometimes alleged to be the cause of methamphetamine, amphetamine, or both being found in urine specimens. Although there is no evidence that appropriate use of a Vicks inhaler will produce concentrations of methamphetamine in urine greater than the cutoff values, the inhaler does contain methamphetamine. The form of the drug however is the l-isomer, which is quite different from the d-isomer of the drug used as an illegal stimulant. Analytical methods are available that separate these isomers and are applied in NIDA-certified laboratories when positive results are blamed on Vicks inhalers (Fitzgerald et al., 1988).

These are just some of the reasons that individuals whose urine has tested positive for an illegal drug give to deny responsibility for the exposure or consumption. Undoubtedly new explanations will be argued in the future. When they are, one can expect that past practice will continue and that each contested or alleged false positive will be investigated by NIDA and the matter evaluated following scientific evaluation by the Drug Testing Advisory Board.

Other test program errors are false negatives, which means that individuals who have recently used a tested drug are not identified. There seems to be no limit to the imaginative methods used by some drug users to avoid detection; these include substitution of drug-free human urine, deliberate adulteration of the urine specimen as discussed earlier, consumption of a drug designed to mask the illicit drug, and deliberate hydration and diuresis using drugs, copious amounts of water, or commercial products that claim to hasten the excretion of a drug or to dilute the urine to a point at which the drug or metabolite falls below the threshold concentration for positive test. Despite efforts such as these, programs that follow the complete NIDA guidelines Standard Operating Procedures from specimen acquisition through specimen integrity checks and laboratory analysis will ordinarily detect any recently consumed NIDA-5 drugs. When they fail to do so, it will ordinarily not be because of failure of analytical methods and technology, but rather because procedural and administrative policies, such as high cutoff levels, will require adulterated specimens to be either rejected before analysis or reported negative. Clearly, the NIDA guidelines are tilted toward avoiding false positives; this cannot be done without enhancing the probability of false negatives, at least to some extent.

When the NIDA guidelines are not followed, poor quality assurance procedures at either the laboratory or the collection site can lead to errors, as can the failure to use appropriate confirmation tests to verify positive initial screening results. In these circumstances, false positive results are a genuine threat to those who are tested. A recent U.S. General Accounting Office report (1993) has made recommendations to simplify NIDA requirements in the interest of cost savings. Their suggestions may have merit but should not be implemented without very careful evaluation of the possible consequences to program quality and safeguards for the employee-donors.

INDIRECT METHODS OF ASSESSING ALCOHOL AND OTHER DRUG USE

In an attempt to avoid some of the technical measurement limitations of the direct methods as well as the controversial legal issues surrounding drug testing specifically (see Appendix A for a detailed treatment of the legal climate of drug testing), the development of indirect methods for assessing alcohol and other drug use has been rapidly growing. Indirect approaches typically involve measuring or observing behaviors or responses that are frequently associated with alcohol and other drug use and inferring such use from what is observed. One approach constructs profiles of personal characteristics or behaviors, including biographical and attitude data, on which alcohol and other drug users and nonusers tend to differ. Another approach identifies behaviors that are associated with alcohol and other drug intoxication or impairment and monitors those behaviors to infer use.

Personal Profiles

As stated above, one approach to assess alcohol and other drug use indirectly is to develop profiles of personal characteristics that differentiate between users and nonusers. These characteristics typically involve demographic and other personal background factors, attitudes and behaviors associated with alcohol and other drug use, and evidence of impairment from use or intoxication.

Integrity Tests

Several efforts at developing indirect measures of alcohol and other drug use based on attitude and personality profiles are outgrowths of paper-and-pencil integrity tests for employee selection (Sackett et al., 1989). These include the London House Personnel Selection Inventory, the Reid Report, and the Stanton Survey. One systematic approach is the London House Drug Abuse Scale (DAS) (Martin and Godsey, 1992). The DAS was developed from a theoretical model based in part on Zuckerman's theory of sensation seeking (Zuckerman, 1971, 1979), which is described as involving four interrelated characteristics: thrill and adventure seeking, experience seeking, disinhibition, and boredom susceptibility. High sensation seekers are viewed as more likely to use illicit drugs and drink heavily, and the trait has been correlated with polydrug use (Zuckerman, 1979).

In addition to sensation seeking, which is viewed as a relatively stable personality characteristic and thus one that refers to general tendencies rather than specific behaviors, the DAS also seeks to measure more specific psychodynamic mechanisms that are posited to influence attitudes toward drug use. Specifically, drug users are thought to be more likely than nonusers to rationalize drug use behavior, to project drug use behaviors onto others, to show more tolerance for drug use behaviors, and to be less likely to favor punitive approaches to drug use behavior (Martin and Godsey, 1992).

The DAS scale includes 20 items, most of which are derived from the psychodynamic mechanisms. Measures of internal consistency range from .68 to .90. The rationale for using DAS scale scores as a selection device is that job applicants will be naturally reluctant to disclose heavy drinking or illicit drug use but that they can be identified by attitudes that are relatively robust to incentives to distort.

A meta-analysis of validation studies with the DAS (Martin and Godsey, 1992) examined 26 studies in which it was the predictor. Criteria included drug and alcohol use (self-report or urinalysis), job performance, and theft. Four potential moderators were examined: (1) type of subject—students, applicants, or employees; (2) method of collecting the criterion—self-report or nonself-report (supervisor ratings, urinalysis, suspensions, or termination); (3) job relevance of the criterion—behavior at work or behavior away from work; and (4) subject matter of the criterion—drug or alcohol use, theft, or job performance.

Results of the meta-analysis showed an overall validity coefficient of .33 (Martin and Godsey, 1992). Studies based on self-reports had higher validities (r = .45) than those based on other types of criteria (r = .25). For self-report studies, applicant and employee samples yielded higher validity coefficients than did student samples. Studies using job-related criteria had higher validity coefficients than those using other criteria. Finally, there were no differences regarding the prediction of different criterion behaviors, such as drug or alcohol use and theft.

The validity of integrity tests for predicting drug and alcohol use was also examined in a meta-analytic study by Viswesvaran et al. (1992). From a data base of 124 integrity test validity studies, several relationships were examined. They first estimated the combined validity of all integrity test items for predicting the criterion of illicit drug and alcohol use. A total of 35 studies with a combined sample size of 24,488 contributed to the analysis. The mean validity was estimated to be .28. In another analysis, these investigators examined the validities of the individual "drug" scales (of the same integrity tests) in forecasting alcohol and other drug use. In 14 correlations with a total sample size of 966, there was an estimated mean validity of .51.

There has been a substantial increase in the use of paper-and-pencil integrity tests, which has stimulated debate about a number of aspects of integrity testing. In particular, there has been significant concern about the possibility that these tests may yield unacceptably large false-positive rates, i.e., they may mistakenly label large numbers of individuals as *dishonest* (American Psychological Association Task Force, 1991; Ekman and O'Sullivan, 1991; Manhardt, 1989; Martin and Terris, 1991; Murphy, 1987, 1993). The same concern applies to these instruments' "drug" scales; that is, a substantial number of individuals can be mistakenly labeled *drug users.*

Although there is now growing evidence that integrity tests demonstrate acceptable levels of validity for predicting both job performance and various forms of problem behavior (including drug use; see Ones et al., in press; Viswesvaran et al., 1992), these tests may still yield an unacceptable number of false positives. This is in part due to the relatively low base rate for drug use in the populations of interest. Murphy (1993) has shown that the proportion of false positives will be high when the base rate is low, even when a highly accurate test is used. Thus, the concern over false positives and the use of integrity tests is not restricted to concerns involving validity, but also reflects the influence of the mismatch between base rates and fail-

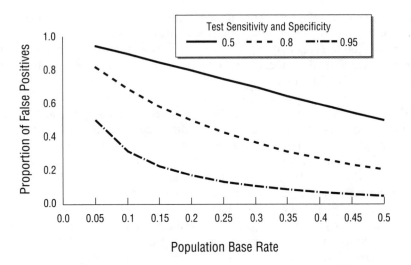

FIGURE 6.2   Proporation of false positives by base rate and test accuracy.

ure rates that might be expected when integrity-type tests are widely used to infer drug use.

For purposes of illustration, Figure 6.2 shows the proportion of false positives expected for various population base rates and various test accuracy levels. The three lines in the figure depict the expected false positive rates for tests differing in sensitivity and specificity. The sensitivity of the test is the likelihood that it will identify an individual as a drug user when he or she is a true drug user. The specificity of the test is the likelihood that it will identify an individual as a nondrug user when he or she is a true nondrug user. The three lines represent tests with a sensitivities and specificities of 0.5, 0.80, and 0.95. For simplicity, the illustration represents tests with equal levels of sensitivity and specificity, although this is not necessarily the case in practice. The trends in the figure demonstrate that false positives will increase as the accuracy of the test (sensitivity and specificity) decreases, and that false positives are considerably higher when the base rate of the behavior of interest (e.g., drug use) is low.

Based on the numbers in Figure 6.2, consider an organization with 1,000 employees, of which 100 (10 percent) are drug users. Using a test with 95 percent sensitivity and specificity[2] would result in correctly identifying 95 of the drug users and 855 of the nonusers. However, 45 employees

---

[2]Note that this level of accuracy is not necessarily representative of the level of accuracy of honesty tests; it probably overestimates the accuracy level associated with typical honesty test.

would be falsely classified as drug users, meaning that 32 percent of the identified users would in fact have not used drugs. If a test with a sensitivity and specificity of 0.8 was used with a base rate of 10 percent, 69 percent of identified drug users would be false positives. The important point is that, for a given level of test accuracy, the value of a test will vary as a function of the base rate (prevalence of drug use) in the population, and that a substantial number of individuals could be mislabeled as drug users, even with a highly accurate test, if the population base rate is low. For a given base rate, mislabeling increases as the accuracy of the test decreases.

Other Personal Profile Measures

Another indirect approach based on attitude theory is that of Lehman and his colleagues (Holcom et al., 1993; Lehman et al., 1992a; Rosenbaum et al., 1992). In this approach, attitude prototype theory (Lord et al., 1984) is used to develop a series of vignettes in which employees are described as using alcohol or illicit drugs at or away from work. Attitude prototype theory predicts how general attitudes about social categories, for example illicit drug users, are applied to specific category members. General attitudes are more likely to guide behavior toward typical rather than atypical category members. Novices, or observers who are not experienced with the category, usually show the typicality effect; experienced observers are more likely to apply their attitudes toward atypical as well as typical members.

Although systems based on attitude prototypes are still in the developmental stage, several pilot studies have been completed that show differences between experienced and novice observers, with experience defined on the basis of the observer's own drug use experience or the number of drug users the observer knows (Lehman et al., 1992b).

In one study with college students, Holcom et al. (1993) asked respondents to classify different alcohol and other drug user types into categories, to develop profiles of different alcohol and other drug user categories by rating each category on a list of positive and negative adjectives, and to express their level of tolerance for different situations involving alcohol and other drug use at work. Results indicated that overall, college students classified alcohol and other drug-user categories according to the perceived harmfulness of the drug, with tobacco use and light drinking at one end of the scale, heavy drinking and marijuana use clustered in the middle, and all other drug use clustered at the most harmful extreme. Experienced observers were more likely to group marijuana with alcohol use; novices had a tendency to group marijuana with other harder drugs.

Consistent with social categorization theory, experienced observers showed more differentiation of alcohol and other drug user classes on the profiling task than did novices. Novices' profiles of user classes were essentially parallel, differing in level of negativity but not in pattern (i.e., shape of negativity rating across user classes). The profiles of experienced observers were more distinct, showing differences in negativity as well as profile pattern. For example, experienced observers tended to use difference levels of negativity. Novices tended to use the same adjectives to describe all alcohol and other drug user classes, but rated them with different levels of negativity. Differences between novices and experienced observers were also found in attitudes, with experienced observers reporting much higher levels of tolerance for alcohol and other drug use at work than did novices.

In a second study of college students, Rosenbaum et al. (1992) presented a series of vignettes describing employee alcohol and other drug use in a variety of situations that varied as to the type of drug used (tobacco, light drinking, heavy drinking, marijuana, cocaine), where drug use took place (at or away from work), whether the user was in a safety-sensitive position, and whether the user was described as having a close working relationship with the observer. Respondents rated each situation with respect to their attitudes (acceptability and normality of the behavior, sympathy for the user) and behavioral intentions toward the user (choosing to work with the user, "covering" for the user). The students' attitudes and behavioral intentions toward alcohol and other drug users were highly dependent on the type of drug used and the context in which the drug use took place. The respondent's personal experience was also highly correlated with tolerance toward alcohol and other drug users; experienced observers were more tolerant than novices of alcohol and marijuana use away from work and of tobacco use both at and away from work. There were no differences for situations involving alcohol or marijuana use at work or of cocaine use at or away from work.

A subset of vignettes from the Rosenbaum et al. (1992) study was then presented to 1,081 municipal employees from a large city in the southwestern United States (Lehman et al., 1992a). Vignettes described tobacco use at work, light and heavy alcohol use away from work, marijuana use at and away from work, and cocaine use away from work. Employees were asked to react to each vignette in terms of their tolerance for the behaviors described and their concerns for safety in the situation. Employees were classified according to their self-reported alcohol and other drug use along two dimensions: whether they reported no use or frequent or problematic alcohol or illicit drug use within the past year, and whether they reported no illicit drug use, some use but not within the past year, or use within the past year.

Results showed that experienced users showed substantially higher tolerance for almost all employee drug use situations, with larger differences for the most extreme behaviors, such as marijuana use at work or cocaine use. Employees who had used illicit drugs during the past year were more tolerant of coworker alcohol and other drug use than were alcohol-only employees and were more tolerant than lifetime but not current users. Results also indicated decreasing tolerance among all groups for more serious forms of drug use, from light to heavy alcohol use to marijuana to cocaine use. However, location of use (at or away from work) and type of job situation (low- or high-risk jobs) were more important than type of drug in some situations. Thus, heavy alcohol use by employees in high-risk jobs was considered less tolerable than marijuana use by employees in low-risk jobs, and marijuana use at work was less tolerable than cocaine use away from work.

Newcomb (1988) used data from a survey of young adults in the Los Angeles area to develop a risk profile of characteristics that were associated with disruptive alcohol and other drug use. A total of 739 young adults between the ages of 19 and 24 were interviewed for the study. Of these, half were currently employed full-time, an additional 14 percent employed part-time, and 33 percent were enrolled in school. Disruptive alcohol and other drug use was defined as any use or being under the influence of illicit drugs or alcohol at work or at school. Newcomb developed two indices of risk factors, one which included gender, marital status, educational plans, cohabitation history, being fired from a job in the past 4 years, having trouble in an intimate relationship (past 3 months), law abidance, liberalism, and any cigarette use (past 6 months); the second index added any cannabis use (past 6 months) and any cocaine use (past 6 months).

These risk factors were selected from variables in previous analyses of the data set that were related to disruptive alcohol and other drug use and for which information was potentially available to an employer. From the set of variables chosen, a multiple regression analysis was run using disruptive alcohol and other drug use as the criterion. Variables that were significant predictors in the multiple regression were chosen for the risk indices.

The prevalence and frequency of disruptive alcohol and other drug use were calculated for each number of risk factors. Results indicated that respondents with few risk factors were very unlikely to engage in disruptive use of alcohol or other drugs; those respondents with many risk factors were very likely to engage in disruptive use. Thus, the extremes of the risk factor indices were more predictive of disruptive use than the middle of the index. Point-biserial correlations between disruptive use and the number of risk factors indicated that disruptive use of any drug was more predictable than disruptive use of any specific drug, including alcohol, marijuana, cocaine, and hard drugs. They also indicated that the risk index that included marijuana and cocaine use did a better job of predicting use than did the index that did not include those drugs. This could be artificial, however, for those willing to admit illicit drug use might be more willing than others to admit disruptive behavior.

A profile of personal and work characteristics predictive of employee alcohol and other drug use was developed by Lehman et al. (1991). In their analyses based on self-report responses from a sample of municipal employees, recent illicit drug use and alcohol or other drug use at work were regressed on sets of predictor variables representing personal background and work domains. The personal background domain included demographic measures such as age, gender, race, and education; personal background measures included religious attendance, arrest history, psychological functioning, and family and peer relations. The job domain included job background variables such as tenure on the job, supervisory status, pay level, job environment, and job category, as well as job attitude variables such as satisfaction, involvement, organizational commitment, job tension, and faith in management.

The results of the Lehman et al. (1991) analyses showed that employees who had recently (in the past year) used illicit drugs were more likely than nonusers to be younger, have an arrest history, associate with peers who were illicit drug users, work in a safety-sensitive job, and work alone or in a small group. Employees who reported using alcohol or illicit drugs at work within the past year were on average younger than their counterparts and more likely to be unmarried, have an arrest history, have low self-esteem, and to associate with peers who use alcohol and other drugs. They were also more likely to work alone or in a small group, to work in a safety-sensitive job, and to have low job involvement.

Summary

Several limitations of the use of profiles to identify alcohol and other drug users should be recognized. Perhaps the most developed use of profiles involves integrity tests used as preemployment selection tools. A number of test batteries are currently in use, and the results of several meta-analyses indicate that they are predictive of alcohol and other drug use as well as of other undesirable employee behavior such as theft and lower productivity. However, use of "drug" scales in selecting employees has a potential for high false-positive rates. Although research has demonstrated significant predictive validities in the 0.25 to 0.51 range, at these validities a high degree of misclassification will occur, the level and direction of misclassifications being affected by population base rates. As illustrated earlier in this chapter, given plausible base rates for alcohol and other drug use, the level of falsely positive misclassification can be substantial even for highly accurate tests.

Regardless of whether or not the preemployment use of "drug" scales is justified, such profiles should not be used to identify current employees who may be users given the level of false-positive classification error associated with these instruments. Taking disciplinary action against a current employee who happens to score high on a "drug" scale has more serious ramifications than using such a test to choose among several job applicants. Moreover, current employees generally are provided a higher degree of due process protection than are applicants (see Appendix B).

Obviously, more research needs to be done on profile scales like those described above in order to develop valid measures. However, it is doubtful that such instruments will ever reach accuracy levels high enough to become useful tools to personnel administrators, given the false-positive rates associated with their use.

Behavioral Indicators

Identifying specific behaviors associated with alcohol- and other drug-induced impairment is the basis for using behavioral indicators to identify users. Such behaviors include overt physical symptoms of intoxication (reddened eyes, slurred speech, impaired motor coordination, odor of alcohol or marijuana), as well as other indicators of impairment, such as decrements in work performance.

Drug Evaluation and Classification Program

The most systematic attempt to identify illicit drug users by using observable behaviors and physiological signals has been the Drug Evaluation and Classification Program (DEC), pioneered by the Los Angeles Police Department. In reaction to increasing evidence of illicit drug involvement among fatally injured drivers and impaired drivers detained by police, a drug recognition procedure was developed that could be performed by a trained police officer to obtain evidence that a suspect was impaired at the time of being detained by police; it also was designed to determine whether the nature of the impairment was consistent with a particular category or subgroup of illicit drug use.

The DEC program is described as a standardized, systematic method of examining a person suspected of impaired driving or some other alcohol- or drug-related offense or both, to determine (1) whether the suspect is impaired and, if so, (2) whether the impairment is drug-related or medically related and, if drug-related, (3) the broad category or combination of drugs likely to have caused the impairment (National Highway and Transportation Safety Administration, 1991). It is stressed that the process is *not* a field procedure but takes place in a carefully controlled environment, does not determine exactly what illicit drugs have been used but seeks to narrow the presence of drugs to certain broad categories, and is not a substitute for a chemical test, which is required to secure evidence to corroborate the suspicion generated by the DEC. However, because the DEC can narrow the probability of drug use to a limited set of drug categories, it can suggest more specific chemical tests than would otherwise be possible.

The DEC program involves a standardized and systematic examination of a suspect's appearance, behavior, performance on psychophysical tests, eyes, and vital signs. The examination includes a breath alcohol test, an interview of the arresting officer, preliminary examination of the suspect, examination of the subject's eyes for horizontal gaze nystagmus, vertical nystagmus, and lack of convergence, divided attention psychophysical tests, examination of vital signs including pulse, blood pressure, and temperature, darkroom examination to check pupil size and response, examination of muscle tone, and examination for injection sites.

The ability of the DEC process to discriminate between different categories of drugs is based on evidence that different drug types have different physiological and behavioral effects. For example, depressants can lead to horizontal gaze nystagmus and lack of convergence in eye examinations and disorientation, sluggishness, and drunklike behavior. Cannabis use, in contrast, is associated with lack of convergence but not horizontal gaze nystagmus, the odor of marijuana, reddened eyes, increased appetite, and impaired perception of time and distance. The utility of the DEC program is that it can provide probable cause to justify a request for a blood or urine sample, it can help the laboratory make decisions about which drugs to test for, and it can provide evidence of impairment that is not available from chemical tests.

Several studies have been completed evaluating the DEC program (Bigelow et al., 1985; Compton, 1986). The study by Bigelow et al. (1985) was a controlled laboratory evaluation of the DEC process conducted at Johns Hopkins University. Using the established DEC process, it was possible to correctly identify 95 percent of drug-free subjects as unimpaired, classify 99 percent of high-dose subjects as impaired, and identify the category of drugs for 92 percent of the high-dose subjects. Identification of low-dose subjects was not nearly so successful.

A second study involved a field-based evaluation of the DEC program (Compton, 1986). In this study, adult suspects arrested by regular traffic officers of the Los Angeles Police Department or the California Highway Patrol for driving under the influence, and who were suspected of being under the influence of a illicit drug or combination of illicit drug and alcohol, were examined by drug recognition experts (DRE), who had been trained and certified in the DEC process. If the DRE concluded that the suspect was under the influence of a drug other than alcohol, the suspect was asked to consent to a blood test. Suspects determined by the DREs not to be under the influence of drugs were released and were not asked for blood specimens. A total of 173 suspects contributed blood specimens (86 percent participation rate).

Results of the evaluation showed that for 94 percent of the suspects identified by a DRE as being under the influence of illicit drugs, a drug other than alcohol was found in the blood. Over 70 percent of subjects yielded detectable levels of more than one illicit drug. In terms of overall accuracy of DRE judgments, all illicit drugs were correctly identified in 49 percent of cases, some (but not all) illicit drugs were correctly identified 38 percent of the time, and the DRE failed to correctly identify any illicit drugs 13 percent of the time. If only one illicit drug was present in a suspect, DREs correctly identified it 53 percent of the time. No data were available on false negatives by DREs because blood specimens were not collected when the DRE failed to find drug impairment.

The DEC program is currently operating in 17 states and the District of Columbia (National Highway Traffic Safety Administration, 1991). Although it is the most systematic attempt to use indirect methods of behavioral assessment to infer drug impairment, it has several limitations that may prevent its widespread use in the workplace. The DEC program seems to be most effective when dealing with highly impaired suspects. Both evaluation studies described above showed limited success with low drug doses. In workplace settings, the highly impaired employee is relatively rare and is likely to be detected by less strenuous methods, such as by a supervisor trained to recognize performance decrements. It is also not known how much of the success rate described for the field evaluation is due to suspect self-reports. When intoxicated suspects are arrested and examined by officials in police headquarters, many of them will confess to drug use when confronted with the suspicion that they have used drugs. These confessions add to the "success" rate of the overall program, even if the DEC process would not have otherwise correctly identified them.

Although it is unlikely that the DEC program can easily be adapted to the workplace, some of its components may be useful in limited workplace situations. For example, for workplaces involving safety-sensitive work situations, EAP personnel could be trained in some of the DEC methods in order to make an assessment of an employee who has been identified as impaired by first-line supervisors. Such techniques could be used to break through employee denial and might lead to successful treatment. However, in order for the techniques to remain useful, they need to be continuously practiced by the practitioner, and few workplaces are likely to provide a sufficient number of cases to be effective. Moreover, the forensic toxicology community has recently expressed some concerns regarding the relatively low importance being given to the role of the laboratory results in the overall DRE process (Field, 1993). The forensic toxicology laboratory results are without a doubt a critical component of the DRE procedures for determining whether drug use may have contributed to the observed impairment.

In summary, although the use of behavioral indicators to indirectly identify users of alcohol and other drugs is a growing field (Heishman and Henningfield, 1990; Ellis, 1992; Perez et al., 1987), this line of research has serious limitations. Indicators based on behavioral impairment may be influenced by a variety of factors other than alcohol or other drug use, such as fatigue, stress, and legally obtained medications. The causal argument, sometimes made, that measures of impairment imply drug use or intoxication is simply not valid.

If, however, the goal is to identify impaired workers to either refer them to treatment or to prevent them from performing a task that may endanger themselves or others, then behavioral indicators provide a more direct means than drug tests of identifying employees unable to perform at required levels. The underlying motivation for many drug-testing programs, although certainly not all of them, is to minimize hazardous behavior and other performance problems. Behavioral indicators may be a better means to this goal than are chemical tests. However, psychomotor tests of impairment have not yet developed to the point at which they are available for widespread use. Given the promise of these tests, further research is a high priority. Another reason to be cautious in the use of such indicators as are now available is the underlying motivation of some organizations to label employees who fail behavioral tests as drug users.

Occupational Alcoholism and Employee Assistance Programs

Behavioral indicators of alcohol and other drug use are widely used through occupational alcoholism programs (OAPs) and employee assistance programs (EAPs). Problem employees are identified by decrements in job productivity, missed deadlines, lower-quality work output, increased absenteeism or tardiness, and accidents (Trice and Roman, 1982; Reichman et al., 1988). Using performance decrements to identify alcohol or other drug-using employees has several problems. One is that performance decrements can be associated with a wide variety of employee problems other than substance use, such as family, health, emotional, and financial problems. The other major weakness of job performance as an indirect indicator of alcohol or other drug use is that only employees whose use has been associated with identifiable job performance decrements are identified. Several studies have suggested that most alcoholic or problem-drinking employees do not cause problems for their employers because only a small percentage suffer performance decrements (Pell and D'Alonzo, 1970; Walker and Shain, 1983). For more details on employee assistance programs, see Chapter 8.

CONCLUSIONS AND RECOMMENDATIONS

This chapter provided a brief review of the critical components of drug-testing programs (i.e., specimen collection, laboratory analysis, interpretation of results) and other indirect methods for detecting drug use. Furthermore, it discussed the technical and procedural strengths and weaknesses of these methods. Based on the substantive issues and the serious nature of the potential negative consequences often associated with the results of such tests, the committee makes the following conclusions and recommendations.

• Methods approved by the National Institute on Drug Abuse (NIDA) for detecting drugs and their metabolites in urine are sensitive and accurate. Urine collections systems are a critical component of the drug-testing process, but they are the most vulnerable to interference or tampering. Positive results, at concentrations greater than or equal to NIDA-specified thresholds, reliably indicate prior drug use. There is, however, room for further improvement along the lines of the recommendations emanating from the 1989 Consensus Report on Employee Drug Testing and the 1992 On-Site Drug Testing Study. Moreover, more could be learned about laboratory strengths and problems if data already collected in the Department of Defense and NIDA blind quality control and proficiency test programs were properly evaluated.

> **Recommendation: To obtain accurate test results, all work-related urine tests, including applicant tests, should be conducted using procedural safeguards and quality control standards similar to those put forth by NIDA. All laboratories, including on-site workplace testing facilities, should be required to meet these standards of practice, whether or not they are certified under HHS-NIDA Guidelines.**

> **Recommendation: The extensive data on the reliability of laboratory drug-testing results that have been accumulated through the DoD and NIDA blind performance testing programs should be analyzed by independent investigators and the findings of their analyses published in the scientific literature.**

• Government standards have improved the quality of laboratory practices; however, their inflexibility and the difficulty of making prompt changes to established government regulations may inhibit the development of new analytical techniques and better experimental-based procedures. Strict regulation of drug-testing procedures and the National Laboratory Certification Programs are nonetheless justified. High-volume, production-oriented drug-testing laboratory operations require the vigilant forensic quality control of routine repetitive procedures, rather than innovative experimental science. Strict regulation need not, however, mean bureaucratic inflexibility that pointlessly increases costs or retards progress, nor should it interfere with research designed to improve current urine testing procedures or efforts to develop reliable tests using specimens other than urine.

> **Recommendation: Within a regime of strict quality control, allowances should be made for variations in procedures so long as they do not compromise standards and they do reflect professional judgments of laboratory directors and forensic toxicologists about what is required to meet individual program needs. No laboratory should be penalized for any practice that is clearly an improvement on or beyond what is required by the HHS-NIDA guidelines. When such innovations are attempted, data on their performance should be systematically collected and shared with NIDA. NIDA should take the lead in disseminating to all laboratories information about such improvements and should provide advice promptly as problems, research results, and new data become available.**

• At present, urine remains the best-understood specimen for evaluation of drug use and the easiest to analyze. Thus, it must for the moment remain the specimen of choice in employee drug-testing programs. However, other specimens have potential advantages over urine in that they involve less intrusive collection procedures or have a longer detection period.

> **Recommendation: Researchers should be encouraged to evaluate the utility of using specimens other than urine, such as head hair and saliva, for the detection of drugs and their metabolites.**

• There has been an unnecessary proliferation of drugs included in the urine test battery. Testing for LSD and sedative drugs, for example, is not always justified.

> **Recommendation: Additional drugs should not be added to the drug-testing panel without some justification based on epidemiological data for the industry and region. The analytical methods used to identify additional drugs should meet existing NIDA technical criteria.**

• Preemployment drug testing may have serious consequences for job applicants. Applicants, unlike most employees, often do not enjoy safeguards commensurate with these consequences. A particular danger of unfairness arises because screening test data are often reported to companies despite the known possibility of a false positive classification errors.

Recommendation: No positive drug test result should be reported for a job applicant until a positive screening test has been confirmed by GC/MS technology. If a positive test result is reported by the laboratory, the applicant should be properly informed and should have an opportunity to challenge such results, including access to a medical review officer or other qualified individual to assist in the interpretation of positive results, before the information is given to those who will make the hiring decision.

• Drug-testing results may reveal drugs taken legally for medical treatment that do not seriously affect an employee's job performance. These drugs may, however, be associated with conditions that the employee for good reasons wishes to keep private.

Recommendation: In the absence of a strong detrimental link to job performance, legally prescribed or over-the-counter medications detected by drug testing should not be reported to employers. Furthermore, such results should not be made part of any employment record, except confidential health records with the employee's permission.

• Alcohol and other drug use by work force members cannot be reliably inferred from performance assessments, since performance decrements may have many antecedents. Conversely, performance decrements are often not obvious despite alcohol and other drug use. More direct measures of the likely quality of worker performance hold promise for determining workers' fitness to perform specific jobs at specific times, regardless of the potential cause of impairment. Efforts to identify such measures, however, are still in their infancy.

Recommendation: If an organization's goal is to avoid work decrement (e.g., accidents, injuries, performance level) due to impairment, then research should be conducted on the utility of performance tests prior to starting work as an alternative to alcohol and other drug tests.

• Integrity testing and personality profiles do not provide accurate measures of individual alcohol and other drug use and have not been adequately evaluated as predictors or proxy measures of use. Using these tests to aid in employment decisions involves a significant risk of falsely identifying some individuals as users and missing others who actually use drugs. The accuracy of these tests is affected not only by their validity but also by the characteristics of the population being tested. Urine tests, by contrast, can be quite accurate in detecting recent drug use.

Recommendation: If an organization treats alcohol and other drug use as a hiring criterion, it should rely on urinalysis testing that conforms with NIDA guidelines to detect use rather than on personality profiles or paper-and-pencil tests.

REFERENCES

American Academy of Forensic Sciences
  1991   Forensic Toxicology Laboratory Guidelines. Society of Forensic Toxicologists, Grosse Point, Mich.
American Psychological Association Task Force
  1991   *Questionnaires Used in the Prediction of Trustworthiness in Preemployment Selection Decisions: An APA Task Force Report.* Washington, D.C.: American Psychological Association.
Baumgartner, W.A.
  1984   *Employee Screening by Hair Analysis: The Answer to Urinalysis Problems.* Los Angeles: IANUS Foundation.
  1989   Hair analysis for drugs of abuse. *Journal of Forensic Science* 34(6):1433.
Bigelow, G.E., W.E. Bickel, J.D. Roache, I.A. Liebson, and P. Nowowieski
  1985   *Identifying Types of Drug Intoxication: Laboratory Evaluation of a Subject-Examination Procedure.* National Highway and Transportation Safety Administration. DOT-HS-807-012. Washington, D.C.: U.S. Department of Transportation.
Boone, J.D.
  1987   Reliability of urine drug testing. *Journal of the American Medical Association* 258:2587.
Cangianelli, L.A.
  1989   The effects of a drug testing program in the Navy. In L.S. Harris, ed., *Problems of Drug Dependence, 1989: Proceedings of the 51st Annual Scientific Meeting, The Committee on Problems of Drug Dependence, Inc.* NIDA Research Monograph 95. Rockville, Md.: National Institute on Drug Abuse.
Caplan, Y.H., and I.S. Dubey
  1992   Workplace drug testing. *Clincial Chemistry News.* Special Issues: Fronteirs in TDM and Clinical Toxicology 18(6):31-33.
College of American Pathologists
  1990   Forensic Urine Drug Testing Inspection Check List. College of American Pathologists, Northfield, Ill.
Compton, R.P.
  1986   *Field Evaluation of the Los Angeles Police Department Drug Detection Program.* National Highway and Transportation Safety Administration. DOT-HS-807-012. Washington, D.C.: U.S. Department of Transportation.
Cone, E., and J.R. Johnson
  1986   Contact highs and urinary cannabinoid excretion after passive exposure to marijuana smoke. *Clinical Pharmacology & Therapeutics* 40:247.

Cone, E., J.R. Johnson, W.D. Darwin, D. Yousefnejad, L.D. Mell, B.D. Paul, and J. Mitchell
1987   Passive inhalation of marijuana smoke: urine analysis and room air levels of delta-9-THC. *Journal of Analytical Toxicology* 11:89.
Cone, E., P. Welsh, J.M. Mitchell, and E.D. Paul
1991   Forensic drug tests for opiates: 1. Detection of 6-monoacetyl-morphine in urine as an indicator of recent heroin exposure; drug and assay considerations and detection times. *Journal of Analytical Toxicology* 15:1.
Crouch, D.J., and T.A. Jennison
1990   Laboratory aspects of forensic urine drug testing. Workshop proceedings, Center for Human Toxicology, University of Utah, Salt Lake City.
Crouch, D. J., D. E. Rollins, T.A. Jennison, and D.E. Moody
1988   Criteria for evaluation of occupational drug screening laboratories. In G.R. Jones and P.P. Singer, eds., *Proceeding of the 24th International Association of Forensic Toxicolgists*. Banff, Canada: Alberta Society of Clinical Forensic Toxicologists.
DeZeeuw, R.F.
1992   *Thin-Layer Chromatographic RF Values of Toxicologically Relevant Substances on Standardized Systems*. Weinham, Germany: Verlagsgsellschaft.
Dubowski, K.M.
1992   *The Technology of Breath Alcohol Analysis*. ADM 92-1728. Washington, D.C.: U.S. Department of Health and Human Services.
Ekman, P., and M. O'Sullivan
1990   Who can catch a lie? *American Psychologist* 46:913-920.
Ellis, G.M.
1992   Drug and Alcohol Abuse in the Transportation Workplace: Research Needs for the Next Decade. Paper presented at a workshop of the Transportation Research Board, National Research Council, Irvine, Calif.
Elsohly, H.N., and M.A. Elsohly
1990   Poppy seed ingestion and opiates urinalysis: a closer look. *Journal of Analytical Toxicology* 14:308.
Federal Register
1972   Proposed special requirements for use of methadone. *Federal Register* 37(April 6):6940.
1988   Mandatory guidelines for federal workplace drug testing programs. *Federal Register* 53(April):69.
1992a   Federal highway administration drug and alcohol testing programs: proposed rules. *Federal Register* 5(241)December 22:59516-59586.
1992b   Specific lists for categorization of laboratory test systems: assays and examinations by complexity. *Federal Register* 57(40)February 28:7245-7258.
1993   Mandatory guidelines for federal workplace drug testing programs. *Federal Register* 58(14)January 25:6062-6072.
Field, M.
1993   Forum. *The DRE* 5(3)Summer.
Finkle, B.S.
1972   Forensic toxicology of drug abuse: a status report. *Analytic Chemistry* 44:9.
Finkle, B.S., R.V. Blanke, and M.J. Walsh
1990   *Technical Scientific and Procedural Issues of Employee Drug Testing*. ADM 90-1684. Washington, D.C.: U.S. Department of Health and Human Services.
Fitzgerald, R.L., J.M. Ramos, S.C. Bogema, and A. Poklis
1988   Resolution of methamphetamine stereoisomers in urine drug testing: urinary excretion of R(-)-methamphetamine following use of nasal inhalers. *Journal of Analytical Toxicology* 12:255-259.

Foltz, R.L., A.F. Fentiman, and R.B. Foltz, eds.
   1980   *GC/MS Assays for Abused Drugs in Body Fluids.* NIDA Research Monograph 32.
           Rockville, Md.: National Institute on Drug Abuse.
Frings, C.
   1986   Drug testing brings chemists back to basics. *Clinical Chemistry News* (September).
Hansen, H.J., S.P. Caudill, and J.D. Boone
   1985   Crisis in drug testing: results of CDC blind study. *Journal of the American Medical
           Association* 253:2382-2387.
Hanson, D.J.
   1986   Drug abuse testing programs gaining acceptance in the workplace. *Chemical Engi-
           neering News* (June 2).
Hawks, R.L., and C.N. Chiang, eds.
   1986   *Urine Testing for Drugs of Abuse.* NIDA Research Monograph 73. Rockville, Md.:
           National Institute on Drug Abuse.
Heishman, S.J., and J.E. Henningfield
   1990   Application of human laboratory data for the assessment of performance in work-
           place settings: practical and theoretical considerations. In S.W. Gust, J.M. Walsh,
           L.B. Thomas, and D.J. Crouch, eds., *Drugs in the Workplace: Research and Evalu-
           ation Data*, Vol. II. NIDA Research Monograph 100. Rockville, Md.: National
           Institute on Drug Abuse.
Holcom, M.L., W.E.K. Lehman, A.L. Rosenbaum, and C.G. Lord
   1993   Drug Involvement and Attitude Structures Concerning Drug Users. Poster presented
           at the annual meeting of the Society of Industrial/Organizational Psychology, San
           Francisco.
Hoyt, D.W., R.E. Finnigan, T. Nee, T.F. Shults, and T.J. Butler
   1987   Drug testing in the workplace: are methods legally defensible? *Journal of the
           American Medical Association* 258:504.
Keegan, A.
   1991   Putting hair to the test. *NIDA Notes* 6(4):10.
Lehman, W.E.K., D.J. Farabee, M.L. Holcom, and D.D. Simpson
   1991   Prediction of Substance Use in the Workplace: Unique Contributions of Demo-
           graphic and Work Environment Variables. Institute of Behavioral Research Techni-
           cal Report, Texas Christian University, Fort Worth.
Lehman, W.E.K., D.J. Farabee, and D.D. Simpson
   1992a   Employee Health and Performance in the Workplace: A Survey of Employees of
           the Housing Authority in a Large Southwest City. Institute of Behavioral Research
           Technical Report, Texas Christian University, Fort Worth.
Lehman, W.E.K., A.L. Rosenbaum, and M.L. Holcom
   1992b   Relationships Between Employee Drug Use and Tolerance for Co-Worker Use. In-
           stitute of Behavioral Research Technical Report, Texas Christian University, Fort
           Worth.
Logan, B.K., H.S. Nicols, G.S. Fernandez, and D.T. Stafford
   1990   The use of HPLC with diode array spectrophotometric detection in forensic drug
           analysis. *Crime Laboratory Digest* 17(1):5.
Lord, C.G., M.R. Lepper, and D. Mackie
   1984   Attitude prototypes as determinants of attitude-behavior consistency. *Journal of
           Personality and Social Psychology* 46:1254-1266.
Manhardt, P.J.
   1989   Base rates and tests of deception. Has I/O psychology shot itself in the foot? *The
           Industrial Psychologist* 26(2):48-50.

Martin, S.L., and C. Godsey
  1992   Assessing the Validity of a Theoretically-Based Predictor of Substance Abuse. Paper presented at the annual meeting of the Society of Industrial Organizational Psychology, Montreal.
Martin, S.L., and W. Terris
  1991   Predicting infrequent behavior: clarifying the impact of false-positive rates. *Journal of Applied Psychology* 76:484-487.
McBay, A.J.
  1986   Problems in testing for abused drugs. *Journal of the American Medical Association* 255:39-40.
Moeller, M.R.
  1992   Drug detection in hair by chromatographic procedures. *Journal of Chromatography* 580:125.
Murphy, K.R.
  1987   Detecting infrequent deception. *Journal of Applied Psychology* 72:611-614.
  1993   *Honesty in the Workplace.* Pacific Grove, Calif.: Brooks/Cole.
National Highway and Transportation Safety Administration
  1991   Drug Evaluation and Classification Program. NHTSA briefing paper, May, U.S. Department of Transportation, Washington, D.C.
National Institute on Drug Abuse
  1990   Conference on analysis of hair for drugs of abuse. NIDA Office of Workplace Testing, Rockville, Md.
  1991   NIDA/DHHS Technical Advisory, March 11. National Institute on Drug Abuse, Rockville, Md.
Needleman, S.B., M. Porvaznick, and D.J. Ander
  1992   Creatinine analysis in single collection urine specimens. *Journal of Forensic Science* 37:1125.
Newcomb, M.D.
  1988   *Drug Use in the Workplace: Risk Factors for Disruptive Substance Use Among Young Adults.* Dover, Md.: Auburn House.
Ones, D.S., C. Viswesvaran, and F.L. Schmidt
  in press Meta-analysis of integrity test validities. *Journal of Applied Psychology.*
Pearson, S.D., K.O. Ash, and F.M. Urry
  1989   Mechanism of false negative cannabinoid immunoassay screens by Visine Eye Drops. *Clinical Chemistry* 35:636.
Peat, M.A., and B.S. Finkle
  1992   Toxicological assay of psychoactive substances in biological fluids. Pp. 95-107 in S.D. Ferrara and R. Giovgetti, eds., *Methodology in Man-Machine Interactions and Epidemiology on Drugs and Traffic Safety.* Padua, Italy: ARFI.
Pell, S., and C.A. D'Alonzo
  1970   Sickness absenteeism of alcoholics. *Journal of Occupational Medicine* 12:198-210.
Perez, W.A., P.J. Masline, E.G. Ramsey, and K.E. Urban
  1987   United Tri-Services Cognitive Performance Assessment Battery: Review and Methodology. Defense Technical Information Center, Alexandria, Va.
President's Commission on Organized Crime
  1986   *The Impact: Organized Crime Today.* Report to the President and Attorney General. Washington, D.C.: U.S. Government Printing Office.
Reichman, W., D.W. Young, and L. Gracin
  1988   Identification of alcoholics in the workplace. *Recent Developments in Alcoholism* 6:171-179.

Rollins, D.E.
1992   On-Site Drug Testing in the Workplace. Unpublished manuscript, Center for Human Toxicology, University of Utah, Salt Lake City.

Rosenbaum, A.L., W.E.K. Lehman, and M.L. Holcom
1992   Using Workplace Vignettes to Elicit Attitudes Toward Employee Substance Use. Institute of Behavioral Research Technical Report, Texas Christian University, Fort Worth.

Sackett, P.R., L.R. Burris, and C. Callahan
1989   Integrity testing for personnel selection: an update. *Personnel Psychology* 42:491-529.

Schramm, W., R.H. Smith, P.A. Craig, and D.A. Kidwell
1992   Drugs of abuse in saliva: a review. *Journal of Analytical Toxicology* 16:1.

Selavka, C.M.
1991   Poppy seed ingestion as a contributing factor to opiate positive urinalysis results. *Journal of Analytical Toxicology* 36(3):685.

Sunshine, I., ed.
1992   *Recent Developments in Therapeutic Drug Monitoring and Clinical Toxicology.* New York: Dekker.

Trice, H.M., and P. Roman
1982   *Spirits and Demons at Work: Alcohol and Other Drugs on the Job.* Ithaca, N.Y.: Cornell University Press.

U.S. Food and Drug Administration
1990   RIA analysis of hair to detect the presence of drugs of abuse. Compliance policy guide 7124.06. U.S. Food and Drug Administration, Washington, D.C.

U.S. General Accounting Office
1993   *Employee Drug Testing: Estimated Cost to Test all Executive Branch Employees and New Hires.* GAO/GGD-92-90. Washington, D.C.: U.S. General Accounting Office.

Viswesvaran, C., D.S. Ones, and F.L. Schmidt
1992   Integrity Tests Predict Drug and Alcohol Abuse on the Job. Poster presentation at the 1992 annual meeting of the American Psychological Society, San Diego, Calif.

Walker, K., and M. Shain
1983   Employee assistance programming: in search of effective interventions for the problem drinking employee. *British Journal of the Addictions* 290-303.

Warner, A.
1989   Inference of common household chemicals in immunoassay methods for drugs of abuse. *Clinical Chemistry* 35:648.

Willette, R.E.
1986   Drug testing programs. In R.L. Hawks and C.N. Chiang, eds., *Urine Testing for Drugs of Abuse.* NIDA Research Monograph 73. Rockville, Md.: National Institute on Drug Abuse.

Zuckerman, M.
1971   Dimensions of sensation seeking. *Journal of Consulting and Clinical Psychology* 36(1):45-52.
1979   *Sensation Seeking: Beyond the Optimal Level of Arousal.* Hillsdale, N.J.: Lawrence Erlbaum Associates, Inc.

7

Impact of Drug-Testing Programs on Productivity

Many employers in the United States have attempted to address the problems they perceive to be related to alcohol and other drug use by establishing drug-testing programs, as described in Chapter 6. What effects do drug-testing policies and programs have on people's productivity at work? Unfortunately, there have been few systematic studies relating these drug-testing programs to workers' productivity, and those that have been done are often flawed in significant ways. This chapter critically reviews the literature that does exist and discusses how the effects of such programs may best be evaluated. It also reviews the literature on the attitudes of workers and job applicants toward such programs and the potential effects of these attitudes on productivity.

We reiterate here an important point that was mentioned in Chapters 1 and 6. It is related to the methods and measures used by the studies reviewed here: most drug-testing programs do not include alcohol among the drugs to be tested. Executive Order #12564 signed by President Reagan in 1986 mandated testing for illicit drugs; subsequently, in 1988 the HHS "Mandatory Guidelines for Federal Workplace Drug Testing Programs" limited the number of drugs to be tested to the following commonly used illicit drug classes: (1) marijuana, (2) opiates (heroin, morphine), (3) cocaine, (4) amphetamine and methamphetamine, and (5) phencyclidine. These guidelines have served as a model for most drug testing programs that have been implemented to date. The only exception to this omission of alcohol is the recent Omnibus Transportation Act of 1991, which requires the Department of Transportation to include alcohol as a target drug in their testing program. To date no evaluation of adding alcohol to the list of drugs to be tested for has been carried out.

TYPES AND USES OF DRUG-TESTING PROGRAMS

Workplace drug-testing programs are of three distinct types: (1) preemployment testing of job applicants; (2) incident-driven or for-cause testing of employees (e.g., post-accident, fitness for duty); and (3) postemployment testing without specific cause, often selected at random from a pool of targeted (usually sensitive) positions (Walsh et al., 1992). In 1988, 3 percent of the employers surveyed by the U.S. Department of Labor (1989) had some type of drug-testing program; by 1990, this figure had risen to 4 percent (Employee Assistance Professional Association, 1991). The majority of this testing has been undertaken by major corporations. Among the largest employers (with more than 1,000 employees) surveyed by the Department of Labor, 43 percent had some type of drug-testing program, whereas only 2 percent of the smallest establishments (with fewer than 50 workers) had such programs. More recent surveys of workplace drug testing indicate that between 50 and 75 percent of medium and large organizations now test current or prospective employees for drugs (American Management Association, 1992; Axel, 1990; Hayghe, 1991).

Preemployment drug testing is the most prevalent form of drug testing: 85 percent of those companies the Department of Labor surveyed with a testing program tested job applicants. Findings from the Monitoring the Future project (Patrick O'Malley, personal communication, 1992) show that increasing proportions of the work force have undergone testing for drug use in recent years: in 1987, 15 percent of men and 6 percent of women surveyed by the follow-up study reported having had a drug test; the corresponding figures in 1991 were 33 and 16 percent. In other words, by 1991, one in three young adult men and one in six women report having been tested. Most of these tests were preemployment drug tests.

Although the surveys reveal that corporate executives and human resources managers believe that drug-testing programs are effective tools for improving workplace safety, health, and productivity, there is little empirical evidence pertaining to their efficacy. To date, most evaluation attempts have consisted of simply monitoring and interpreting trends in laboratory tests results.

The main impetus for the rapid diffusion of these programs appears to have evolved from the preeminence given by the Reagan and Bush administrations to their "war on drugs" policies, from which the concept of a "drug-free workplace" first emerged, the substantial amount of publicity given to recent tragic accidents, and numerous government regulations and directives. Favorable court rulings have also substantially contributed to making drug testing common in corporate America.

Over the past decade, incumbent presidents and Congress have not only authorized drug testing by public and private employers, but also have required or encouraged it in some workplaces. Their actions provide legal authority for drug testing that overrides all contrary authority except the U.S. Constitution. The scope of workplace drug testing is limited by certain state and federal constitutional restrictions, particularly in the public sector and in postemployment settings; these limits, however, are generous and allow a broad range of employees to be tested using a wide range of reliable methodologies. A detailed treatment of the legal issues surrounding drug testing is provided in Appendix B. The argument here is that the policies of previous administrations, the legislature, and the judicial systems have all contributed to establishing drug testing as a major component of the nation's "war on drugs."

Unfortunately, to date, little consideration if any, has been given to assessing the impact of such programs on public health. Although this chapter is concerned with the effectiveness of workplace drug-testing programs on productivity, the reviewed literature still provides valuable information to policy makers. The emphasis on workplace productivity rather than public health or social welfare affects the evaluation method and criteria used in this chapter. In evaluating the efficacy of drug-testing programs, the researcher's perspective will influence what are regarded as acceptable program objectives, which in turn will determine the proper criteria for evaluating program effectiveness. Walsh et al. (1992) point out that, from a public health perspective, the primary question is whether drug intervention programs prevent or postpone any death, disease, disability, or dysfunction associated with the use or abuse of drugs.

From business or human resource management perspectives, the prevailing question is different from that of the public health perspective. In a business context, the primary concern is whether such programs allow the corporation to function more efficiently in a competitive market. Acceptable evaluation criteria are whatever business decision makers consider relevant productivity indices (e.g., absenteeism, work output, safety and health).

Job-site drug-testing programs have some promise in this respect. About three-fourths of adult men (16 years and older) and over half of adult women are in the labor force (Bureau of the Census, 1989). A sizable proportion of a worker's waking hours are spent at work, and a common sense of identity often exists within the work setting, where coworkers share norms and values. Workers are also subject to powerful influences that encourage conformity that can be used constructively to tackle problem behaviors such as alcohol and drug abuse. Formal and informal channels for communicating messages about drug abuse and treatment abound. Workplace drug programs thus have the potential for extensive social benefits. At the same time, such programs may have social costs. Some have argued, for example, that business drug intervention programs such as preemployment testing may aggravate society's drug problem by making those in need of assistance (e.g., applicants testing positive who are denied a job) unemployable.

IMPACT OF DRUG-TESTING PROGRAMS

Preemployment Drug Testing

Preemployment testing is not only the most common form of drug-testing currently in place in organizations, but it has also received the largest amount of attention from the research community. One of the earliest evaluation studies attempting to assess the efficacy of preemployment drug testing that appeared in the published literature was carried out by Lewy (1983), who reported that 13 of 500 hospital job applicants tested positive for one or more of 5 drug classes (benzodiazapine, barbiturates, amphetamines, phencyclidine, and opiates). Based on this limited descriptive information and the cost of testing, the author concluded that preemployment drug testing is not a financially viable selection procedure. A significant limitation of the study is that the investigator did not test for the most prevalent illicit drugs (marijuana and cocaine) and made no attempt to assess the relationship between test results and performance.

Parish (1989) also attempted to evaluate the effectiveness of an applicant drug-testing program at a large hospital. This study focused on the important question, which had not yet been addressed in the literature, of whether preemployment drug test results were associated with job performance indicators. All employees hired over a 6-month period were tested for illicit drug use. The drug test results were kept confidential and, after 1 year of employment, job performance measures were extracted from personnel files. The 22 employees who had tested positive were found to have had a 28 percent higher turnover rate and a 64 percent higher rate of receiving disciplinary warnings. Twenty-five percent of the identified drug users received poor performance evaluations from their supervisors, compared with 5 percent of those who tested negative. Despite these observed disparities, no statistically significant relationship was detected between drug test results and job performance characteristics. The author commented that the null results were probably due, at least in part, to the small number of cases in the drug-positive group, an observation that has since been confirmed by other reviewers (Normand et al., 1990; Zwerling et al., 1990). These cautions are well taken. Given the low power of the statistical tests used, the brief tenure of the employees, and the complete absence of hired applicants testing positive for cocaine, the study's failure to reject the null hypothesis provides little reason to believe that preemployment drug use cannot predict some employment behavior.

Blank and Fenton (1989) carried out a similar predictive study with U.S. Navy recruits who were screened for illicit drugs before being sent to recruit training. Only those who tested positive for marijuana alone or negative for all drugs were retained. The 500 recruits who tested positive for marijuana were compared with a matched group of approximately 500 recruits who tested negative for all drugs. The results showed that 43 percent of the marijuana positives but only 19 percent of the negatives had been discharged from the Navy after 2.5 years. Despite this dramatic difference, the study should not be read as establishing the efficacy of drug testing as a selection procedure, even in the naval context. When evaluating the predictive value of an employee selection procedure, it is essential that the research sample include applicants who are typical of the population to which the results will be generalized and that the procedure be assessed in a way that is consistent with its operational use (Society for Industrial and Organizational Psychology, 1987). In the Blank and Fenton study, the use of a matched control group of 500 recruits resulted in a prevalence rate of 50 percent in the studied sample, which is substantially higher than what would be expected in the population of interest (i.e., Navy recruit applicants). The inflation of the prevalence rate upwardly biases the estimated predictive validity coefficient (i.e., the correlation between test results and turnover). Furthermore, the drug-positive group consisted only of identified marijuana users, whereas most organizations with a preemployment drug-testing program screen applicants on a wide variety of illicit substances. More importantly, recruits who tested positive for marijuana at selection, though retained by the Navy, were subject to follow-up and occasional random testing. Failing a subsequent drug test was grounds for dismissal. Thus, at least some of the turnover was probably a direct result of ongoing efforts to detect and discharge drug-using sailors and was not necessarily based on actual performance decrements or behavioral problems that might have resulted from the use of drugs. Moreover, since recruits who had tested positive for marijuana before induction were more likely to be tested subsequently then controls, a higher rate of dismissal for subsequent drug use would not show that they were more likely than the control group members to have used drugs after induction.

A large-scale attempt to assess the predictive efficacy of preemployment drug testing was conducted at the Boston general mail facility (Zwerling et al., 1990). The authors of this prospective study tested 4,964 job applicants in the Boston division of the U.S. Postal Service at the time of their preemployment medical examinations. Data from the urinalysis were collected for research purposes only and had no bearing (with the exception of positive opiates) on hiring or other employment decisions. Outcome measures were later obtained from personnel files (subjects were followed up, on average, for 406 calendar days). Of those tested, 2,537 applicants accepted the postal job offer. A proportional hazards model was used to analyze the data and to statistically control for age, sex, smoking, exercise status, race, and job classification. Identified marijuana users showed increased risks (relative risk ratio) of termination (1.56) (i.e., positive marijuana employees were 1.56 times more likely than negatives to turnover), accidents (1.55), injuries (1.85), disciplinary actions (1.55), and absenteeism (1.56) when compared with employees who tested negative. Cocaine positives showed an increased risk of absenteeism (2.37) and injuries (1.85).

One problem with this study is that the representativeness of the study sample (and therefore the generalizability of the results) was compromised by arbitrarily deleting whole applicant subgroups from the analyses (e.g., Hispanics, Native Americans, employees in professional or technical positions). If these individuals belong to the population of job applicants, then excluding them from the study sample limits the generalizability of the results and biases the parameter estimates. Furthermore, the authors elected to operationalize drug test results into discrete categories (e.g., marijuana, cocaine) rather than defining it as it is typically operationalized (positive on any drug versus negative on all drugs). Also, the use of statistical control techniques for potential confounding factors is questionable (Lord, 1967; Cochran and Rubin, 1973; Reichardt, 1979) when the predictive value of a selection device is being assessed.

Normand and Salyards (1989) reported the results of a large-scale longitudinal study that assessed the contribution of preemployment drug testing to the prediction of future job success. In this study, 5,465 U.S. Postal Service job applicants at 21 sites across the country were tested for use of illicit drugs as part of their preemployment medical examination. Test results were kept confidential and had no bearing on any subsequent personnel actions. Job outcome measures for 4,396 applicants who were hired were extracted from personnel records at four different time points (see Figures 7.1 and 7.2). After having been on the job for an average of 8.2 months, employees who tested positive were found to be absent at a rate 45 percent higher than those who tested negative (4 percent of scheduled work hours versus 3 percent). The drug-positive group also showed a 40 percent higher dismissal rate compared with the group testing negative for drugs (13 compared with 10 percent). A follow-up study indicated that, after an average of 1.3 years on the job, the observed absence and turnover differences between the two groups had increased substantially (Normand et al., 1990). The positive group showed a 59 percent higher rate of absenteeism (7 compared with 4 percent) and a 47 percent higher rate of firing (15 compared with 11 percent) compared with those testing negative. Despite a

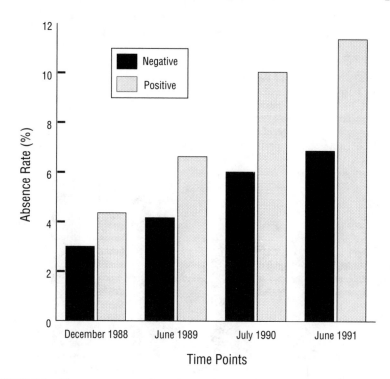

FIGURE 7.1 Absence rates at four time points. NOTE: employee tenure: 8.2 months, 1.3 years, 2.4 years, and 3.3 years.

high level of statistical power in this study (the probability of detecting even weak effects exceeded 0.95 in this study), no significant associations were detected between drug test results and accidents and injuries.

In July 1990, after having been on the job for an average of 2.4 years, both the absenteeism and turnover disparities across the two groups had further increased: the positive group's absenteeism and firing rates were found to be 66 and 69 percent higher, respectively, than those of the negative group (Normand and Salyards, 1991). Finally, after 3.3 years on the job, the disparity in absenteeism rates plateaued at 66 percent, whereas the disparity in firing rates had increased to 77 percent (Normand and Salyards, 1992). As part of this latest follow-up, the investigator examined more specific indicators of job absence. A notable finding was that the observed disparities in absenteeism rates across the two groups were mirrored when annual absence frequencies were examined (30.61 compared with 18.75). Furthermore, more specific analyses by type of leave (sick leave, leave without pay, and absent without official leave—AWOL) showed that the

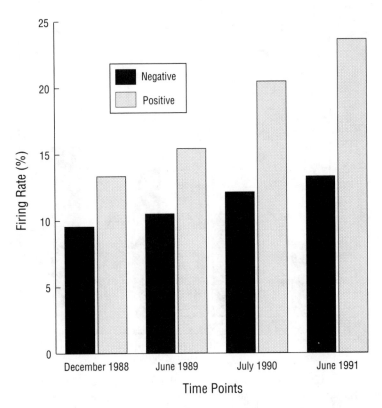

FIGURE 7.2   Firing rates at four time points.   NOTE: employee tenure: 8.2 months, 1.3 years, 2.4 years, and 3.3 years.

disparities across groups were greatest for AWOLs, the most dysfunctional leave type. This latest update also extracted information pertaining to disciplinary infractions (Figure 7.3) and employee assistance program referrals (Figure 7.4). Results indicated that the employees who tested positive for drugs at preemployment were much more likely to be formally disciplined (a risk ratio of 2.44) and to experience problems requiring the intervention of an employee assistance program (EAP) (a risk ratio of 2.67). Further analyses revealed that the most common disciplinary action was due to attendance infractions and that the most commonly diagnosed EAP assessment problem at induction was alcohol-related. Employees who tested positive were 3.47 times more likely to be referred to an EAP for drinking problems and 5.69 times more likely to be referred for drug abuse problems as those who tested negative. A similar pattern was observed when medical claims data were examined (see Figure 7.5). The drug-positive employees were

3.42 times more likely as drug-negative employees to file medical claims having alcohol or drug-related diagnosis. Accident and injury rates continued to show no difference.

The generalizability of the results of this study may be limited by the peculiarities of the work setting. That is, the positive rates and outcome measures distributions may not necessarily be reflective of other organizational settings. Until more empirical studies of this kind are carried out, one will not be able to determine with a high degree of accuracy to what extent these results can be generalized to other organizations. One factor that further complicates the generalizability issue is the change in prevalence rates of illicit drug use over time. The proportion of people in the general population who use illicit drugs has been declining relatively quickly since 1980. Such fluctuations in the prevalence of drug use are bound to affect the rate of positive preemployment drug-test results and consequently the effectiveness of preemployment drug-testing programs.

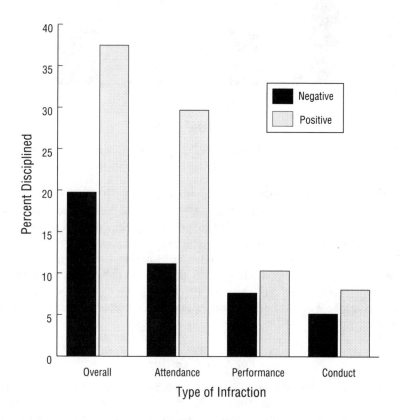

FIGURE 7.3 Disciplinary actions: drug-test results by infraction.

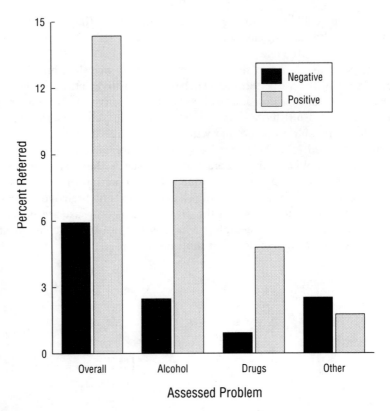

FIGURE 7.4 EAP referrals: drug-test results by problem identification.

This study also highlights the importance of the perspective in which statistics are presented. For example, a 77 percent higher rate of firing after 3 years may suggest great benefits to preemployment drug screening and the policy of not hiring positive testers. However, as depicted in Figure 7.2, 76 percent of those who tested positive at preemployment had not been fired after 3 years, compared with 86 percent of those testing negative. This represents a 10 percent absolute difference between groups in retention rates, which appears to be less drastic than the reported 77 percent higher rate of firing.

For-Cause Testing

Only two published studies are available that attempt to evaluate the effectiveness of for-cause drug-testing programs (Crouch et al., 1989; Sheridan and Winkler, 1989). Each of these studies appeared in a nonrefereed publi-

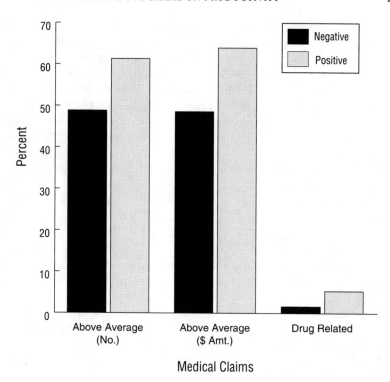

FIGURE 7.5 Drug-test results by medical claims information: number, dollar amount, and drug-related claims.

cation. Crouch et al. (1989) compared employees (N = 12) who tested positive in a for-cause drug-testing program to a control group (N = 47) selected from the total employee pool who had similar demographic characteristics at the Utah Power and Light Company. Retrospective employment information was collected over a 2-year period. The mean number of sick hours accumulated by the drug-positive group was 75.3 compared with the control mean of 55.8. Employees testing positive used an average of 63.8 hours of unexcused leave compared with 18.7 hours for the control group. An analysis of vehicle accidents revealed that the identified drug users were significantly more likely to be involved in an accident compared with the matched control group. These differences were all found to be statistically significant. Surprisingly, a comparison of the medical expenditures used by each group indicated that the control group's use of medical benefits ($719) actually exceeded that of the drug-positive group ($504).

Findings from a similar study conducted at Georgia Power Company (Sheridan and Winkler, 1989; Winkler and Sheridan, 1989) compared employees who tested positive in a for-cause drug-testing program to a control group on the use of medical benefits, absenteeism, and accidents. Drug-positive and control groups were matched on sex, age, ethnicity, job category, and length of service in an attempt to control for nonrandom selection of subjects. When compared with their controls, individuals testing positive used significantly more medical benefits ($1,377 compared with $163), showed greater absenteeism (165 compared with 47 hours of yearly absenteeism), and had a higher rates of vehicular accidents (23 compared with 11 percent).

These two studies, however, are fraught with both conceptual and methodological difficulties. From a conceptual view point, it is not clear whether the objective of these studies was to evaluate the impact of a for-cause drug-testing program or the impact of individual drug use on productivity indices. Because both studies attempted to isolate, through matching techniques, the effect of testing positive from potential individual confounding factors, the intent appears to be to assess the impact of drug use on outcome measures, rather than to isolate the effect of the for-cause drug-testing programs on outcome measures.

Methodologically, however, the matching technique used is inadequate to this task. Matching has serious, well-recognized methodological weaknesses (Campbell and Erlebacher, 1975; Campbell and Stanley, 1966; Cochran and Rubin, 1973; Craig and Metze, 1979; Kerlinger, 1986; Reichardt, 1979) that are exacerbated in these studies for two reasons. First, the drug-tested group may have been selected in part by behaviors related to the dependent variables and, second, drug use, which was a basis for separating the groups, is no doubt correlated with a number of variables on which the subjects are not matched and that are plausibly related to the dependent variables. Thus, these two studies cannot tell us whether for-cause drug testing deters drug use or affects an organization's productivity, and they provide no reliable information on the effects of drug use on job-related performance measures.

Random Drug Testing

The committee was not able to locate any published studies that examine the effects of random drug testing on the productivity of the work force. The published literature on the effects of random drug testing consists mostly of descriptive reports of trends. Deterrence effects of random testing programs are often inferred from observed decreases in positive drug test rates, which frequently follow the implementation of such programs (Osborn and Sokolov, 1989; Taggart, 1989). However, the evaluation of random drug-testing programs is complicated by the fact that very few, if any, corporations have implemented such programs in isolation. Most corporations with random drug-testing programs have also implemented applicant and/or for-cause drug-testing programs. This makes it difficult to isolate the effect of random drug testing on productivity. The trend studies done to date have not overcome these difficulties, for they lack the kinds of controls that would allow one to confidently attribute observed changes in drug-use patterns to the implementation of random drug-testing programs. Furthermore, even if a reduction in drug use could be attributed to the implementation of a random drug-testing program, this would not in itself be evidence that the program has affected productivity. More research and more sophisticated research is clearly needed. Information on the relative effectiveness of the various components of a universal drug-testing program (i.e., applicant, for-cause, and random drug-testing programs) would be useful to business and could have substantial policy relevance.

Workplace Drug Testing and Productivity

What can we conclude from the extant research on the efficacy of drug-testing programs? Contrary to what certain popular publications or newsletters may indicate, there are few empirically based conclusions that may be reached concerning the effectiveness of drug-testing programs in improving workplace productivity. The two for-cause drug-testing evaluation studies published to date suffer from serious methodological problems that preclude any scientific assessment of the impact of for-cause testing on work force productivity, and no evidence evaluating the effects of random drug testing on worker productivity has yet appeared in the published literature. Enough studies of preemployment drug-testing programs have been published with sufficiently consistent results that we can conclude that preemployment drug-test results are, in at least some job settings, valid predictors of some job-related behaviors. Those who test positive for drugs before employment are, as a group, likely to have higher rates of absenteeism, turnover, and disciplinary actions than those who test negative (Blank and Fenton, 1989; Normand et al., 1990; Zwerling et al., 1990).

In addition, it appears that preemployment drug-test results are also predictive of subsequent alcohol and drug problems. Salyards (1993) reported that job applicants who tested positive were 3.47 times more likely to be referred to an EAP for drinking problems and 5.69 times more likely to be referred for drug abuse problems as those testing negative at preemployment. Furthermore, drug-positive individuals were 3.42 times more likely as other employees to file medical claims involving an alcohol- or drug-related diagnosis. Blank and Fenton (1989) found that 14 percent of marijuana-positive Navy recruits were discharged for drug- or alcohol-related problems compared with 1 percent of those who tested negative.

These figures do not necessarily mean, however, that preemployment drug testing is a cost-effective selection program. Finding that job applicants' drug-test results are predictive of critical job behaviors means that employers can select, on average, more productive workers if they attend to drug test information than if that information is not used to make hiring decisions. However, as with any other type of selection program, the predictive efficacy of drug test results depends on a few critical selection parameters. In particular, the prevalence of drug use among potential job applicants has to be sufficiently large to yield meaningful measures of association between test results and the outcome measure and to justify the cost of testing (see Chapter 6 for discussion on low base rate). Thus a test that is cost-effective and predictively valid at one point in time may cease to be or, conversely, may become even more useful, if the pattern of drug use in the larger population changes.

Another important characteristic of most of the preemployment drug studies we have reviewed is that they have used analytical drug-testing procedures that conform with the guidelines of the National Institute on Drug Abuse. Many private organizations (especially smaller employers) that test today use less stringent testing procedures and methods that introduce sources of error that can be expected to make their programs less efficacious than the programs that have been studied to date (Murphy and Thornton, 1992a).

It is also possible for employers to overweight preemployment drug-test results. In the best studies done to date, employers chose applicants using the cues they ordinarily apply without reference to evidence of drug use. The research shows that, among this group, those who tested positive performed worse by certain job-related criteria than those who showed no evidence of recent drug use. The studies do not show that positive testers performed worse than those who would have replaced them had they been rejected on the basis of drug-test information. In particular, there is a danger that, if drug-test results trump other signs that warn of job difficulties, negative drug testers will be preferred to positive testers who exceed them on job-related criteria. A major gap in the extant research is its failure to examine the interaction of recent drug usage and other job-related applicant characteristics. Although the studies show preemployment drug testing to be predictively valid, they also indicate that many applicants who test positive could be hired without producing any job-related difficulties.

CONCEPTUAL INCONGRUITIES IN RESEARCH METHODS

Conceptual Issues

As stated at the beginning of this chapter, considerable confusion surrounds the basic evaluation research issue of how to assess the efficacy of drug-testing intervention programs. Most studies we reviewed claim to be investigating the same basic issue (i.e., the efficacy of drug-testing programs on productivity), and many employ similar designs. In many instances, however, the methods used to compare the work outcomes of drug-positive employees with those found to be drug-negative (or a matched drug-negative control group) are conceptually distinct from one another and reflect divergent research purposes. This state of affairs can be attributed to a lack of clarity in defining the research purpose.

Central to any scientific investigation is an analysis of the problem situation and a clear-cut formulation of the research purpose. Broadly speaking, a research study may be designed primarily for the purpose of explaining or predicting phenomena (e.g., see Cook and Campbell, 1979). In explanatory research, the emphasis is on identifying variables and understanding the processes by which they influence the phenomenon of interest. Establishing that covariation among variables exists is not sufficient. What is sought is an explanation as to why variables covary (Blalock, 1968). The hope is that by understanding the conditions that influence these phenomena, researchers and policy makers will be in a better position to recommend courses of action that will help to alleviate individual, organizational, and social woes. The task is difficult to accomplish. Most problems in the social and behavioral sciences have multiple and entangled causes that are often difficult to identify, isolate, and measure. Because the number of possible causal patterns among variables is virtually infinite, it is necessary to rely on theory to provide guidance and direction (James et al., 1982) in attempts to explain why observed differences exist. Theory confirmed by data can provide powerful explanations.

In predictive research, the emphasis is on studying the degree of covariation among variables and using this information to make predictions about subjects' future behavior or performance. Predictive research does not require a theoretical framework to proceed, even though theory may play a role in the initial development or selection of predictor variables and may be useful in generating finer predictions. Prediction is particularly important in practical applications, for example, the selection of applicants for employment, college entrance, and training programs. Prediction studies are descriptive by nature—they describe differences and examine their potential impact on aggregate outcomes.

The appropriateness of the methods used to assess the efficacy of an intervention program depends on the goals or purpose of the programs and the evaluation. If the primary objective for implementing drug-testing programs is to enhance work force productivity, what is crucial to the evaluation of preemployment testing is the predictive validity of drug test results (Society for Industrial and Organizational Psychology, 1987). If the drug test results are found to be valid predictors of critical job outcome measures, the average quality of new employees is likely to improve by implementing a selection program that takes drug test results into account. Evidence that such a program is predictively valid (i.e., that it enhances the average quality of the selected workers) means that the *program* has an effect on aggregate measures (e.g., mean value) of the outcome variables— not that *drug use* has an effect on the outcome variables. This is equally true of assessments of postemployment, for-cause, and random drug-testing programs. To evaluate their efficacy is to assess the impact of implementing the programs on productivity measures and not the impact of individual drug use on productivity measures. Within this framework, controlling for potential individual confounding variables (e.g., Crouch et al., 1989; Sheridan and Winkler, 1989; Winkler and Sheridan, 1989; Zwerling et al., 1990, 1992) is irrelevant and potentially erroneous.

There seems to be an implicit notion in the evaluation literature on drug intervention that negative employment behaviors or outcomes must be shown to be due to the effects of drug use, separate from other "extraneous" influences, in order to establish the efficiency of a drug intervention program. This might possibly explain why so many drug intervention evaluation studies employ matching or statistical control procedures. The notion that drug use must be causally linked to critical employment criteria (otherwise why control for the effects of other influences?) goes well beyond the requirements for establishing the efficacy of drug intervention programs on productivity. As we note elsewhere in this report (see Chapter 5), it may be that drug use is more of a symptom of problematic job behavior than a cause, at least for the early stages of drug involvement.

These comments are not intended to detract from the importance of carrying out studies that attempt to untangle the complex causal relationship between drug use and problem behavior at work or elsewhere. Indeed, even though program evaluation and understanding human behaviors are different research issues, there is an important practical intersection. The better we understand the relationship between drug use and problem behavior, the more likely we are to be able to design an efficacious intervention program. In doing so, we can limit the unfairness that results from false negative predictions that have negative consequences for individuals. Moreover, in certain situations, it may be wrong or even illegal to employ valid selection programs. Thus there are reasons for research on drug-testing programs to control for individual variables. The reasons, however, are not to ascertain whether drug-testing programs have predictive validity but rather to further specify the conditions under which individual drug use influences individual performance. Because of conceptual confusion, statistical and matching techniques tend to be used for the former purpose.

The type or nature of drug-testing programs (preemployment, for-cause, or random) is another factor that is critical to the selection of an adequate evaluation strategy, because different types of drug-testing programs have different objectives. Program objectives determine the research purpose, which in turn dictate the choice of the study design and methods (e.g., variables to be measured, their operationalization, and statistical models) to be used. Unfortunately, most organizations that implement such testing programs do not articulate their program objectives clearly. This complicates matters for a researcher charged with evaluating the effectiveness of these programs. The lack of congruency between research purpose and method is an underlying source of much of the current conceptual and interpretational confusion regarding acceptable strategies for assessing the efficacy of drug intervention programs. To deal with this problem, researchers must secure clear statements of the program goals before designing their studies, and they must specify the goals that have motivated their evaluations in writing their research reports.

Cost-Effectiveness of Drug-Testing Programs

Two distinct audiences use the results of cost-effectiveness evaluations of intervention programs: policy makers and program administrators (or organizational decision makers). These groups need different types of information in order to make informed decisions. Policy makers, for example, are particularly concerned with the costs and benefits associated with various drug intervention programs (e.g., treatment modalities, testing) for society as a whole, while organizational decision makers need program-specific information pertaining to the costs and benefits of programs in their organizations or organizations like theirs.

Business decision makers want to know whether drug intervention programs enhance productivity, and if so, whether the consequent financial benefits justify program expenditures (relative to the costs of not intervening or to implementing another intervention). Unlike the cost of illness studies that are reviewed in Chapter 5, cost factors such as criminal activities, social welfare, incarceration, and early death were not typically included in utility models implemented by business. It is not that these factors are unimportant, but, from a business perspective, the interest is on relatively short-term return on investment at the organizational level. This is in contrast to policy decision makers, who are more interested in the long-term economic impact of broad policy change on society's welfare.

Only two peer-reviewed studies (Normand et al., 1990; Zwerling et al., 1992) have reported empirical estimates of the costs and benefits associated with implementing a drug-testing program. Both of these were carried out within the U.S. Postal Service and dealt with preemployment drug testing. In both instances the findings revealed that preemployment drug testing was a cost-efficient selection program. However, both studies neglected to include some important parameters into their models (e.g., variable cost, corporate taxes). Since there have been almost no empirical studies of the cost-effectiveness of drug-testing programs, it appears that decisions by organizations to adopt such programs have often been made without a well-grounded consideration of the likely benefits associated with their implementation. To the extent that governmental pressure has induced such programs, this is particularly likely to be the case.

There is a substantial body of literature that deals with the difficult issue of translating the statistical impact of organizational intervention programs into financial productivity indicators (i.e., dollars). Researchers in human resource management and related fields have applied the methods of utility analysis to estimate the probable benefits of programs ranging from ability testing to improved performance appraisal and feedback (see Boudreau, 1991; Jones and Wright, 1992; and Judiesch et al., 1992 for recent reviews of utility estimation techniques).

Both the utility and fairness of preemployment drug testing as a selection device depend in part on the type of employment errors that result from implementing such programs. Two types of errors are of concern. First, as discussed in Chapter 6, false positive classification error (mislabeling an individual as a drug user when in reality he or she is not a user) not only is disconcerting but also reduces the efficacy of the selection process. In the case of drug testing, it is well established that, when performed by a competent (NIDA-certified) laboratory, the rate of false-positive classification is virtually zero. But the superficial screening tests used by some businesses without confirmation increase the probability of false-positive classification error substantially. Second, and numerically more important, are what can be thought of as false-negative prediction errors. There will always be a number of applicants who test positive who would have been successful in their jobs had they been hired; to judge by the findings reported in the studies reviewed in this chapter, these falsely negative prediction errors will constitute the majority of drug-positive job applicants. False negative prediction errors also affect the efficacy of drug-testing programs, and minimizing them will increase a program's benefit-cost ratio.

This discussion of false-positive and false-negative errors should not obscure a central fact: the use of a valid selection program increases the proportion of successful new hires over what would be obtained had the selection program not been implemented. The prevalence of errors does affect the magnitude of the gains from a cost-benefit standpoint, so totally apart from fairness there are reasons to work to minimize them.

EFFECTS OF DRUG TESTING ON
ATTITUDES AND MORALE

Another issue that merits discussion is the impact of drug-testing programs on the attitudes and morale of applicants and employees. Despite its increasing frequency, employee drug testing is still controversial. Several authors (e.g., Crant and Bateman, 1989; Murphy et al., 1990, 1991; Stone and Kotch, 1988) have suggested that workers and job applicants may react negatively to drug testing. Although different studies yield different estimates of the frequency of negative reactions, it is common for 40 to 50 percent of those surveyed to express reservations about employee drug testing (Hanson, 1990; Konovsky and Cropanzano, 1993; Murphy et al., 1990).

Attitudes toward drug testing may affect the behavior of applicants and incumbents, especially if drug testing involves policies or procedures that are objectionable to large numbers of individuals (Chadwick-Jones et al., 1982; Goodman and Friedman, 1971). In particular, attitudes toward practices such as drug testing may affect an individual's job search and job choice and his or her subsequent satisfaction with the job and the organization (Murphy and Thornton, 1992b; Schwab et al., 1987).

Murphy and Thornton (1992b) present evidence that individuals with negative attitudes toward drug testing are less likely to apply to, and may be less likely to accept, jobs in organizations that test for drugs. Their study suggests that attitudes toward drug testing and the probability that attitudes would affect subsequent job search behavior were largely unrelated to grades and academic qualifications, which implies that highly qualified applicants are as likely as less qualified applicants to be influenced in their job choices by their attitudes toward testing. Given the frequency of negative reactions to drug testing and the possible consequences of those attitudes, it is important to examine the ways in which specific characteristics of drug-testing programs affect attitudes and to explore ways in which negative reactions to drug testing might be minimized. The apparent efficacy of preemployment drug testing could be illusory if testing programs bias applicant pools so as to overrepresent those with few job options.

Influence of Job Characteristics

Reactions to employee drug testing vary substantially, depending on the job in question (Murphy and Thornton, 1992b; Murphy et al., 1991). In general, the higher the likelihood that impaired job performance could pose a danger to an individual, his or her coworkers, and the public, the higher the level of approval for drug testing. Thus, drug testing is likely to be seen as more acceptable for airline pilots than for accountants. Murphy et al. suggest that drug testing will also meet with higher levels of approval if the job involves activities or functions that are believed to be substantially impaired by drug use. Finally, there is evidence that drug testing is more common and more likely to be accepted in lower-level jobs than in managerial and executive jobs (Murphy and Thornton, 1992a).

Influence of Program Characteristics

There is considerable evidence that the policies and practices that define employee drug-testing programs can substantially affect reactions to drug testing. First, employee drug testing may be seen as an invasion of privacy, which is likely to lead to negative reactions (Stone and Stone, 1990). Urine testing is an especially sensitive procedure; the need to provide urine samples strikes many people as offensive, and the need to do so in front of witnesses or under tightly monitored conditions may seem particularly offensive. Privacy-related concerns might also be more salient in situations in which drug tests provide information about behavior outside the workplace. For example, it is well known that an individual who is a chronic user of marijuana can test positive for days or even weeks after having stopped using the drug, and that marijuana use that is completely divorced from the work setting can nevertheless lead to a positive drug test.

Research on attitudes toward drug testing and on perceptions of justice and equity in organizations (e.g., Konovsky and Cropanzano, 1993; Murphy et al., 1990) suggests that there are three factors that substantially affect the likelihood of negative reactions. First, drug-testing programs vary in the extent to which they are seen as reasonable. Testing programs that are restricted to high-risk occupations, or that are clearly and convincingly justified by management, are not likely to be a significant source of controversy. Second, drug-testing programs vary in the extent to which their overall orientation is seen as punitive. Testing programs that result in severe or irrevocable sanctions (e.g., dismissal) are more likely to be seen in a negative light than programs that are designed to help people deal constructively with substance abuse (e.g., by recommending counseling). Finally, drug-testing programs that involve consultation between labor and management are less likely to be seen in a negative light than those that are unilaterally imposed by management.

Limitations of Research on Reactions to Drug Testing

In evaluating research on attitudes toward drug testing, there are two reasons for caution in making broad generalizations. First, the majority of the studies in this area have employed convenience samples, usually college students. The attitudes of college students might differ in a number of ways from those of a general work force population (Murphy et al., 1991). Second, these studies often employ simulation methods (e.g., asking students to go through a simulated job interview) whose external validity is unclear (for an exception, see Murphy and Thornton, 1992b). The fact that an individual is willing to turn down a job offer in an experimental simulation does not necessarily predict behavior in real job interviews.

One of the few studies that has investigated the reactions of work force members is the High School Senior follow-up surveys (Patrick O'Malley, personal communication, 1992). These follow-up surveys show that, in general, most young adults are supportive of both preemployment and postemployment drug testing. In 1991, 65 percent "approved" or "strongly approved" of urine tests as a condition for getting a job like their own job, and 60 percent approved of urine tests as a condition for keeping a job such as their own. These figures reflect increases of about 15 percent in approval since 1987; for getting a job, the 1987 figure was 49 percent, and for keeping a job, the 1987 figure was 46 percent.

Approval rates have consistently been slightly higher among those who had actually been required to take a urine test. In 1991, among those who had been tested, either pre- or postemployment, 78 percent approved of preemployment testing compared with 61 percent of those who had not been tested. Postemployment testing was approved by 70 percent of those who had been tested, compared with 57 percent of those who had not been tested. These differences may reflect the types of people who get tested, positive experience with drug testing, or cognitive dissonance resulting from consent to a previously disapproved procedure.

On the basis of the research literature reviewed in this chapter, the committee provides the following conclusions and recommendations.

CONCLUSIONS AND RECOMMENDATIONS

• The empirical evidence pertaining to the efficacy of preemployment drug testing indicates that such programs may be useful to employers in choosing wisely among job applicants. However, regardless of the magnitude of the correlations between drug use and dysfunctional job behavior measures, the practical effectiveness of any drug-testing program depends on other parameters such as the prevalence of drug use in the population tested. The presence of significant relationships between drug use and workplace performance measures does not necessarily mean that an effective drug-testing program will substantially improve work force performance, and a program that substantially improves performance with some employees or in some job settings may do little to improve performance with other employees or in other job settings.

• Despite beliefs to the contrary, the preventive effects of drug-testing programs have never been adequately demonstrated. Although, there are some suggestive data (e.g., see the military data in Chapter 3) that allude to the deterrent effect of employment drug-testing programs, there is as yet no conclusive scientific evidence from properly controlled studies that employment drug-testing programs widely discourage drug use or encourage rehabilitation.

Recommendation: Longitudinal research should be conducted to determine whether drug-testing programs have deterrent effects.

•   Many studies of alcohol and other drug use by the work force have been flawed in their design and implementation. Organizations that conduct their own drug studies can, by encouraging their researchers to publish in professional journals, enhance quality control and contribute to a knowledge base that will enable them to deal more effectively with future alcohol and other drug problems.

•   Different objectives have been suggested for work site drug-testing and diverse alcohol and other drug intervention programs. These include improving workers' performance, preventing accidents, saving on health costs, and working toward a drug-free society by deterring drug use. The effectiveness of alcohol and other drug intervention programs cannot be adequately evaluated unless the goals of such programs are clear.

Recommendation: Organizations should clearly articulate their objectives prior to initiating alcohol and other drug intervention programs and should regularly evaluate their programs in light of these objectives.

Among job applicants and workers, testing for drugs other than alcohol is already common and generally accepted. Of young men in a 1991 general population survey of high school graduates, 33 percent reported that they had been tested, 61 percent reported that they approved of preemployment testing, and 60 percent reported that they approved of postemployment testing. Approval rates were even higher among those who had been tested.

•   Very little is known about what happens to job applicants who are not hired or to employees who are fired as a consequence of a positive drug test.

Recommendation: Research should be conducted on the impact of drug-testing programs with attention not only to those who remain within the organization as well as to those who are not hired or are dismissed. In particular, more information is needed about the impact of drug-testing programs on the health and productivity of the work force.

Recommendation: In light of the relatively low rates of alcohol and other drug abuse among the work force (see Chapter 3), the moderate predictive validity of testing programs (see Chapter 7), and the fact that many factors other than drug use may cause performance deficiencies seen in drug users (see Chapter 5), drug-testing programs should not be viewed as a panacea for curing workplace performance problems. Nonetheless, drug-testing for safety-sensitive positions may still be justified in the interest of public safety.

REFERENCES

American Management Association
1992   *1992 AMA Survey on Workplace Drug Testing and Drug Abuse Policies.* New York: American Management Association.
Axel, H.
1990   *Corporate Experiences with Drug Testing Programs.* New York: The Conference Board.
Blalock, H.M.
1968   Theory building and causal inferences. In H.M. Blalock and A.B. Blalock, eds., *Methodology in Social Research.* New York: McGraw-Hill.
Blank, D.L., and J.W. Fenton
1989   Early employment testing for marijuana: demographic and employee retention patterns. Pp. 139-150 in S.W. Gust and J.M. Walsh, eds., *Drugs in the Workplace: Research and Evaluation Data.* Rockville, Md.: National Institute on Drug Abuse.
Boudreau, J.W.
1991   Utility analysis for decisions in human resource management. Pp. 621-746 in M. Dunnette and L. Hough, eds., *Handbook of Industrial and Organizational Psychology,* Vol. 2. Palo Alto, Calif.: Consulting Psychologists Press.
Bureau of the Census
1989   *Statistical Abstract of the United States, 1988.* Washington, D.C.: U.S. Department of Commerce.
Campbell, D.T., and A. Erlebacher
1975   How regression artifacts in quasi-experimental evaluations can mistakenly make compensatory education look harmful. Pp. 597-617 in E.L. Struening and M. Guttentag, eds., *Handbook of Evaluation Research.* Beverly Hills, Calif.: Sage Publications.
Campbell, D.T., and J.C. Stanley
1966   *Experimental and Quasi-Experimental Designs for Research.* Chicago: Rand McNally.
Chadwick-Jones, J.K., N. Nicholson, and C. Brown
1982   *The Social Psychology of Absenteeism.* New York: Praeger.
Cochran, W.G., and D.B. Rubin
1973   Controlling bias in observational studies: a review. *Sankhya, The Indian Journal of Statistics* 35:417-446.
Cook, T.D., and D.T. Campbell
1979   *Quasi-Experimentation: Design and Analysis Issues for Field Settings.* Chicago: Rand McNally.
Craig, J.R., and L.P. Metze
1979   *Methods of Psychological Research.* Philadelphia, Pa.: W.B. Saunders.

Crant, J.M., and T.S. Bateman
   1989   A model of employee responses to drug-testing programs. *Employee Responsibili-
           ties and Rights Journal* 2:173-190.
Crouch, D.J., D.O. Webb, L.V. Peterson, P.F. Buller, and D.E. Rollins
   1989   A critical evaluation of the Utah Power and Light Company's substance abuse pro-
           gram: absenteeism, accidents, and costs. Pp. 169-193 in S.W. Gust and J.M. Walsh,
           eds., *Drugs in the Workplace: Research and Evaluation Data.* Rockville, Md.:
           National Institute on Drug Abuse.
Employee Assistance Professional Association
   1991   *EAPA Exchange* October:23-25. Employee Assistance Professional Association,
           Alexandria, Va.
Goodman, P., and A. Friedman
   1971   An examination of Adams' theory of inequity. *Administrative Science Quarterly*
           16:271-288.
Hanson, A.
   1990   What employees say about drug testing. *Personnel* July:32-36.
Hayghe, H.V.
   1991   Anti-drug programs in the workplace: are they here to stay? *Monthly Labor Review*
           114:26-29.
James, L.R., S.A. Mulaik, and J.M. Brett
   1982   *Casual Analysis: Assumptions, Models, and Data.* Beverly Hills, Calif.: Sage
           Publications.
Jones, G.R., and Wright, P.M
   1992   An economic approach to conceptualizing the utility of human resource manage-
           ment practices. Pp. 271-300 in G. Ferris and K. Rowland, eds., *Research in Person-
           nel and Human Resources Management*, Vol. 10. Greenwich, Conn.: JAI Press.
Judiesch, M.K., F.L. Schmidt, and M.K. Mount
   1992   Estimates of the dollar value of employee output in utility analysis: an empirical
           test of two theories. *Journal of Applied Psychology* 77:234-250.
Kerlinger, F.N.
   1986   *Foundations of Behavioral Research*, 3rd ed. New York: Holt, Rinehart, and
           Winston.
Konovsky, M.A., and R. Cropanzano
   1993   Justice considerations in employee drug testing. In R. Cropanzano, ed., *Justice in
           the Workplace: Approaching Fairness in Human Resource Management.* Hillsdale,
           N.J.: Erlbaum. (In press.)
Lewy, R.
   1983   Preemployment qualitative urine toxicology screening. *Journal of Occupational
           Medicine* 25:579-580.
Lord, F.M.
   1967   A paradox in the interpretation of group comparisons. *Psychological Bulletin* 68:304-
           305.
Murphy, K.R., and G.C. Thornton, III
   1992a   Characteristics of employee drug testing programs. *Journal of Business and Psy-
           chology* 6:295-309.
   1992b   Development and validation of a measure of attitudes toward employee drug testing.
           Educational and Psychological Measurement 52:189-201.
Murphy, K.R., G.C. Thornton, III, and D.H. Reynolds
   1990   College students' attitudes toward employee drug testing programs. *Personnel Psy-
           chology* 43:615-631.

Murphy, K.R., G.C. Thornton, III, and K. Prue
1991   The influence of job characteristics on the acceptability of employee drug testing. *Journal of Applied Psychology* 76:447-453.

Normand, J., and S.D. Salyards
1989   An empirical evaluation of preemployment drug testing in the United States Postal Service: interim report of findings. Pp. 111-138 in S.W. Gust and J.M. Walsh, eds., *Drugs in the Workplace: Research and Evaluation Data.* Rockville, Md.: National Institute on Drug Abuse.
1991   Applicant Drug Testing: Update of a Longitudinal Study. Paper presented at the 1991 Annual Convention of the IPMA Assessment Council, Chicago, Illinois.
1992   Applicant Drug Testing: An Update of the Empirical Validation Evidence. Paper presented at the 7th annual conference of the Society for Industrial and Organizational Psychology, Montreal.

Normand, J., S.D. Salyards, and J.J. Mahoney
1990   An evaluation of preemployment drug testing. *Journal of Applied Psychology* 75:629-639.

Osborn, C.E., and J.J. Sokolov
1989   Drug use trends in a nuclear power company: cumulative data from an ongoing testing program. In S.W. Gust and J.M. Walsh, eds., *Drugs in the Workplace: Research and Evaluation Data.* NIDA Research Monograph 91. Rockville, Md.: National Institute on Drug Abuse.

Parish, D.C.
1989   Relation of the pre-employment drug testing result to employment status: a one-year follow-up. *Journal of General Internal Medicine* 4:44-47.

Reichardt, C.S.
1979   The statistical analysis of data from nonequivalent group designs. Pp. 147-205 in T.D. Cook and D.T. Campbell, eds., *Quasi-Experimentation: Design and Analysis Issues for Field Settings.* Chicago: Rand NcNally.

Salyards, S.D.
1993   Preemployment drug testing: associations with EAP, disciplinary, and medical claims information. *PharmChem Newsletter* 21(1):1-4.

Schwab, D.P., S.L. Rynes, and R.J. Aldag
1987   Theories and research on job choice. In K. Rowland and G. Ferris, eds., *Research in Personnel and Human Resource Management,* Vol. 5. Greenwich, Conn.: JAI Press.

Sheridan, J.R., and H. Winkler
1989   An evaluation of drug testing in the workplace. In S.W. Gust and J.M. Walsh, eds., *Drugs in the Workplace: Research and Evaluation Data.* NIDA Research Monograph 91. Rockville, Md.: National Institute on Drug Abuse.

Society for Industrial and Organizational Psychology
1987   *Principles for the Validation and Use of Personnel Selection Procedures,* 3rd ed. College Park, Md.: Division of Industrial-Organizational Psychology, American Psychological Association.

Stone, D.L., and D.A. Kotch
1988   Individuals' attitudes toward organizational drug testing policies and practices. *Journal of Applied Psychology* 74:518-521.

Stone, E.F, and D.L. Stone
1990   Privacy in organizations: theoretical issues, research findings, and protection mechanisms. In G. Ferris and K. Rowland, eds., *Research in Personnel and Human Resource Management,* Vol. 8. Greenwich, Conn.: JAI Press.

Taggart, R.W.
  1989   Results of the drug testing program at Southern Pacific Railroad. In S.W. Gust and
          J.M. Walsh, eds., *Drugs in the Workplace: Research and Evaluation Data*. NIDA
          Research Monograph 91. Rockville, Md.: National Institute on Drug Abuse.
U.S. Department of Labor
  1989   *Survey of Employer Anti-Drug Programs*. Washington, D.C.: U.S. Department of
          Labor.
Walsh, D.C., L. Elinson, and L. Gostin
  1992   Worksite drug testing. *Annual Review of Public Health* 13:197-221.
Winkler, H., and J. Sheridan
  1989   An Analysis of Workplace Behaviors of Substance Abusers. Paper presented at the
          National Institute on Drug Abuse conference on Drugs in the Workplace: Research
          and Evaluation Data, Bethesda, Md.
Zwerling, C., J. Ryan, and E.J. Orav
  1990   The efficacy of preemployment drug screening for marijuana and cocaine in predict-
          ing employment outcome. *Journal of the American Medical Association* 264:2639-
          2643.
  1992   Costs and benefits of preemployment drug screening. *Journal of the American
          Medical Association* 267:91-93.

8

Employee Assistance Programs

Everyday social settings and relationships figure importantly in the development and prevention of and recovery from alcohol and drug problems (Bacon, 1973). Next to the family, the workplace is probably the most important setting for shaping and constraining alcohol and other drug-related expectations and behavior (Beattie et al., 1992). This chapter examines three aspects of workplace responses to alcohol and other drug use. First, it briefly reviews some of the most popular activities and programs focused on prevention that have potential to impact alcohol and other drug use. The discussion then turns to employee assistance programs (EAPs). The chapter concludes by examining treatment issues as they relate to program entry, and treatment follow-up, and work site reentry.

PREVENTION ACTIVITIES

Organizations have attempted to minimize the effects of alcohol and other drug use on work settings through policy design and various health promotion activities. Among the most prominent workplace prevention activities are health promotion/wellness programs that have attempted to alter individual risk factors, such as smoking, obesity, and untreated hypertension, that are often associated with alcohol and other drug use.

Fielding and Piserchia (1989) examined data from the Office of Disease Prevention and Health Promotion's 1985 National Survey of Worksite Health Promotion Activities. This survey involved telephone interviews with representatives of 1,358 work sites randomly selected from the 1984 Dun and Bradstreet list of businesses that had work sites with 50 or more employees. The response rate was over 80 percent. Of the responding companies, 66 percent reported offering one or more types of health promotion activities, including health risk assessments, smoking cessation, blood pressure control, exercise/fitness, weight control, nutrition education, stress management, back care, and accident prevention. The average number of activities offered was under three, for those companies that offered any. Participation in wellness programs was not very high, and most activities were offered only once or intermittently, not regularly or continuously.

Work site wellness programs are quite varied (Roman and Blum, 1988; Blum et al., 1990). The services that are described as wellness or health promotion programs range from establishing a smoking policy, to offering an occasional health education class or newsletter, to a comprehensive array of interventions that include health risk screening, follow-up counseling, a menu of health improvement interventions, and organization-level activities designed to provide an environment supportive of health (Heirich et al., 1992).

Health Promotion and Wellness Programs

A number of investigators have voiced the hypothesis that wellness or health promotion programs can help reduce the consumption of alcohol and other drugs (Room, 1981; Nathan, 1984; Case, 1985; Moskowitz, 1989; Shain, 1990). However, there is no substantial body of literature that explores whether wellness programs can reduce the use of alcohol and other drugs or identifies specific wellness services that might be effective in preventing alcohol and other drug use (Sonnenstuhl, 1988). Although there is a considerable literature reporting on work-site wellness programs, the literature is largely descriptive. Studies tend to use self-selected subjects and often have no control or comparison groups. Typically, short-term program results—because of the frequency of relapse in these targeted behaviors (e.g., smoking, weight loss)—tell us little about long-term behavioral change. Another characteristic of these studies is that most empirical evaluations are performed on comprehensive programs. These programs typically target a variety of risk factors (e.g., smoking, alcohol use, overweight, hypertension) associated with health promotion, making it difficult to assess the effectiveness of individual components in successfully reducing specific health risk factors (e.g., smoking, alcohol use). Nonetheless, some studies have reported positive evaluation results of specific prevention services in addressing specific risk behaviors. For example, studies have shown a short-term reduction in alcohol consumption after participation in wellness classes or seminars. However, no studies have demonstrated persistent, long-term effects.

Rohsenow et al. (1985) provided stress management training to a group of 15 heavy social drinkers among college students and compared results with a control group of 21 students. They found a short-term reduction in drinking, but a return to baseline by 5.5 months. Shain et al. (1986) reported the results of a 6-hour work-site wellness seminar designed to increase knowledge and awareness of health issues that was attended by some 56 percent of the work force. The heaviest drinkers reported reduction in their weekly consumption of alcohol after participation. However, there were no data to validate self-reports, no comparison or control group, and no measures of long-term maintenance of reported changes. A second study involved a 15-hour course in relaxation and stress management. Heavy drinkers maintained their levels of consumption, but moderate drinkers showed significant decreases. No such decreases were found in a comparison group. There was again no long-term follow-up to ascertain that these changes were maintained over time.

In another study, Shain (1990) surveyed public transportation workers and found that 12 percent of the work force (17 percent of the drinkers) reported concern about their drinking level, as well as about other health risks. Those concerned about their drinking had more health concerns generally than those not concerned about their drinking. The concerned heavy drinkers tended to be overweight and inactive, often got less than 6 hours of sleep, and reported being stressed at work. Nearly three-fourths of them smoked, and over one-third reported having used illicit drugs. This suggests that health promotion programs may be able to raise and address drinking issues by first addressing other health issues and then demonstrating the relevance of drinking to health.

One study utilized a quasi-experimental design to compare four different types of work site wellness programs implemented in four demographically similar manufacturing plants. The study tested the effectiveness of the four program models at reducing obesity, cigarette smoking, and high blood pressure over a 3-year time period. The four models were (1) *fitness center*: an in-plant fitness center equipped with muscle-toning and aerobic equipment and staffed by athletic trainers; (2) *health education*: regular offering of health education classes and media information about health risks; (3) *outreach and counseling*: health education classes and media information coupled with one-to-one and small-group interventions, managed by wellness counselors who regularly contacted and counseled employees with health risks; and (4) *outreach, counseling, and plant organization*: the services just listed, plus plant-wide support services and activities to encourage healthful behaviors (Erfurt et al., 1991).

The study reported after a 3-year follow-up that many more people took part in health improvement interventions when personal outreach and counseling were provided to the employees with health risks (Erfurt et al., 1990). At the two sites that did not provide personal outreach and counseling (the fitness center site and the health education site), impact on blood pressure control for hypertensive employees was minimal, and the overweight employees gained weight. At the two sites that provided personal outreach and counseling, blood pressure was significantly reduced among hypertensive employees, and overweight employees lost weight. There was a decrease in the prevalence of smoking at all four sites (paralleling national trends), but the decrease was greater at the sites with outreach and counseling, and the relapse rate was lower (Erfurt et al., 1991). Similar findings on the positive impact of follow-up contact and support have been reported in other studies of wellness program services for various health risks (Gregg et al., 1990; Perri et al., 1984; King et al., 1988; Taylor et al., 1990). One recent study (Gomel et al., 1993) randomly assigned 28 work sites to one of four intervention groups: (1) health risk assessment, (2) risk factor education, (3) behavioral counseling, and (4) behavior counseling plus incentives in an attempt to evaluate the relative efficacy of these work-site health promotion programs on various disease risk factors. The results showed that higher rates of continuous smoking cessation and weight loss were observed for the two behavioral counseling conditions after 3-, 6-, and 12-month follow-up.

Effects of Interventions on Work-Related Outcome Measures

From a business perspective, in addition to improving the health status of employees, employers are also concerned about whether such intervention programs have any impact on work-related outcome measures. Several studies suggest that an effective work site wellness program can reduce absenteeism and employee benefit claims and can show a positive cost-benefit ratio.

Gibbs et al. (1985) examined insurance claims for employees who participated in Blue Cross and Blue Shield of Indiana's employee health promotion program, compared with nonparticipating employees at the same work site. Program components included health risk screening, assessment, and feedback; group programs for nutrition, weight loss, smoking cessation, and fitness; and individual counseling for alcohol and drug abuse. Participants had higher claims in the 6-month period after the program began, but costs declined in relation to nonparticipants for subsequent periods. Over a 5-year period after the commencement of the program, participants averaged 24 percent lower health care costs than nonparticipants. The cost of operating the program was about $100 per employee per year. Savings due to reductions in health care claims exceeded program costs by a factor of

1.45. The longer time period evaluated in this study is an improvement over previous studies, but the self-selection of participants is a design weakness likely to exaggerate the beneficial effects of participation.

Bertera (1990) examined absenteeism changes associated with a comprehensive health promotion program. He compared 41 intervention sites with 19 demographically equivalent control sites in the same company. The program included smoking cessation, fitness, weight management, cholesterol control, stress management, and healthy back programs. There were group meetings and individual counseling as well as self-directed materials, competitions, and incentive programs.

Data on disability days (days lost due to illness) were collected for blue-collar employees for a 1-year baseline (preprogram) period and 2 program years. Similar data were not available for white-collar employees. The employees at the intervention sites experienced a 14 percent reduction in disability days by the end of 2 years, compared with a 6 percent decline at the control sites. This produced a return of $2.05 per dollar invested by the end of the second year. This study is particularly strong because it compares changes for all employees at the experimental and control sites, not just self-selected participants.

Bly et al. (1986) explored the relationship between exposure to a work site health promotion program and health care costs and utilization. The experience of employees exposed to a comprehensive program of health screening, lifestyle improvement programs, and work site changes to support healthier lifestyles was compared over a 5-year period with employees at other work sites in the same company that did not have this program. To account for baseline differences, analyses of covariance produced adjusted means for inpatient hospital costs, admissions, hospital days, outpatient costs, and other health costs. Mean annual inpatient cost increases were about $43 for the experimental group and $76 for the control group, and the experimental group also had lower rates of increase in hospital days and admissions. This study had a strong research design, comparing sites that did and did not have access to the program. It also covered a substantially longer time period than most of the other studies, lending credence to the results.

As the above review suggests, apart from drug-testing programs, few work site prevention efforts have been directed at illicit drugs. Most health promotion programs or drug prevention programs have targeted alcohol and smoking as the primary drugs of interest. The evaluation studies reviewed above indicate that such programs can be effective, especially when a follow-up component is incorporated into the intervention program. Some believe that such programs have a spillover effect on illicit drug use. However, methodological weaknesses associated with these studies temper our ability to make a strong statement regarding their overall efficacy in preventing the use and abuse of alcohol and other drugs. The literature on drug-testing programs, which may have a preventive (e.g., deterrence effect) effect on alcohol and other drug use, was reviewed in Chapter 7.

EMPLOYEE ASSISTANCE PROGRAMS

Employee assistance programs are designed to assist in identifying and aiding employees who need assistance because of behavioral, health, and job performance problems attributable to alcohol and other drug abuse, health, emotional, marital, family, financial, legal, stress, and other personal concerns. There are a variety of types of services that are labeled EAPs, some of which represent very minimal offers of assistance to employees. In response to such diversity in programs, the Employee Assistance Professional Association (EAPA) has set standards defining what functions are needed to provide comprehensive EAP services. Ideally, alcohol and other drug problems should be addressed through EAPs that include: making expert consultation and training available to supervisors and others so that they can better identify and help resolve a subordinate's or coworker's behavioral, health, or job performance problems; confidential and timely problem assessment services; referrals for appropriate diagnosis, treatment, and other assistance; the establishment of links between workplace and community resources that provide these services; follow-up services; and education and information on the prevention of alcohol and other drug problems. In light of the growing popularity of "managed care," and since assessing the level of care needed is one of the main activities of the EAPs, it is important that functional groups (i.e., managed care and EAP) work in close collaboration in order to ensure that the level of care provided to employees will maximize their chances of recovery. A detailed examination of the various types of EAPs and their history is presented in Roman and Blum (1992).

The set of activities that might be seen as part of EAPs is fairly well defined and accepted by practitioners in the field. Although employees are encouraged to seek out EAP services (self-referral), the program's case-finding strategy is based on job performance. Supervisors are trained in methods of constructive confrontation and referral to the EAP and are discouraged from attempting to counsel employees regarding their personal problems or overlooking problems until they become so severe that disciplinary action is required. Constructive confrontation involves assembling the evidence of deteriorated performance, confronting the employee with that evidence, describing what will be required to bring job performance back to an adequate level, and referring the employee to the EAP for assistance with any underlying problem that is affecting work performance.

Types of Data Available

Data on the spread of EAPs in major private-sector corporations were initially generated through Executive Caravan field surveys conducted by the Opinion Research Corporation (Roman, 1979). In 1972, 25 percent of Fortune 500 corporations had some form of program for providing constructive assistance to employees with drinking problems; subsequent Executive Caravan surveys revealed that these proportions grew to 34 percent in 1974, 50 percent in 1976, and 57 percent in 1979, by which point the survey was querying specifically about the presence of EAPs (Roman, 1982). There are no post-1979 national survey data on the prevalence of EAPs among the Fortune 500 corporations. Informal estimates indicate, however, that nearly all Fortune 500 corporations currently have an EAP. There is great variation, however, in the level of investment in EAP services and in the implementation of the EAPs. These variations are not only evident across corporations but are also observed within corporations across different operating units.

In 1985, a computer-assisted telephone survey of 1,358 private-sector work sites with 50 or more employees (86 percent response rate) was conducted by the Research Triangle Institute for the U.S. Department of Health and Human Services. The survey revealed that 24 percent of the work sites offered employees an EAP (Kiefhaber, 1987). Work site size was significantly associated with the availability of an EAP: 15 percent of work sites with fewer than 100 employees had an EAP, compared with 28 percent of work sites with 100 to 249 employees, 35 percent of work sites with 250 to 749 employees, and 52 percent of work sites with 750 or more employees. A national survey conducted in 1992 (Blum et al., 1992) indicated that almost half of all full-time, non-self-employed workers worked in settings that provided EAPs. The probability of an employee working for an employer that provides an EAP is directly related to the size of the employer.

In the early 1970s, the federal government mandated EAPs for all its civilian employees, but two research studies that involved interviews and on-site assessments of the nature of these programs in samples of federal installations revealed very uneven implementation (Beyer and Trice, 1978; Hoffman and Roman, 1984a, 1984b). In recent years, federal government units with EAPs have increased due in part to the Reagan administration initiative for a drug-free workplace. Federal civilian employees are supposed to be covered by EAPs, but each federal department or agency is responsible for finding the funds to support the implementation of the service, and the mandate to establish EAPs is underenforced.

With the exception of the nuclear power industry and some sectors of the transportation industry in which federal mandates have recently required the implementation of EAPs, the adoption and implementation of EAPs in the private sector has been almost exclusively voluntary. Thus, comparisons of private- and public-sector programming is problematic because of the mandated nature of the latter.

Utilization of Services

A study of 439 EAP sites (Blum et al., 1992; Blum and Roman, 1992), emphasizing caseload compositions for alcohol and other drug problems provides valuable information on EAP utilization and outcome measures. On average, about 30 percent of the caseloads in the EAPs studied stem from employees' problems with alcohol and other drugs. In addition, many cases recorded by EAPs as marriage and family problems, the largest single caseload category, involve the alcohol and other drug abuse of spouses or other family members. An average of 6 percent (median equals 4 percent) of employees used the EAPs studied in a 12-month period.

Data from a 1991 national survey (Blum et al., 1992; Blum and Roman, 1992) of full-time employees who are not self-employed indicate that 15 percent of those who work for organizations with EAPs have contacted it about an employee they supervise. Among covered employees, 48 percent said they knew someone at work who had used the EAP. More than 8 percent of the employees who were covered by EAPs had used it sometime in the past for a problem of their own, and 6 percent had used the EAP for a family member's problem. One should note that there is obviously some overlap among those who used the EAP for themselves, their family members, or their subordinates. The data on use reported in this section is therefore not representative of utilization for a given period of time. Rather it is accumulated usage over the period the EAP was in existence in a given work site and is limited by the tenure of a worker at the work site.

Results also reveal that the assessments of EAP counselors of their clients' problems typically identified an average of 2.1 problem categories per client. The most prevalent problem category is psychological and emotional problems, with 44 percent of the clients in this category. Marital problems applied to 28 percent, whereas "other family problems" was diagnosed for 31 percent of the clients. Alcohol and other drug problems are the next most prevalent problem categories; the EAP counselors indicated that 16 percent of the clients had problems with alcohol, 3 percent had problems with cocaine or crack, and 4 percent had problems with other drugs (Blum et al., 1992; Blum and Roman, 1992).

The EAP caseloads also include employees who have come to the EAP because of alcohol or other drug problems among their family members. Almost 21 percent of the EAP clients fall into this category, two-thirds of them being troubled by the alcohol problems of their family members and the other one-third by family members' use of drugs other than alcohol.

Thus, although only a minority of employees in EAP caseloads have alcohol or other drug problems of their own, when employees seeking help with problems with alcohol and other drugs of their family members are added, the caseload attributed to alcohol and other drug use is considerable. Moreover, alcohol and other drug cases take on the average more time at intake and referral, as well as in after-care and follow-up, than do cases of other types (Blum et al., 1992).

Evidence of Effectiveness

In 1984 Kurtz et al. reviewed the literature on EAP effectiveness and found a paucity of evidence. They identified 16 studies that used job performance outcomes as criterion measures. Absenteeism was used more often than other criteria and showed improvements in all the studies in which it was evaluated. Other variables on which improvements were shown include accidents, grievances, disciplinary actions, and the use of sick time.

However, all of the studies had design problems. The typical methodology was a one-group pretest/posttest design. Most of the studies showed improvements in the measured variables, but the absence of a control group means that one cannot rule out alternative workplace factors (e.g., disciplinary procedures) or external factors (e.g., pressure from spouse) as possible causes of the observed improvements. This is a particular problem when newly established EAPs are evaluated, for they may be one of a number of actions designed to improve working conditions. A few studies used as comparison groups those who refused EAP services, but these workers are likely to be different in important respects from those willing to take advantage of EAPs. Compounding the problems posed by missing or inadequate control groups are short follow-up periods in most studies and unclear subject selection procedures in others. In addition, the impact of EAP activities was typically confounded with treatment effect when treatment was provided by external service providers.

Since 1984, additional EAP studies have been published, but there is as yet no definitive study of the impact of EAP participation on employee work performance, absenteeism, or health claims. However, Smith and Mahoney (1989) present insightful results from a study conducted at McDonnell Douglas Corporation, in which EAP clients who received psychiatric treatment or treatment for alcohol and other drug use were compared with employees in the same company who did not use the EAP but who also received psychiatric or alcohol and other drug use treatment during the same time period. Data were compared for the year of program entry or treatment and up to 3 years after.

Results showed that the EAP clients—both psychiatric treatment and alcohol and other drug use treatment—had lower absenteeism (34 percent and 44 percent fewer days lost, for employees with psychiatric problems and alcohol and other drug use, respectively) during the 4-year study period than did the clients who sought out treatment without using the EAP. And there was a reduction in turnover of 60 percent for psychiatric clients and 81 percent for alcohol and other drug use clients. Medical claims were also lower, both for the impaired employees and for their dependents. The study estimated over $4 million in reduced medical claims (in 1988 dollars) over the 3-year follow-up period and over 6,000 fewer days of absenteeism.

Unfortunately, the study has certain deficiencies that weakens its conclusions. Sample sizes and selection criteria are not clear. More critically, the study provides no information to demonstrate the comparability of the EAP and non-EAP samples. In one respect it is clear that the groups were not comparable: something brought the EAP clients to the EAP. Without more information about the members of the two groups, we cannot conclusively ascribe the differences in outcomes between the groups to the EAP intervention.

One of the earlier EAP studies (Foote et al., 1978) compared changes in six work performance measures by EAP clients across EAPs in four different companies. The measures were absenteeism, disciplinary actions, grievances, workplace accidents, visits to the medical department, and use of sick leave benefits. The study also computed ratios of client performance on each measure to company norms for each client group. The study found that changes in these measures after EAP intervention were not the same across companies. Those EAPs whose clientele was characterized by significant deteriorations in work performance (with performance well below the company norm) showed improvements in client performance after intervention. Programs whose clients were not performing below the company norm did not show such improvement. These data, however, are not necessarily evidence of differential effectiveness, for they are consistent with the classic regression artifact. The study, nonetheless, suggests that (1) not all EAPs are the same and (2) the kinds of clients seen by the EAP may have a major impact on performance measures following EAP intervention. Dealing with this latter problem suggests the need for true field experiments in which access to EAPs would be randomized, ideally at the individual level but more realistically by work site in multisite companies.

The general question of whether EAPs are effective at improving work performance is not, however, a promising path for investigation. EAPs are not all the same and should not be expected to produce the same results. Although a company might ask whether the use of its specific EAP increases work performance, a more promising focus for the research community is on the effects of specific EAP activities and services, not the presence or absence of EAPs. Several studies have been done on specific aspects of employee assistance programs.

Specific Activities and Services

Supervisor Training

Perhaps the most unusual feature of EAPs is the use of job performance as a means for identifying, confronting, and referring for treatment employees with alcohol and other drug abuse problems. Because work organizations have formalized mechanisms for observing employee performance and setting standards for such performance and, most important, because they can sanction unacceptable behavior (Googins, 1990), they constitute an unusual resource for the area of alcohol and other drug abuse intervention. The key to activating this resource lies in the ability and willingness of supervisors to use company-provided mechanisms for confronting alcohol- and other drug-abusing employees who have performance problems. Identification based on job performance and constructive confrontation of employees so identified are part of the core technology of EAPs (Roman, 1988).

The research surrounding the role of the supervisor can be examined within two primary areas: supervisor training and supervisor intervention.

In light of the pivotal role given supervisors within the EAP framework, training supervisors has had a high priority since the early conception of the EAP (Trice and Belasco, 1968; Trice and Roman, 1972). In a recent survey based on a national sample of EAPs (Schneider et al., 1990), over 92 percent of respondents agreed that "an EAP must conduct supervisor training to be considered a quality EAP," and over 87 percent of the respondents reported that they had conducted supervisor training sessions within the last year. A study initiated in 1984 on EAPs of medium- to large-size organizations found that supervisory training had improved in 45 percent of the work sites by 1988 (Blum et al., 1988, 1992).

However, there are also data indicating the reluctance of supervisors to engage in the identification and referral process. Trice and Roman (1972) and Googins and Kurtz (1980, 1981) identify a number of barriers that commonly impede supervisor intervention, including: ignorance of the EAP and its procedures; attempts by supervisors to solve workers' problems themselves; the perception that referring employees might reflect poorly on the referring supervisor; and fear of harming the employee and his or her family. Googins, in his study of supervisors, identified three specific barriers to referring problem employees to the EAP: (1) supervisors' attitudes toward perceived effectiveness of the EAP; (2) factual knowledge of the EAP; and (3) attitudes toward the supervisor role. Many of these factors have also recently been found to be important factors in influencing employees' propensity to use the services of an EAP (Sonnenstuhl and Trice, 1986; Harris and Fennell, 1988; Steele and Hubbard, 1985).

In a similar study, Hoffman and Roman (1984a) collected data from 84 supervisors and found that supervisors' attitudes toward an EAP and their supervisory style were significantly associated with supervisor perceptions of the extent to which referred workers were helped.

A study by Blum and Roman (1989) indicated that supervisory involvement in EAP referrals is much greater than EAP professionals perceive. This study also indicated that supervisors and managers were eager to spend time in training sessions learning how best to refer cases to and use the EAP. The propensity of managers to use EAPs is highly related to how familiar they are with the EAP and how accessible it appears (Milne et al., 1992), both of which may be increased through training.

Only recently has the impact of supervisor training been the subject of research. Schneider and Colan (1993), in NIDA-funded research on the effects of supervisor training, report significant differences between trained and untrained supervisors. Supervisors who received training showed significantly increased levels of knowledge of the EAP at a 1-year follow-up as well as more consultations with and referrals to the EAP than did an untrained control group. The tendency of the trained group to make significantly more referrals was also reflected in the number of referrals for alcohol and other drug problems (Schneider and Colan, 1993).

Impact of Supervisor Training

The job performance model developed by the EAP relies on the supervisor to identify troubled employees on the basis of deteriorating job performance and then to intervene with constructive confrontation (Trice and Roman, 1978). Several studies have examined in detail the effectiveness of the constructive-confrontation strategy and generally conclude that this strategy leads to increased employee acceptance of treatment and a subsequent improvement in overall job performance (Hilker et al., 1972; Trice and Beyer, 1984).

Constructive confrontation or supervisor referrals have been consistently reported as highly effective, although one must be cautious in accepting this conclusion because of repeated flaws in methodology and design (Kurtz et al., 1984). Heyman (1976), for example, reporting on employees from five different work organizations with varying degrees of coercion, found a significant relationship between constructive confrontation and improved work performance "for those whose pre-program performance had deteriorated." Freedburg and Johnston (1979) found virtually the same findings in their study of Canadian workers.

Trice and Beyer (1984) interviewed supervisors who had referred employees with alcohol problems to the EAP within the previous 3 years. The supervisors reported that 74 percent of these employees showed subsequent improvements in work performance. These results were compared with reports of a different sample of supervisors who had not made a referral to the EAP, but who were asked about how they had handled an employee with some other type of behavioral problem. This latter group reported a lower rate of improvement. This study did not address directly the question of whether supervisory confrontation and referral produce better results than self-referral or referral by coworkers, family, or some other source (i.e., whether the "stick" is effective). The 74 percent improvement estimate almost certainly overvalues referrals both because of regression artifacts and because respondents might have thought positive outcomes reflected positively on their actions. The difference between the percentage improvement estimates of referring and nonreferring supervisors is a better estimate of the help that referral provided.

A study that looked at objective work performance outcomes was conducted through the EAP of the Los Angeles City Department of Water and Power (Amaral and Cross, 1988). The study included 43 EAP clients with alcohol problems—21 were mandatorily referred to the EAP by their supervisors and 22 were voluntary referrals (informal supervisor referrals, self-referrals, and medical department referrals). The study examined sickness absenteeism for both groups in the year before program entry and the year after. There was a 49 percent increase in sickness absenteeism for the voluntary referrals, but a 33 percent decrease (approaching the norm for the entire group) for mandatory referrals. The authors argue that the additional monitoring and potential job jeopardy resulting from a mandatory supervisory referral produced the difference.

It is not clear from the study report whether these samples included all clients with alcohol problems entering the EAP during the target year, or whether some selection criteria were applied. The two groups were relatively comparable in that they both had excess absenteeism (above the work group norm) in the year prior to entering the EAP. A more detailed description of the two groups would have been useful to rule out other potential confounding factors. However, the primary weakness of this study is the small sample size.

Macdonald et al. (1989) conducted a study of 163 clients of EAPs in five work sites to examine rates of continued employment. In this study, job loss was not related to type of referral (voluntary or formal) or source of referral. However, no information was provided as to what constituted a "formal" referral and whether this included either a form of job jeopardy or any further monitoring after referral.

In sum, the literature on constructive confrontation and referral by supervisors provides some limited evidence that supervisor referrals are effective in improving job performance compared with self-referral or failures to refer. The question of whether it is worth training supervisors in confrontation and referral techniques is easier to study than the question of whether an EAP is helpful. It is difficult to randomly assign employees in private-sector workplaces to receive or not receive EAP services. It is relatively easy, however, to design a study in which randomly sampled supervisors are given special instruction in constructive confrontation and referral techniques, and then to compare the work groups of supervisors who did and did not receive such training. However, if an EAP is not effective, referral may have no effects or confrontation and referral may affect employee performance for reasons that have nothing to do with the EAP services that follow. The extant literature does not allow us to determine whether confrontation and referral are effective only in interaction with EAP services or whether confrontation has value in and of itself.

Follow-Up Counseling and Support

The workplace is in a unique position to help employees address problems associated with alcohol and other drug use, as well as other personal problems. It not only holds leverage to move an employee toward seeking appropriate help, but it can also provide long-term support in helping the client recover. No other system outside the family (or the legal system) has the kind of ongoing contact that allows this. Certainly treatment facilities are not able to maintain such long-term relationships.

There has been little attention to this aspect of EAPs in the literature. While EAP staff in general affirm the importance of providing long-term support, many are not in fact able to provide it. Their attention is fully occupied in addressing new cases and moving them into appropriate treatments.

A number of studies have been conducted on the effects of follow-up counseling for other health risks; some have already been reviewed above in the section on wellness programs. One study has been published that examined this component of service for EAPs. Foote and Erfurt (1991) randomly assigned all clients with alcohol and other drug abuse problems entering an EAP in 1985 into two groups: 161 who received regular care and 164 who in addition to regular care received routine follow-up services over the subsequent year by a specially hired EAP counselor. The EAP was jointly operated by labor and management and served a primarily male blue-collar manufacturing work force.

The study found that, during the year after EAP intervention, the experimental group had 15 percent fewer hospitalizations for treatment of alcohol and other drug abuse than the control group and a 24 percent reduction in alcohol and other drug abuse-related health benefit claims (combining claims for treatment and disability). The difference in disability claims was statistically significant when outliers (the two clients with the highest claims in each group) were removed. Differences in health care claims, while large, were not statistically significant. Health benefit claims for diagnoses other than alcohol and other drug abuse were higher for the experimental group. A multivariate analysis controlling for age, race, severity, and number of follow-up visits found that being in the special follow-up group was significantly associated with reductions in alcohol and other drug abuse disability, alcohol and other drug abuse treatment costs, and relapse leading to hospitalization for alcohol and other drug abuse. There was no effect on absenteeism or health benefit claims other than substance abuse.

Unfortunately, the study's 1-year follow-up period was too short to evaluate truly long-term effects. The higher rate of nonalcohol and other drug abuse health benefit utilization in the experimental group may have reflected greater attention to long-term health problems that would lead to lowered health benefit utilization in subsequent years—a finding that has been reported elsewhere (Smith and Mahoney, 1989). In addition, the study needs to be replicated among other types of employees and work sites with other types of management practices and benefit structures. Finally, there was some organizational difficulty in implementing the experimental protocol, so that many employees in the experimental group did not receive the intended amount of follow-up. Results may have been underestimated for this reason.

The major strength of this study was in the random allocation of all EAP clients, so that there is a low probability that hidden biases resulted from the process of selection into the study groups. The two groups were comparable, and we can have a high degree of assurance that differences in outcomes resulted from the additional follow-up counseling given to the experimental group.

Level of Care

Another issue that has received considerable attention in the EAP field is the level of care needed for the treatment of alcohol and other drug abuse. Level of care ranges from inpatient hospitalization to self-help groups. Health maintenance organizations (HMOs) have tended to restrict access to inpatient or residential care in favor of outpatient treatment, and as HMOs have attracted more and more enrollees, many EAP staff have found themselves restricted in their ability to refer clients to more intensive treatment.

Walsh et al. (1991) considered this question of treatment options in a study of 227 EAP clients with alcohol problems. The study subjects were largely white male blue-collar workers from a manufacturing environment. Employees were excluded from the study if they required medically supervised detoxification (e.g., a history or symptoms of delirium tremens or grand mal seizures during withdrawal), or if they required medical attention for a serious illness, posed an immediate danger to themselves or others, needed psychiatric care, or were leaving the work force. A total of 65 percent of newly identified alcohol-abusing clients entering the EAP during the intake period met the inclusion criteria, and 93 percent of those eligible consented to participate and were randomly assigned to one of three experimental groups.

The three groups were (1) inpatient hospitalization (about 3 weeks) followed by Alcoholics Anonymous (AA) attendance, (2) AA only, and (3) "choice," in which the client decided in consultation with the EAP staff what the treatment plan would be. Clients for whom the initial group assignment did not work were shifted into other treatment options, but remained in the initial study group for analysis purposes. All clients were seen weekly by the EAP during the year after initial treatment. The groups were followed by the research team for a total of 2 years.

All three groups showed significant improvement in job measures, when compared to pretreatment information, and there were no significant differences among the groups. The number of hours missed from work dropped by more than one-third, comparing the 6 months before intake with the last 6 months of follow-up 2 years later.

On drinking-related measures, however, the hospital group showed significantly better rates of continuous abstinence and sobriety than the other two groups, with the AA-only group generally showing the poorest results. A majority of the AA-only group (63 percent) were subsequently hospitalized for alcoholism treatment during the study period due to relapse. Comparable rehospitalization figures for the other groups were 23 percent for the hospital group and 38 percent for the choice group. By the end of the study, total costs for the treatment of alcoholism were only about 10 percent lower for the AA-only group than for the hospital group due to the greater amount of relapse in the AA group.

The study showed substantial improvements in job performance measures for the EAP clients. These are presumed to be due to a combination of treatment effects and follow-up counseling and monitoring through the EAP. These effects cannot be disentangled, because all of the groups received the same follow-up support since the purpose of the study was to examine varieties of treatment, not EAP follow-up support. However, the similarity of results across treatment groups suggests that the specific treatment modality may be less significant in producing work performance improvements than the longer-term support and monitoring provided by the EAP.

The study's core finding is that, in the population studied, there is little money to be saved by withholding inpatient treatment in favor of self-help modalities; relapse rates are much higher without the initial hospitalization for intensive treatment. A weakness of the study is that it did not include a test of outpatient treatment as an initial modality. The growth in outpatient services as primary treatment occurred after the study began. Like the EAP follow-up study, this study should be replicated with subjects who are not primarily white male blue-collar workers.

Summary

The weight of evidence from EAP evaluation studies (pretest-posttest designs) suggests that the work performance and health benefit utilization levels of EAP clients return toward normal after intervention. However, the evidence does not conclusively address the magnitude of the independent contribution (effects) of EAPs to the observed improvements.

Definitive studies of EAP effectiveness have yet to be conducted. Despite this, there is growing evidence from studies of specific EAP components that: (1) constructive confrontation and referral by supervisors may improve outcomes, (2) long-term follow-up support by EAP staff may improve outcomes, and (3) initial referral of alcoholic employees to intensive inpatient treatment followed by AA attendance produces better outcomes than referral to AA without other treatment when the EAP provides long-term support and monitoring of the clients.

In studying EAP effectiveness, one should not assume that EAPs are generic across work sites. Although there are standards in terms of components that a good EAP must have, EAPs should and do vary. Different EAP designs are needed to accommodate differences in organizational structures, employee demography, methods of dealing with good or poor performance, benefit packages, supervisor training and authority, and the organizational experience with different types of human resource innovations. Customizing EAPs to take account of such differences leads to a greater or lesser emphasis on different aspects of core and supporting EAP technologies as well as different types and levels of investment in EAP components. Moreover, different EAPs are at different phases of maturity in terms of the completeness of implementation. Indeed, implementation is never complete, given turnover in the employee population, changes in the external environment, and alteration of EAP staffing and organization.

Thus it is misguided to ask whether the (generic) EAP is effective. We should seek instead to understand how EAPs contribute to a range of different outcomes in a range of different settings. This requires more high-quality critical case studies of EAPs, perhaps with some common criteria of programmatic effectiveness. In these studies, care must be taken to secure adequate control groups, and attention should be paid to the effects of particular EAP techniques and services. Ultimately, one may develop theoretical understandings that allow more generic statements about what is likely to work in particular types of settings.

TREATMENT

Great strides have been made in the development of effective treatments for abuse of alcohol and other drugs. There remain, however, major problems in public perceptions of treatment efficacy. Even among members of the medical profession, the idea that addiction is untreatable because virtually all addicts relapse is common. Thus physicians are often reluctant to refer patients for treatment because they believe that the results will inevitably be poor. There is also a strong tendency to think of total and permanent abstinence from alcohol and other drug use as the only sign of successful treatment when diminution in alcohol and other drug use may itself be a valuable outcome. Alcohol and other drug use disorders are a complex group of chronic conditions that vary not only according to the substance or substances abused, but also according to individual factors such as psychiatric comorbidity, heredity, gender, race, ethnicity, education, and occupation. Different types of patients require different treatment modalities. Overall, the treatment for alcohol and other drug use disorders produces about as much improvement as the treatment of other chronic medical disorders.

One fundamental cause of the mistaken perception that treatment for these disorders is ineffective is the tendency to view them as acute problems controllable by will power. Yet from the medical perspective, alcohol and other drug abuse and dependence are chronic disorders much like arthritis or diabetes. They develop gradually and they have a course characterized by remissions and relapses, although there is often overall progression over time. Treatments reliably produce relief of symptoms and improvements in function, but not cures. The efficacy of treatment for alcohol and other drug use disorders has been reviewed in a recent Institute of Medicine report (Gerstein and Harwood, 1990) and in other recent publications (McLellan et al., 1992), and so is not reviewed here. The work site has important linkages to treatment, with employees directly accessing treatment through EAPs, when they exist, or indirectly, via third-party payment. The workplace is an important element in the treatment arena because of the third-party benefits it may provide, the constraints it may place on payment for treatment, and the role it may play in treatment entry and treatment participation, employment maintenance, and relapse prevention.

Entering Treatment

Self-Referral

Self-referral to treatment is difficult to define because it has not been operationalized and examined scientifically. Even the notion of self-referral is questionable since many hidden pressures are exerted on individuals. Thus a client may enter therapy only to escape coercion from a supervisor or pressure from family and friends. One study found that the impetus for self-referral emerged from a social network, and the decision to self-refer resulted from a complex network of formal and informal controls. In some cases, supervisors urged the employees because of poor work performance; in others, coworkers were involved (Trice and Sonnenstuhl, 1988).

Supervisor Referral

As discussed with regard to EAPs, constructive confrontation is one of the mechanisms thought to arouse readiness for treatment in employees. This strategy uses deteriorating job performance to identify alcohol- and other drug-abusing employees. Organizational and occupational policies direct supervisors to confront suspected employees with impaired performance, to emphasize the negative consequences of its continuation, and to offer support for an EAP assessment. Constructive confrontation proceeds in steps. First, performance problems are discussed with the employee, and the individual is urged to seek help. If improvement does not follow these informal discussions, more formal disciplinary procedures are invoked. The constructive part of the informal discussion (1) expresses concern for the employee's welfare, (2) emphasizes that group membership may be maintained if conformity is restored, and (3) suggests that alternative routes are available to regain satisfactory performance.

Constructive confrontation has been shown to be successful in improving work performance when used as intended. When the components of constructive confrontation were measured, it was found that concrete offers of help and persistence led employees to accept treatment, but the confrontational element could lead to refusing help and leaving the company. The combined results suggest that the balanced use of both constructive and confrontational elements produced positive outcomes with problem drinkers, whereas the use of confrontational elements alone tended to produce negative results (Trice and Sonnenstuhl, 1988).

In contrast to the positive results produced by constructive confrontation, formal discipline produced unfavorable outcomes. Hence, written warnings, suspensions, and discharges were negatively associated with work performance following intervention. A combination of constructive confrontation and treatment outside the company generated greater performance improvements than either of these two alone (Trice and Sonnenstuhl, 1988).

Advantage of Early Detection and Referral

Although there are productivity-based arguments for efforts to detect alcohol and other drug use in the workplace, a clinician might focus solely on the potential benefits to the patient. The available outcome studies suggest that better outcomes are associated with earlier treatment (Institute of Medicine, 1989), and factors such as employer pressure toward continuation in treatment can favorably influence prognoses.

Addiction is a complex disorder that responds to treatment at any point along the line in its progression. The notion that one must "hit bottom" before recovery no longer seems accurate (Runge, 1990). Treatment of alcoholism is more effective in the early stages of the addictive process, when the clients are socially stable and have not yet developed adverse medical or social consequences (Heather, 1989). However, the effectiveness of early intervention in altering the course of the disease is still debatable, and critics have voiced concern over labeling and creating self-fulfilling prophesies.

Although it is premature to judge the value of early intervention, there is reason to believe it is beneficial (Heather, 1989). A few studies have recruited drinkers who either were not seeking treatment or had been heavy drinkers for a relatively short period of time in an attempt to evaluate the effectiveness of early intervention. Skutle and Berg (1987) investigated early intervention in problem drinkers, and evaluated four behavioral treatment methods in an outpatient setting with clients who had been problem drinkers for less than 10 years and had no prior treatment, tolerance, dependence, liver damage, or medical illness. All treatment groups were comparable at admission and showed a similar decrease in drinking behavior after treatment. After the initial decrease, the level of consumption remained lower during the 3-, 6-, and 12-month follow-up periods. Other life problems also decreased. Hence, minimal intervention (4 to 16 hours) can be recommended for early problem drinkers with relatively low consumption at intake. Clients with higher consumption appeared to profit less.

In the Malmo Project in Sweden (see Babor et al., 1986), Kristenson identified 585 heavy drinkers through elevated serum gamma glutamyl transferase (GGT) and intervened in half of the group by giving them a thorough evaluation and follow-up until their GGT returned to normal. A control group was sent a letter that their GGT was elevated, advised to restrict intakes, and told to repeat the GGT in 2 years. The GGT values of both groups decreased significantly; however, the control group had more sick days, more hospitalization, and twice as many deaths. Hence, simple early intervention based on regular feedback had a significant effect on drinking habits and physical health.

The Edinburgh Royal Infirmary Project in Scotland (see Babor et al., 1986) investigated the effects of brief intervention in problem drinkers identified in a general hospital as having a current problem. The intervention group had 30-50 minutes of counseling and received a booklet with advice about reducing drinking. The control group received nothing. After 1 year, only

35 percent of the intervention group had alcohol problems compared with 62 percent of the control group. Thus, there is evidence that both early interventions in problem drinking and inexpensive interventions of a minimal sort can have substantial positive effects.

Treatment Follow-up and Work Site Reentry

Plan for After-Care

Although the initial phase of alcohol and other drug treatment is designed to teach clients abstinence skills, the maintenance of these skills and their generalization to new situations and environments is a continuing issue (McCrady et al., 1985). Hence, after-care oriented toward the maintenance of abstinence and therapeutic gains is an important component of treatment. Indeed, it may well be the active ingredient in the achievement of long-term sobriety.

The term *after-care* has assumed a number of different meanings and encompasses a variety of intervention strategies. After-care treatments vary in modality (individual, family/couples/groups), organization, time parameters, therapeutic orientation, purpose, and attendance expectations, but as a concept after-care has two important components. First, it involves therapeutic activities designed to maintain gains achieved in the initial phases of treatment rather than procedures that attempt to develop new skills. Second, it can be an important complement to many different forms of initial treatment. After-care may follow outreach activities, emergency treatment, inpatient treatment, intermediate care, or outpatient treatment. Although after-care is a critical part of treatment, there are few studies that evaluate its effectiveness (Ito and Donovan, 1986).

Effectiveness of After-Care

Ito and Donovan (1986) reviewed studies of the effectiveness of after-care on treatment outcomes. They concluded that it contributes significantly to positive outcomes in alcoholic clients and that it does so independently of patient prognostic variables (residential stability, interpersonal relationships, social activity, health, employment, and drinking status). After-care is also important to the early detection of and intervention in relapse. Its effectiveness appears to lie not so much in preventing slips but rather in preventing minor slips, that are almost inevitable, from developing into full-blown relapses. Patients in after-care may obtain help in dealing with the stresses that lead to slips and with the stresses that slips create. However, in order for this to occur, the clients' slips must come to the attention of after-care workers. Hence, it is important for a program to provide a clear expectation that slips will be acknowledged immediately so that appropriate interventions can be made.

Common sense indicates that attendance at after-care is crucial to long-term outcomes; however, its effects have been difficult to evaluate scientifically. Foote and Erfurt (1988) reviewed a number of studies that investigated the effectiveness of after-care and found mixed results. Some studies report no relationship between outcome and follow-up attendance, whereas others found a positive relationship. However, all of the studies had serious shortcomings in their designs. Follow-up periods were short; there was selection bias in those who attended after-care; and often there was an absence of collateral information. Thus Foote and Erfurt concluded that most after-care studies were relatively uninformative about the power of after-care to improve recovery rates.

Ito and Donovan (1986) found three major predictors of after-care attendance: (1) the autonomy perceived by the patient during inpatient treatment, (2) the distance traveled to after-care, and (3) the cognitive functioning of the patient. They report that after-care attendance can be increased by telephone calls, orientation lectures, and behavioral contract scheduling.

Foote and Erfurt also discussed the need for a nontraditional proactive approach to after-care in which the provider reaches out to the client. In this approach, the provider seeks out the patient until the problem is solved— yet this seldom happens. Indeed, Foote and Erfurt found that little attention was paid to the process of getting patients to participate in after-care. Patients were often "encouraged" to attend after-care; however, stronger intervention than encouragement is needed. One of the major problems may be that after-care is not given in the best settings. The authors argue that it should be located at the work site because of the work organization's financial interest and its ability to monitor employees. They also feel that the use of the relapse prevention model at the work site deserves attention.

However, there are few guidelines pertaining to EAP follow-up activities and a dearth of studies concerning the effectiveness of EAP follow-up. Although it is clear that EAPs and work sites should pay more attention to follow-up and after-care, additional research is needed to determine the best, most cost-effective ways to do this (Foote and Erfurt, 1988).

EAPs have placed their energies in case finding, intake, and referral; most have devoted little time to relapse prevention. Follow-up for many is either nonexistent or limited to the duration of treatment and one or two visits after return to work. Hence, EAPs may not be preventing relapses as much as they are teaching clients how to use the treatment system more frequently and effectively. Currently, most EAPs have neither the time nor the staff to deal with follow-up and relapse prevention since the model focuses so heavily on case discovery and initial treatment. Yet since EAPs have a close relationship with the work site, they are in an excellent position to provide meaningful follow-up. Foote and Erfurt concluded that EAPs and work sites should pay more attention to follow-up and after-care, a conclusion the committee endorses.

In summary, much of the thrust of the EAP effort has been on the detection of new cases as opposed to the follow-up of those who have received treatment. Given the marked propensity for relapse and the EAP's important link with the work site, much more emphasis should be placed on follow-up. Thus recovery should be viewed as a process rather than an event with workplaces, EAPs, and treatment providers all playing important roles in aiding clients' recoveries over the long term.

CONCLUSIONS AND RECOMMENDATIONS

- Recovery from alcoholism and other drug use disorders is a process that can take months or years of continuing care. The continuing abuse of alcohol or other drugs is a chronic disorder, and the evidence suggests that the ameliorative effects of brief treatments without follow-up are seldom sustained over the long run. Employee assistance programs (EAPs) are well situated to oversee that follow-up, which is essential to a long-term recovery.

Recommendation: Because of high dropout rates in substance abuse treatment programs, EAPs should monitor treatment participation and provide for long-term follow-up.

- EAPs are not generic across work sites. EAPs should and do vary across work sites and over time. Thus, it is misguided to ask whether the generic EAP is an effective program.

Recommendation: EAPs should be evaluated in terms of the amount and quality (including process evaluation) of the services they provide and not just by patient count. Researchers should seek to understand how EAPs contribute to a range of different outcomes in a range of different settings. This requires more high-quality critical case studies of EAPs, perhaps with some common criteria of programmatic effectiveness. Care must be taken to secure adequate control groups, and, rather than attempting to evaluate the overall effectiveness of supposedly static programs, attention should be paid to the effects of particular EAP services and their dynamic nature.

- Given the measurement limitations of drug test results in assessing drug abuse or dependence (see Chapter 6), not all individuals testing positive require or are likely to benefit from treatment, counseling, or other administrative actions that might be triggered by a positive drug test result. Blanket rules referring all positive-testing employees to treatment can be costly to employers without providing commensurate benefits to them or their employees. Care is required to determine the appropriate course of action in the event of a positive test.

Recommendation: Persons reviewing test results should be required to demonstrate expertise with respect to toxicology, pharmacology, and occupational medicine. Standards should be set and continuing education and certification should be required. Such individuals should be involved in the interpretation of the results of drug-testing programs, and in the case of positive postemployment tests, should assist other professional staff in interpreting the seriousness of revealed drug use and provide guidance in determining the best course of action for coping with any drug problems (e.g., evaluation referral to proper medical specialist if needed).

REFERENCES

Amaral, T.M., and S.H. Cross
  1988   Cost-Benefits of Supervisory Referrals. Paper presented at the 17th ALMACA Annual Conference, Los Angeles, Calif.
Babor, T.F., E.B. Ritson, and R.J. Hodgson
  1986   Alcohol related problems in the primary health care setting: a review of early intervention strategies. *British Journal of Addiction* 81:23-46.
Bacon, S.D.
  1973   The process of addiction to alcohol: social aspects. *Quarterly Journal of Studies on Alcohol* 34:1-27.
Beattie, M.C., R. Longabaugh, and J. Fava
  1992   Assessment of alcohol-related workplace activities: development and testing of your workplace. *Journal of Studies on Alcohol* 53:469-475.
Bertera, R.L.
  1990   The effects of workplace health promotion on absenteeism and employment costs in a large industrial population. *American Journal of Public Health* 80:1101-1105.
Beyer, J.M., and H.M. Trice
  1978   *Implementing Change: Alcoholism Policies in Federal Work Organizations.* New York: The Free Press.
Blum, T.C., and P.M. Roman
  1989   Employee assistance programs and human resource management. *Research in Personnel and Human Resource Management* 7:259-312.
  1992   A description of clients using employee assistance programs. *Alcohol Health and Research World* 16:(2)120-128.
Blum, T.C., P. Roman, and N. Bennett
  1988   A Longitudinal Analysis of Internal EAPs. Paper presented at the annual meetings of the Association of Labor-Management Administrators and Consultants on Alcoholism, Los Angeles, Calif..

Blum, T.C., P.M. Roman, and L. Patrick
1990   Synergism in worksite adoption of employee assistance and health promotion activities. *Journal of Occupational Medicine* 32:461-467.

Blum, T.C., J.K. Martin, and P.M. Roman
1992   A research note on EAP prevalence, components and utilization. *Journal of Employee Assistance Research* 1(1):209-229.

Bly, J.L., R.C. Jones, and J.E. Richardson
1986   Impact of worksite health promotion on health care costs and utilization. *Journal of the American Medical Association* 256:3235-3240.

Case, J.B.
1985   Integrating EAPs with health education efforts. In S.J. Klarreich, J.L. Francek, and C.E. Moore, eds., *The Human Resources Management Handbook.* New York: Praeger Publishers.

Erfurt, J.C., A. Foote, M.A. Heirich, and W. Gregg
1990   Improving participation in worksite wellness programs: comparing health education classes, a menu approach, and follow-up counseling. *American Journal of Health Promotion* 4:270-278.

Erfurt, J.C., A. Foote, and M.A. Heirich
1991   Worksite wellness programs: incremental comparison of screening and referral alone, health education, follow-up counseling, and plant organization. *American Journal of Health Promotion* 5:438-448.

Fielding, J.E., and P.V. Piserchia
1989   Frequency of worksite health promotion activities. *American Journal of Public Health* 79:16-20.

Foote, A., and J.C. Erfurt
1988   Posttreatment follow-up, aftercare, and worksite re-entry of the recovering alcoholic employee. Pp. 193-204 in M. Galanter, ed., *Recent Developments in Alcoholism,* Vol. 6. New York: Plenum Press.
1991   Effects of EAP follow-up on prevention of relapse among substance abuse clients. *Journal of Studies on Alcohol* 52:241-248.

Foote, A., J.C. Erfurt, P.A. Strauch, and T.L. Guzzardo
1978   Effectiveness of Occupational Employee Assistance Programs: Test of an Evaluation Method. Institute of Labor and Industrial Relations, University of Michigan, Ann Arbor.

Freedburg, E.J., and W.E. Johnston
1979   Changes in drinking behavior, employment status, and other life areas for employed alcoholics 3, 6, and 12 months after treatment. *Journal of Drug Issues* 9:523-534.

Gerstein, D.R, and R.J. Harwood, eds.
1990   *Treating Drug Problems,* Vol. I. Committee for the Substance Abuse Coverage Study, Institute of Medicine. Washington, D.C.: National Academy Press.

Gibbs, J.O., D. Mulvaney, C. Henes, and R.W. Reed
1985   Work-site health promotion: five-year trend in employee health care costs. *Journal of Occupational Medicine* 27:826-830.

Gomel, M., B. Oldenburg, J.M. Simpson, and N. Owen
1993   Work-site cardiovascular risk reduction: a randomized trial of health risk assessment, education, counseling, and incentives. *American Journal of Public Health* 87(9):1231-1238.

Googins, B., and N. Kurtz
1980   Factors inhibiting supervisory referrals to occupational alcoholism intervention program. *Journal of Studies on Alcohol* 4(11):1196-1208.

1981   Discriminating participating and non-participating supervisors in occupational alcoholism programs. *Journal of Drug Issues* 11(2):199-216.

Googins, B., with J. Gonyea and M. Pitt-Catsouphes
1990   Linking the Worlds of Family and Work: Family Dependent Care and Workers' Performance. A Report to the Ford Foundation. School of Social Work, Boston University.

Gregg, W., A. Foote, J.C. Erfurt, and M.A. Heirich
1990   Worksite follow-up and engagement strategies for initiating health risk behavior changes. *Health Education Quarterly* 17:455-478.

Harris, M., and M. Fennell
1988   Perceptions of an employee assistance program and employees' willingness to participate. *Journal of Applied Behavioral Science* 24(4):423-438.

Heather, N.
1989   Psychology and brief intervention. *British Journal of Addiction* 84:357-370.

Heirich, M.A., J.C. Erfurt, and A. Foote
1992   The core technology of worksite wellness. *Journal of Occupational Medicine* 34(6):627-637.

Heyman, M.
1976   Referral to alcoholism programs in industry: coercion, confrontation and choice. *Journal of Studies on Alcohol* 37(7):900-907.

Hilker, R., F.E. Asma, and R. Eggert
1972   A company-sponsored alcoholic rehabilitation program: ten-year evaluation. *Journal of Occupational Medicine* 14:769-771.

Hoffman, E., and P.M. Roman
1984a   Effects of supervisory style and experiential frames of reference on successful organizational alcoholism policy implementation. *Journal of Studies on Alcohol* 45:260-267.
1984b   The effect of organizational emphasis upon the diffusion of information about innovations. *Journal of Management* 7:277-292.

Institute of Medicine
1989   *Prevention and Treatment of Alcohol Problems: Research Opportunities.* Washington, D.C.: National Academy Press.

Ito, J.R., and D.M. Donovan
1986   Aftercare in alcoholism treatment: a review. Pp. 435-456 in W.R. Miller and H. Health, eds., *Treating Addictive Behaviors: Process of Change.* New York: Plenum Press.

Kiefhaber, A.
1987   *The National Survey of Worksite Health Promotion Activities.* Washington, D.C.: Office of Health Promotion and Disease Prevention, U.S. Department of Health and Human Services.

King, A.C., C.B. Taylor, W.L. Haskell, and R.F. DeBusk
1988   Strategies for increasing early adherence to and long-term maintenance of home-based exercise training in healthy middle-aged men and women. *American Journal of Cardiology* 61:628-632.

Kurtz, N.R., B. Googins, and W.C. Howard
1984   Measuring the success of occupational alcoholism programs. *Journal of Studies on Alcohol* 45:33-45.

Macdonald, S., W. Albert, M. Maynard, and P. French
1989   Survival analysis to explore the characteristics of employee assistance program (EAP) referrals that remain employed. *The International Journal of Addictions* 24:113-122.

McCrady, B.S., D.L. Dean, E. Dubrevil, and S. Swanson
1985   The problem drinkers project: a programmatic application of social-learning based treatment. Pp. 417-471 in G.A. Marlatt and J.R. Gordon, eds., *Relapse Prevention.* New York: Guildord Press.
McLellan, A.T., D. Metzger, A.I. Alterman, J. Cornish, and H. Urschel
1992   How effective is substance abuse treatment? Compared to what? In C.P. O'Brien and J. Jaffe, eds., *Advances in Understanding the Addictive States.* New York: Raven Press.
Milne, S.H., T.C. Blum, and P.M. Roman
1992   Factors Influencing the Implementation of an Employee Assistance Program as a Human Resources Innovation. Paper presented at the Southern Management Association Annual Meetings, New Orleans, La.
Moskowitz, J.M.
1989   The primary prevention of alcohol problems: a critical review of the research literature. *Journal of Studies on Alcohol* 50:54-88.
Nathan, P.
1984   Alcoholism prevention in the workplace: three examples. Pp. 387-405 in P.M. Miller and T.D. Nirenberg, eds., *Prevention of Alcohol Abuse.* New York: Plenum Press.
Perri, M.G., R.M. Shapiro, W.W. Ludwig, C.T. Twentyman, and W.G. McAdoo
1984   Maintenance strategies for the treatment of obesity: an evaluation of relapse prevention training and posttreatment contact by mail and telephone. *Journal of Consulting and Clinical Psychology* 52:404-413.
Rohsenow, D.J., R.E. Smith, and S. Johnson
1985   Stress management training as a prevention program for heavy social drinkers: cognitions, affect, drinking, and individual differences. *Addictive Behaviors* 10:45-54.
Roman, P.M.
1979   The emphasis on alcoholism in employee assistance programs: new perspectives on an unfinished debate. *Labor Management Journal on Alcoholism* 9:186-191.
1982   Employee programs in major corporations in 1979: scope, change and receptivity. Pp. 177-200 in J. Deluca, ed., *Prevention, Intervention, and Treatment: Concerns and Models.* Alcohol and Health Monograph No. 3. Washington, D.C.: U.S. Government Printing Office.
1988   Growth and transformation in workplace alcoholism programming. Pp. 131-158 in M. Galanter, ed., *Recent Developments in Alcoholism*, Vol. 6. New York: Plenum Press.
Roman, P.M., and T.C. Blum
1988   Formal intervention in employee health: comparisons of the nature and structure of employee assistance programs and health promotion programs. *Social Science and Medicine* 26:503-514.
1992   Drugs, the workplace, and employee-oriented programming. Pp. 197-244 in D.R. Gerstein and H.J. Harwood, eds., *Treating Drug Problems*, Vol. II. Committee for the Substance Abuse Coverage Study, Institute of Medicine. Washington, D.C.: National Academy Press.
Room, R.
1981   The case for a problem prevention approach to alcohol, drug and mental problems. *Public Health Reports* 96:26-33.
Runge, E.G.
1990   Intervention: raising the bottom. *Journal of South Carolina Medical Association* 86:19-21.

Schneider, R., and N. Colan
  1993   The effectiveness of EAP supervisor training: an experimental study. *Human Resource Development Quarterly*, in press.
Schneider, R., N. Colan, and B. Googins
  1990   Supervisor training in employee assistance programs: current practices and future directions. *Employee Assistance Quarterly* 6(2):41-55.
Shain, M.
  1990   Health promotion programs and the prevention of alcohol abuse: forging a link. Pp. 163-179 in P.M. Roman, ed., *Alcohol Problem Intervention in the Workplace: Employee Assistance Program and Strategic Alternatives*. Westport, Conn.: Quorum Press.
Shain, M., H. Suurvali, and M. Boutilier
  1986   *Healthier Workers: Health Promotion and Employee Assistance Programs*. Lexington, Mass.: Lexington Books.
Skutle, A., and G. Berg
  1987   Training in controlled drinking for early-stage problem drinkers. *British Journal of Addictions* 82:493-501.
Smith, D.C., and J.J. Mahoney
  1989   McDonnell Douglas Corporation Employee Assistance Program Financial Offset Study, 1985-1988. Presented at the 18th EAP Annual Conference, Baltimore, Md.
Sonnenstuhl, W.J.
  1988   Contrasting employee assistance, health promotion, and quality of work life programs and their effects on alcohol abuse and dependence. *Journal of Applied Behavioral Science* 24:347-363.
Sonnenstuhl, W.J., and H.M. Trice
  1986   *Strategies for Employee Assistance Programs: The Crucial Balance*. Ithaca, N.Y.: ILR Press.
Steele, P.D., and R.L. Hubbard
  1985   Management styles, perceptions of substance abuse, and employee assistance programs in organizations. *Journal of Applied Behavioral Science* 21:271-286.
Taylor, C.B., N. Houston-Miller, J.D. Killen, and R.F. DeBusk
  1990   Smoking cessation after acute myocardial infarction: effects of a nurse-managed intervention. *Annals of Internal Medicine* 113:119-123.
Trice, H., and J. Belasco
  1968   Supervisor training about alcoholics and other problem employees. *Quarterly Journal on Alcohol* 29(2):382-389.
Trice, H.M., and J.M. Beyer
  1984   Work-related outcomes of the constructive-confrontation strategy in a job-based alcoholism program. *Journal of Studies on Alcohol* 45:393-404.
Trice, H.M., and P.M. Roman
  1972   *Spirts and Demons at Work: Alcohol and Other Drugs on the Job*, 1st ed. Ithaca, N.Y.: ILR Press.
  1978   *Spirits and Demons at Work: Alcohol and Other Drugs on the Job*, 2nd ed. Ithaca, N.Y.: ILR Press.
Trice, H.M., and W.J. Sonnenstuhl
  1988   Constructive confrontation and other referral processes. Pp. 159-170 in M. Galanter, ed., *Recent Developments in Alcoholism*, Vol. 6. New York: Plenum Press.
Walsh, D.C., R.W. Hingson, D.M. Merrigan et al.
  1991   A randomized trial of treatment options for alcohol-abusing workers. *New England Journal of Medicine* 325:775-782.

APPENDIXES

A

Methodological Issues

This appendix is included to achieve two goals. The first is to alert readers unfamiliar with social research methodology to technical terms encountered in this report and to crucial methodological issues that arise in an attempt to collect and evaluate evidence relating to the causes and effects of alcohol and other drug use, the effects of drug-screening programs, and the effects of efforts designed to treat or prevent alcohol and other drug use by the work force. The second is to provide potential researchers in industry and elsewhere with guidelines concerning the strengths and weaknesses of alternative strategies for the collection of evidence. The paucity of good scientific research on many aspects of alcohol and other drug use in the workplace suggests that even generic guidelines may be useful.

SCIENTIFIC JUDGMENT AND RESEARCH DESIGN

The way in which a study is conducted is referred to as the *design* of the study. The design of a study in large measure determines the extent to which the results contribute compelling evidence for or against a hypothesized causal relation. A stronger (or better) design is one in which an observed association (between drug use and job performance, for example) is less subject to alternative or artifactual explanations. For example, a survey that asks workers about their wages and their drug use and finds the two directly related does not necessarily imply that high wages lead to increased drug use because the study's design does not rule out other plausible explanations for the finding. Drug users may exaggerate their self-reported wages, people who use drugs may work harder to pay for them (rather than work less so as to spend more time in drug activities), and so on. In contrast, an experiment that found a reduction in positive drug tests at a large number of randomly selected work sites that implemented a particular prevention policy compared with smaller or no reduction at other randomly selected work sites would be subject to few alternative explanations.

The extent to which a scientific hypothesis is considered "established" does not involve proof in the sense found in logic or mathematics, but rather reflects the degree of consensus in the relevant scientific community that a series of studies supporting the hypothesis has been designed so that alternative explanations are unlikely.

The definitive single study is an ideal that in some areas does not even admit of realization. Scientific consensus develops instead through a series of studies in which later research avoids the flaws of earlier work but may introduce problems of its own. It is the consistency of findings across studies with different strengths and weaknesses that allows the cumulative results of such studies to provide strong evidence for or against a hypothesis. When research findings are inconsistent, the flaws in individual studies preclude confident judgments.

TYPES OF STUDY DESIGNS

Epidemiologic (Observational, Nonexperimental)

In epidemiologic study designs, researchers systematically observe variables related to human health, but they do not intervene to manipulate exposure to these variables. The potential power of systematic observation is illustrated by astronomy, one of the oldest and most successful of the observational sciences.

There are three major types of epidemiologic designs: case-referent (or case-control) studies, cross-sectional surveys, and prospective panel (or cohort) studies. Case-referent studies are retrospective in that they begin with diseased persons (e.g., drug abusers) and then seek to identify aspects of their personal histories that differentiate them from nondiseased persons (nonabusers) in a control group. The cross-sectional survey is similar to the case-referent design except that all population members are eligible for sampling and the survey process itself separates diseased from nondiseased individuals. The case-referent design is necessary when the prevalence of a disease is so low that sampling from a population will yield too few instances of the disease for reliable analysis. Finally, the prospective panel design involves following a population or a population sample over time to study the relation between risk factors measured at an earlier point in time and subsequent disease occurrence.

Drug-Use-Related Issues by Epidemiologic Designs

In this section, we briefly delineate a number of issues frequently encountered in epidemiologic research.

Incidence of drug use: given a defined population of persons at a particular point in time, what is the probability that a member of that population will use drugs during a subsequent period of time?

Prevalence of drug use: given a defined population of persons at a particular point in time, what is the probability that a member of the population is a current drug user?

Risk factors for drug use: a risk factor for drug use is a characteristic of some individuals or subgroups of a population that is associated with an increased risk (relative to others in the population) of becoming a drug user. Whether or not a consistently observed risk factor is a causal determinant of drug use is difficult to establish with epidemiologic studies. Experimental studies involving randomized change in risk factors are better suited to establishing causation. However, it is often impractical to study causal relations experimentally, and judgments of causality must be derived from epidemiologic observations.

Possible consequences of drug use: epidemiologic studies concerned with the consequences of drug use rely on comparisons between current or former drug users and nonusers.

Treatment effectiveness: the effectiveness of treatment and prevention programs is generally addressed by experiments, but surveys can also address this issue. In particular, regional variation in the type and extent of drug treatment programs can be related to the level and rate of change of drug use in communities, cities, and states.

Strengths and Weaknesses

The major weakness of epidemiologic designs is that observed associations are often causally ambiguous due to factors that confound the relationship. A plausible causal relationship may be in fact due to the joint effects of unmeasured, or poorly measured, "third" variables (spuriousness); reverse causation; measurement artifacts or other explanations that the epidemiologic design does not allow the researchers to rule out. For example, a positive association between self-reported drug use and wages might be due to the joint effect of educational attainment on both variables (spuriousness); to the increased opportunity to purchase drugs that comes with higher income (reverse causation); or to exaggerated reports of wages by drug users (measurement artifact). Similarly, preemployment drug-screening programs may induce drug users with a keen interest in the job for which they are applying to abstain for a period prior to the drug test. Thus, only drug users not very interested in the job might test positive. In that case, good job performance by those who passed a screening test and poor performance by those who failed (assuming they were hired anyway) would tell us little about the impact of drug use on job performance, since we would be wrong in supposing that those who had tested negative were not using drugs, and it might be lack of motivation which explained the poor performance of those who tested positive. (The results would, however, inform employers about the utility of a drug test as a preemployment screening device for identifying poor employment risks. It would just misinform them about why it was useful.)

There are a number of techniques that researchers can use in an effort to determine if an observed association in an observational study is due to confounding. Statistical modeling with multivariate equations can be used to adjust for the joint effects of measured third variables; however, such modeling requires accurate measurement of third variables or the use of measurement models that estimate and adjust for well-behaved error in observed variables. Suppose, for example, that drug use is higher in one plant than another. Multivariate adjustment of drug use rates by age and sex may indicate that the difference is due to work force demographics rather than some other plant characteristic.

Longitudinal observations can counter confounding due to reverse causation because the temporal sequence of changes in the hypothesized cause and effect variables can be observed. For example, observing that low self-esteem during the seventh grade predicts drug use in the twelfth grade is more convincing evidence that the trait leads to drug use than an observed association between self-esteem and drug use in the twelfth grade. If all we observed was the twelfth grade association, we could not rule out the possibility that using drugs caused the low self-esteem. Statistical modeling of cross-sectional observations can also address confounding due to reverse causation, but such "simultaneous equation" models require strong assumptions about the absence of other causal effects among variables in the model. Finally, the plausibility of measurement artifacts can be reduced through the use of multiple indicators; for example, drug use could be measured by self-report, peer report, and biochemical methods. If all measures of drug use yield the same conclusion about the relation of drug use with another variable, then the plausibility that each is due to a measurement artifact is low.

The major strength of epidemiologic studies is that they can address important questions that are difficult or expensive to address experimentally. For example, only the short-term consequences of acute drug exposures can be addressed in experiments with human beings. The long-term consequences of chronic use must be studied epidemiologically in humans or experimentally in animal models. Thus, some of the most important issues concerning drug use among the work force must be addressed with epidemiologic studies that minimize the potential for confounding through the use of longitudinal designs, careful measurement procedures, and appropriate statistical modeling.

Quasi-Experiments: Strengths and Weaknesses

The defining characteristic of a quasi-experiment is the *non*randomized manipulation of the causal (or independent) variable. Such designs in the workplace are likely to involve the assignment of work sites to conditions. For example, if one of a company's two plants begins drug testing and the other does not, the plant that started drug testing may be regarded as the experimental plant and the other as the control. Indeed, even if there were no control plant, the institution of the testing program could itself be treated as a quasi-experiment. There are many different models for quasi-experiments, and they have different strengths and weaknesses. Generally, a quasi-experimental design will be stronger (i.e., in the sense of ruling out other plausible explanations) if outcome data are available over time both before and after the experiment manipulation, if there are many units in the experimental and control conditions, and if within units there are many subjects exposed to the experimental and control conditions. These quasi-experimental designs are the most commonly used design strategies employed by applied researchers who attempt to evaluate the impact of new organizational programs. With regard to work force drug use, they can be used efficiently to assess the effectiveness of work-site drug use intervention programs (e.g., educational, drug testing) or work-site drug treatment programs.

The major weakness of quasi-experiments is that the assignment of persons or work sites to experimental conditions may be confounded with other factors. For example, work sites eager to implement prevention programs may have other characteristics that will lead to a decline in drug use (even in the absence of implementing the program under evaluation), so comparisons with control sites may be misleading. Or a company may be motivated to implement a prevention program when its workers' drug use seems to have hit crisis proportions. Since exceptionally high rates of drug use may result in part from factors such as a temporary period of high stress, postintervention measurements may reveal improvement that in fact reflects a return to baseline that would have occurred absent the intervention.

A major strength of quasi-experiments is that the potential limitations associated with variants of these experiments are well known. For example, longitudinal observation and statistical modeling can deal with the possibility that future outcomes are consistent with preintervention trends. So-called deviation from secular trend designs (or regression discontinuity) uses a series of preintervention baseline measurements to establish a behavior trend line and then determine whether measures of postintervention behavior differ significantly from the behavior that a simple projection of the trend would have predicted (Dwyer, 1993). A design like this controls for unmeasured factors that affect both the level and trends in drug use for a particular work site. It also increases power and guards against numerous, but not all, sources of confounding. For example, it does not control for events around the time of the intervention that might explain changes in behavior. A firm that established through drug testing over time that its workers were abusing cocaine and also established a program to combat cocaine use around the time of Len Bias's death would not know whether a steep drop in cocaine use was due to its program or the publicity that Bias's death engendered about the dangers of cocaine use. This kind of threat could be partially controlled, however, by adding sites that did not institute anticocaine programs at the same time. If Bias's death was not associated with a drop in cocaine use at the control sites or if it was associated with a significantly lower drop, this competing historical explanation becomes less plausible. When a quasi-experimental design includes a number of experimental and control sites and has outcome data from these sites for a substantial period before and after the intervention, it is a particularly strong design for making causal inferences. In some circumstances, the real-world richness of the units studied may even make it superior to the more limited true experiments.

Randomized Trials and Laboratory Experiments: Strengths and Weaknesses

The defining characteristic of a randomized trial or experiment is the random assignment of persons or work sites to experimental and control conditions. Typically the results of well-designed true experiments provide the strongest evidence to either support or refute a hypothesis. Typical work-site drug use questions that can be addressed with such designs include assessing the effectiveness of work-site drug use prevention programs, work-site drug abuse treatment programs, and the effectiveness of drug abuse treatment programs for individuals as well as to identify the effects of drug use on individual performance.

The major strength of the randomized design is that it renders the spuriousness and reverse causation explanations of association unlikely alternatives to the hypothesized causal relation under study. This is because, if randomization is properly carried out, one can have confidence to a known degree of statistical probability that the units receiving the treatment are like the units serving as controls with respect to the myriad unmeasured factors that might affect the behavior of interest. Consider, for example, a field experiment in which, of 500 workers under treatment for drug abuse, 250 are randomly assigned to follow-up treatment and the other 250 are not offered follow-up. If the former group improves more than the latter, one can be confident to a known degree of statistical probability that the improvement was not due to factors, such as a greater desire to keep the job, that distinguished the follow-up group from the other and was also plausibly related to treatment success. One could not have such confidence if the workers chose whether they wanted follow-up treatment or if assignments to follow-up were made on some nonrandom basis, such as by offering follow-up to the day shifts but not to the evening or swing shifts.

Despite their great strength in eliminating threats posed by confounding variables, randomized experiments are not a perfect methodology, nor are they always a feasible or even best way to search for causal relationships. They are still subject to measurement artifacts, and they can be prohibitively expensive or otherwise impractical. Large-scale experiments can also fail because of an inability to control the exposure of assigned groups to the experimental or the control treatment. In the example we have used, for instance, workers not offered follow-up aid may search it out on their own, and an effective intervention may appear to be without effect. Also, one may not know what it is about an experimental treatment that is effective, so experimental results may be misleading. In the drug treatment experiment we posit workers assigned to follow-up may feel they are especially valued by their employers, or those not assigned to treatment may feel undervalued. These feelings rather than follow-up or lack of it may affect future drug use in these groups, meaning that the experiment is no guide to what would happen if everyone or no one received follow-up treatment.

The possibility of problems like these, however, should not disguise the great strengths of randomized field experiments. The more important problems associated with them are practical. Random assignment to treatment, for example, can be extraordinarily hard to implement. A supervisor told to assign workers to experimental or control groups might, for example, cheat and assign those he thinks are most likely to benefit from the treatment to that condition, or workers may informally trade places if controls to ensure against this are not in place. If deviations like these are known, they can to some extent be corrected for statistically, but some of the power of the randomized experiment is lost.

Cost, too, is a factor. In particular, when treatments are randomized across units, like factories, other than across individuals, as they may be when it is feared that morale problems would result if individuals within units were treated differently, only a small number of units may be assigned to the two conditions. Yet the strength of randomization depends on the random assignment of a sufficiently large number of units to weaken substantially the possibility that confounding factors would coincidentally vary with the random assignment. When only a small number of units are randomly assigned to conditions, the design should be considered quasi-experimental, and methods appropriate to quasi-experiments should be utilized (e.g., deviation from secular trend design).

Laboratory studies can generally randomize individuals to conditions and thus achieve substantial internal validity by using large numbers of participants. The major practical drawback of laboratory research generally lies not in the threat that confounding variables pose for causal inference but rather in limited *external validity*. Because laboratory conditions are usually quite different from conditions in the world in which people live, use drugs, and work, it is often unclear how far one may generalize from what occurs in the laboratory to what occurs in the world of work. If, for example, smoking two marijuana cigarettes degrades the performance of a 19-year-old student responding to a speed addition test, it does not mean that two marijuana cigarettes would adversely affect the performance of a 35-year-old driving a truck who has smoked marijuana daily for 10 years.

PRACTICAL IMPORTANCE VERSUS
STATISTICAL SIGNIFICANCE

Consumers of research, who are unfamiliar with the technical language of statistics, often misconstrue the term *significant*. When a finding is labeled *statistically significant* or simply *significant*, it seems reasonable to conclude that the finding is of practical or scientific importance—but this conclusion may be wrong. Moreover, the fact that a relationship is *highly significant* does not mean that it is large in magnitude. All statistical significance means is that it is unlikely (to some specified degree) that a relationship as large or larger than the one observed could arise by chance if no relationship between the variables investigated existed. When large samples are studied, relationships may be statistically significant without having important policy implications.

The potential practical importance of a relationship is communicated by the magnitude of the actual difference, assuming the difference is statistically significant and so cannot be plausibly attributed to chance. But even when a study is of potential practical importance, it still may not provide a sound basis for policy decisions. All of the aspects of the study design must be considered. An observed effect in a study may be statistically significant and sufficiently large to be of practical importance, but if the design is so flawed that many alternative explanations of the observed difference are plausible, then the study is a weak basis for policy decisions. Finally, even well-designed studies that identify substantial significant relationships do not necessarily mean that an intervention is justified. This further depends on the cost of the intervention, the prevalence of the problem to be prevented or solved, and the costs the problem imposes.

To appreciate the interaction of these various factors, consider a company that is thinking of initiating a drug use prevention program and wisely decides to study the program's likely effects before investing heavily in its implementation. It finds that, among workers exposed to the program, 39 percent are using drugs after 6 months; among workers not exposed to the program, 40 percent of the workers are using drugs after 6 months. If there are enough workers in the exposed and unexposed groups, the difference may be statistically significant, suggesting that the program actually affects workers' drug use, but the effect is so weak that instituting the program would not be beneficial, unless its costs were truly minuscule, as for example, a program that consisted of posting a few "Just Say No" signs on company premises. Alternatively, suppose the effects were large—say 20 percent of exposed workers were using drugs after 6 months—compared with 40 percent of unexposed workers, but only 10 workers were in each group. The difference, although large, would not be statistically significant; before instituting the program the company would want to test more workers to be sure that the results were not due to chance factors. If, after exposing more workers to the treatment and control conditions, a large effect still remained, other aspects of the design might still lead the company to question the advisability of relying on the research. If, for example, the treatment had been delivered to workers with low-stress jobs while control group members had been selected from among workers with high-stress jobs and no preintervention baselines had been established, the design would not rule out the possibility that it was a job stress rather than a treatment effect that had been identified. Finally, suppose a well-designed study yielded large, significant differences between the treatment and control groups. Now the company could have confidence that it had identified a successful treatment that could be expected to substantially reduce drug use in its work force. This would still not mean that the company would necessarily want to initiate the program. If the program were expensive, if it reduced only the use of marijuana, and if the company had no reason to believe that marijuana use was impairing the performance of its workers, then the company could reasonably find that the cost of the program was not justified.

RESEARCH DESIGN ISSUES SPECIFIC TO
DRUG USE IN THE WORKPLACE

There are a number of problems, that, although not unique to studies of drug use in the workplace, are sufficiently common as to merit special mention. First, there are frequent misconceptions regarding what is the proper unit of analysis and the role of temporal sequence of events in establishing causality. Moreover, problems of error in measurement are important because the confounding effects of poorly measured variables will not be adequately adjusted when multivariate models are used in epidemiologic and quasi-experimental analyses (Dwyer, 1983). Understanding the characteristics of such errors is crucial in efforts to use multivariate models

Unit of Analysis

The unit of intervention, and thus of statistical inference, in workplace prevention studies is often whole companies or work sites within companies. Special problems arise in these circumstances. These include a lack of statistical power due to the small number of units studied and the need for multiple baseline observations to increase the power to detect deviations from secular trends. The appropriate statistical model when large social units are randomized to conditions is not always obvious, and in some recent reports from large community prevention trials the models used have been misspecified. The only direct estimate of sampling variability in such studies comes from between-community or between-company differences. Multiple observations over time can be used to reduce error in measures, but they cannot skirt the fundamental "degrees of freedom" problem that is inherent in a small number of experimental units (Dwyer, 1993).

Temporal Sequence and Causality

Researchers interested in how early exposure to some drugs affects the later use of other drugs often use longitudinal data to address issues of temporal sequence and causality. They may find, for example, that children who use cigarettes or alcohol at one point in time are more likely, than those who do not, to go on to use marijuana. The observation of such a sequence does not, however, imply that cigarette and alcohol use increase the risk of marijuana use. It may be that the use of all these drugs is influenced by the same set of social and psychological factors, and that their association arises from these underlying factors rather than from a causal sequence. Sorting out causal relationships is important. If, for example, the relationship between early alcohol use and later marijuana use is spurious, removing access to alcohol could conceivably increase the use of marijuana rather than prevent its use.

Measurement Errors of Drug Use Indicators

Just determining who is using what drugs in which contexts is difficult. Drug tests are the basic measure of drug use in many studies and in most drug screening and treatment programs. They are powerful methodological tools in that they give consistent readings and they can accurately identify the presence of known drugs or their metabolites in tested specimens. It is tempting to interpret the high levels of reproducibility of urine tests results for certain drugs as evidence of validity of those tests. However, the validity of a test is the extent to which it measures what it is intended to measure. What a urinalysis drug test measures is the presence of drugs and/or their metabolites in urine as an indication of recent drug use. As discussed in Chapter 6, when performed according to current professional standards, the sensitivity and specificity of those tests in detecting recent drug use is very high. However, measurement problems do arise when researchers use such test results as a measure of constructs the test was not intended to measure. For example, urine testing does not provide accurate estimates of the prevalence of drug use in specified populations (see Chapter 3), it does not provide a good measure of the individual drug use involvement (i.e., use, abuse, dependence), and it is not a good measure of impairment (see Chapter 6). Urinalysis test results are not sensitive or specific measures of those latter constructs. Furthermore, drug testing is not always possible, and when it is, even if the sample of those tested is not biased by a need for cooperation, measurement of metabolic residues is problematic when the half-life of residues is shorter or longer than the time period of interest. Moreover, given the low prevalence of positive tests in many populations, it remains plausible that rare and unidentified causes of false positives are operating.

Self-report measures of drug use and abuse are obviously suspect when respondents realize that admitting drug use may have adverse personal consequences, but even when there are no threatened adverse consequences, social norms may affect answers. Thus, several studies have found systematic underreporting of such behaviors as cigarette use among pregnant women, cocaine use among patients at a county hospital, drug use among arrestees, and drug use at work sites. In some instances, consistent bias in self-reports may allow valid comparisons between groups or over time. However, persons in drug use prevention programs may be more likely to underreport than controls, and temporal changes in social norms concerning drug use may change the extent of underreporting or overreporting over time. One useful source of more information on this subject is a research monograph (Rouse et al., 1985) entitled *Self-Report Methods of Estimating Drug Use: Meeting Current Challenges to Validity*. Perhaps the most general conclusion that can be supported is that most people appear to be reasonably truthful (within the bounds of capability) under the proper conditions. The "proper conditions" of course are the key words. When respondents believe they are guaranteed anonymity or confidentiality, when they accept the scientific or practical value of the survey, when they accept the legitimacy of the survey, and when they are not fearful of adverse consequences, then the evidence suggests that they tend to be generally truthful. More relevant to the present report, there is every reason to be cautious about self-report surveys that are conducted at a work site. Common sense suggests that employees, when asked about their substance use at a workplace, may have concerns about the uses to which the data could be put. Hence, there may be some considerable incentive for drug users to underreport their drug-using behaviors.

In addition to problems of intentional underreporting, there are other potential problems with the validity of survey data, including issues of population coverage and response rates. Particularly with respect to estimation of trends, an important consideration is consistency over time. If response rates or coverage were to change, that could produce spurious changes in apparent prevalence rates.

The best protection against all these threats to validity is to be aware of them and to deal with them as forthrightly as possible. The major point to be made for present purposes is that, when the circumstances allow the respondent to consider the questions reasonable and justified in terms of purpose, and when the respondent can feel reasonably certain that the answers will not be used against him or her, then self-reports can be sufficiently valid for research and policy purposes. When those conditions are not met—which is often the case in work site related research—there may well be very substantial underreporting.

Psychological tests designed to assess individual drug use also have serious measurement limitations. As discussed in detail in Chapter 6, psychological tests designed to reveal current or predict future drug use have been shown to have moderate levels of validity. Combining this moderate validity with the relatively low prevalence of drug use in work site populations means that if psychological tests are used to identify drug users, false positive rates can be expected to be high. Thus, employers are unlikely to find psychological tests to be practical instruments for eliminating drug users from the ranks of employees or from applicant pools.

CONCLUSION AND RECOMMENDATION

• The most powerful methodology for evaluating the effectiveness of workplace alcohol and other drug-intervention programs is the randomized field experiment. The implementation of new work site alcohol and other drug-intervention programs or significant changes in existing programs provide propitious occasions for experimental assessment.

Recommendation: To enhance scientific knowledge, organizations instituting new work-site alcohol and other drug intervention programs should proceed experimentally if possible. Funding agencies should make field experiments a priority, and should consider providing start-up aid to private companies that are willing to institute programs experimentally and subject them to independent evaluation.

REFERENCES

Dwyer, J.H.
   1983   *Statistical models.* New York: Oxford University.
   1993   Estimating Statistical Power in the "Deviation From Secular Trend" Design. NIDA Research Monograph (in press).
Rouse J.J., N.J. Kozel, and L. G. Richards, eds.
   1985   *Self-Report Methods of Estimating Drug Use: Meeting Current Challenges to Validity.* NIDA Research Monograph No. 57. Rockville, Md.: National Institute on Drug Abuse.

B

The Legal Environment of Drug Testing

The law today mandates and defines permissible drug-testing programs. All drug testing by public bodies and some drug testing by private entities is done pursuant to legal authority or command. This authority may not only mandate testing, but may also constrain the conditions under which drug testing proceeds and the consequences that can attach to positive results. There are also limits on what the law can authorize or mandate with respect to drug testing. These limits are established by courts in suits that challenge the legal authority or constitutionality of drug-testing programs. Finally, the law, either through statutes, regulations, or court decisions, may control what private entities can do on their own initiative by way of drug testing. This appendix addresses these matters as we describe the legal environment in which drug testing occurs today.

SOURCES OF AUTHORITY

Over the past decade, the President and the Congress have not only authorized drug testing by public and private employers, but have also required or encouraged it in some workplaces. Their actions provide legal

This appendix is based on a paper commissioned by the Committee on Drug Use in the Workplace from David Wasserman of the Institute for Philosophy and Public Policy, University of Maryland, and James Jacobs of the School of Law, New York University.

authority for drug testing that overrides all contrary authority except the U.S Constitution.

Executive Order 12564 (1986) introduced the concept of a "drug free workplace" and set in place many of the features of workplace drug testing that have now become standard for public and regulated private employers. It required all federal agencies to adopt employee drug-testing programs, which included mandatory testing for employees in "sensitive" positions involving law enforcement, public health and safety, and national security, with the extent of testing and the criteria for testing being left to the discretion of each agency head. It also permitted the testing of employees in other positions: (1) when there was reasonable suspicion that the employee was using illegal drugs; (2) in an examination regarding an accident or unsafe practice; and (3) as part of, or as a follow-up to, counseling or rehabilitation for illegal drug use through an employee assistance program.

Under the executive order, visual monitoring of the giving of a urine specimen was not permitted unless there was reason to believe that the employee would alter or substitute the specimen. The order also mandated procedures to protect the confidentiality of test results. In addition, it required each agency to establish a comprehensive employee assistance program involving education, counseling, and rehabilitation.

In Section 503 of the Supplemental Appropriations Act of 1987, Congress required federal contractors as well as agencies to guarantee a drug-free workplace; although drug testing was not mandatory, it was recommended. Section 503 also required all federal agencies to draft detailed testing plans to be reviewed by the U.S. Department of Health and Human Services (DHHS), thereby promoting the uniformity of federal testing procedures. The DHHS "Mandatory Guidelines for Federal Workplace Drug-Testing Programs" contain stringent procedural safeguards that have now become standard: requirements for the collection of urine specimens, the avoidance of sample mix-ups, the certification of and quality control measures for testing laboratories, and the confirmation of positive test results.

In 1988 Congress passed the Drug Free Workplace Act (DFWA), which required all federal contractors with contracts of $25,000 or more to certify to the appropriate contracting agency that they are maintaining a drug-free workplace. If they failed to do so, the contract could be canceled. Contractors were not required to implement a drug-testing program, but could do so in order to demonstrate compliance.

In 1991 standards for industries regulated by the U.S. Department of Transportation (DOT) were unified and consolidated in the Omnibus Transportation Employee Testing Act (OTETA) of that year. OTETA mandates drug and alcohol tests for all individuals who hold or apply for "safety-sensitive" jobs in the transportation industry. Public- and private-sector employers must set up drug programs in conformity with the DOT regulations.

LEGAL CONSTRAINTS

Any program of workplace drug testing must operate within legal constraints—not all testing programs are legally permissible. It is important, however, to remember that legal constraints are not necessarily binding for all time, even when they are constitutionally based. Changing technology, changing perceptions of the drug problem, and changes in the perceived relationship between drug use and workplace performance may all influence legal decision makers, be they judges or legislators, in determining what should be permitted. This committee's report, in contrast, is time bound. We can only recount what as of this writing seem to be the constraints that the law places on workplace drug-testing programs.

In surveying the law as it currently exists, three important distinctions emerge. First is the public-private distinction. Drug testing done by a government agency or by a private business in compliance with a government mandate will face legal constraints that will not bind a private firm that chooses to test for drugs at its own initiative. Second is the distinction between preemployment and postemployment drug testing. Generally speaking, both governmental agencies and private businesses are freer to test potential employees for drug use than they are to test those already employed. Third is the distinction between state and federal law. Drug-testing programs that are permissible under federal law may nonetheless be impermissible under the law of a particular state. However, state law will not prevent the federal government from testing its own employees in conformance with federal law, nor can it preclude employers within the state from complying with federally mandated drug-testing programs.

The Fourth Amendment

The public-private distinction is important because drug testing normally involves the taking and examination of material from a person's body that is not normally exposed to public scrutiny and so is considered a search under the Fourth Amendment to the U.S. Constitution. This amendment prohibits unreasonable searches and seizures by governmental agents and, subject to certain exceptions, limits governmental searches to those made pursuant to a warrant upon a showing of "probable cause." The Fourth Amendment does not, however, restrict the actions of private individuals or organizations so long as they are acting on their own initiative and not in response to some governmental mandate.

Universal or routine workplace drug testing obviously fails to satisfy the warrant and probable-cause requirements of the Fourth Amendment. If the amendment were applied to drug testing as it is applied in ordinary criminal investigations, routine drug testing when conducted by public officials or by private parties acting in response to a legal mandate, such as the Omnibus Transportation Employee Testing Act of 1991, would not be permitted. The "probable-cause" language of the Fourth Amendment has, however, been held inapplicable to administrative searches that serve primarily a regulatory rather than a law enforcement purpose, so long as the search does not contravene the Fourth Amendment's more general preclusion of "unreasonable searches." The reasonableness or unreasonableness of an administrative search depends on the balance between the governmental interests served by the search and its intrusiveness.

A special rule for administrative searches was first carved out by the Supreme Court in 1967 in *Camera v. Municipal Court* (387 U.S. 523, 1967), which held that city housing inspectors could secure warrants to conduct areawide searches for housing code violations without having probable-cause to believe that any building or buildings were in violation of the code. In abandoning the probable-cause requirement for warrants, the Court pointed to several factors clearly present in the *Camera* case: a neutral plan that limited discretion and possible bias in conducting searches, very limited intrusion in conducting the searches, and a showing of a compelling government need for the plan in the absence of less intrusive alternatives. However, since *Camera*, "[t]he 'tests' have been reformulated, qualifications have been stripped away, and the elements have been applied ever less strictly" (Schulhoffer, "On the Fourth Amendment Rights of the Law-Abiding Public," 189 *Supreme Court Review* 87, 94). In particular, in certain circumstances not only is there no need to justify searches with a showing of probable-cause, but also the warrant requirement itself has been abandoned. Among the contexts in which the Supreme Court since *Camera* has upheld searches without probable-cause and/or without a warrant are: an inspection program of federally licensed firearms dealers (*United States v. Biswell*, 406 U.S. 311, 1972); an inspection by the Occupational Safety and Health Administration to determine compliance with workplace safety regulations (*Marshall v. Barlow's Inc.*, 436 U.S. 307, 1978); safety inspections of mines and stone quarries (*Donovan v. Dewey*, 452 U.S. 594, 1981); a search of the handbag of a student suspected of smoking (*New Jersey v. T.L.O.*, 459 U.S. 325, 1985); an inspection of an automobile junkyard done with crime control goals in mind (*New York v. Burger*, 482 U.S. 691, 1987); and stops at roadblocks set up to control drunk driving (*Michigan Dept. of State Police v. Sitz*, 496 U.S. 444, 1990). Finally, in a pair of cases decided in 1989, *Skinner v. Railway Labor Executive's Association* (489 U.S. 602, 1989) and *National Treasury Employees Union v. Von Raab* (489 U.S. 656, 1989), the Court added drug testing to this list.

Skinner and Von Raab

In *Skinner* the Supreme Court was faced with a challenge to the constitutionality of the Federal Railroad Administration's (FRA) mandatory and permissive alcohol- and drug-testing procedures. Testing for drugs and alcohol was mandatory after a major train accident involving (1) a fatality, (2) the release of hazardous materials accompanied by evacuation or reportable injury, or (3) damage to railroad property of $500,000 or more. Furthermore, blood and urine samples had to be collected after an "impact accident," one that resulted in a reportable injury or in damage to railroad property of $50,000 or more. Finally, a railroad had to test after "any train incident that involves fatality to any on-duty railroad employee." If an employee declined to give a blood sample, the railroad could presume impairment, absent persuasive contrary evidence.

The Court, in a 7-2 decision, upheld the regulations. The majority began by holding that a search conducted by a private railroad under the auspices of a federal regulatory agency constituted state action under the Fourth Amendment. The Court next found that both the collection of blood, urine, and breath and the subsequent chemical analysis of these substances constitute searches for Fourth Amendment purposes. But, having found that the testing program was a search within the meaning of the Fourth Amendment, the Court analyzed the FRA's drug-testing requirements under the reasonableness test used for administrative searches rather than by reference to the law enforcement standard of probable-cause or a lesser standard of reasonable suspicion.

The administrative search standard required the reviewing court to balance the governmental interest served by the testing program against its intrusiveness. Just as the adoption of this balancing test was significant, so was the way the Court weighed the factors in the case before it. In assessing the infringement of privacy involved in blood, urine, and breath testing, the Court pointed out that railroad employees already consent to significant restrictions on their freedom of movement and that "any additional interference with a railroad employee's freedom of movement that occurs in the time it takes to procure a blood or breath sample for testing cannot, by itself, be said to significantly infringe on privacy interests." While the urine test raised greater privacy concerns, the fact that urine collection did not involve visual monitoring and that it took place in a medical setting led the Court to conclude that the infringement of privacy was not significantly greater. Finally, the Court argued that, since railroads have long been a heavily regulated industry, their employees must expect greater intrusion. "Though some of the privacy interests implicated by the toxicological testing at issue reasonably might be viewed as significant in other contexts, logic and history show that a diminished expectation of privacy attaches to information relating to the physical condition of covered employees and to this reasonable means of procuring such information" (489 U.S. 602, 628).

Perhaps the most significant indicator in *Skinner* of how the Court might rule in future cases was its assessment of the government's interests served by testing. The Court deferred substantially to the FRA's claim of alcohol or drug problems on railroads, although there was only weak factual support for that claim in the FRA's data on accidents over a 20-year period. Almost all drug-related railroad accidents were alcohol-related, but the Court, like the agency, spoke of "alcohol and drugs" in a single breath: ". . . the government's interest in testing without a showing of individualized suspicion is compelling."

Employees subject to the tests discharge duties fraught with such risks of injury to others that even a momentary lapse of attention can have disastrous consequences. Much like persons who have routine access to dangerous nuclear power facilities, employees who are subject to testing under the FRA regulations can cause great human loss before any signs of impairment become noticeable to supervisors or others (489 U.S. 602, 628).

The dissenters argued that the approach that led the Court to accept postaccident drug testing in this case would likely lead to a broad acceptance of drug testing in many contexts. Their point seems to be supported by the Court's holding in *Von Raab*, the companion case to *Skinner*.

In *Von Raab*, a union of federal employees and a union official challenged the U.S. Customs Service's drug-testing program, which made drug tests a condition of promotion or transfer to positions that met one or more of three criteria: (1) direct involvement in drug interdiction or the enforcement of related laws, (2) the carrying of firearms, or (3) the handling of classified materials. Employees who tested positive for drugs and offered no satisfactory explanation were subject to dismissal. However, test results could not be turned over to any other agency, including criminal prosecutors, without the employee's consent.

The Customs Service characterized drug interdiction as its primary enforcement mission and argued that "there is no room in the Customs Service for those who break the laws prohibiting the possession and use of drugs." While no serious drug problem had been uncovered within the Customs Service, the implications of such a problem, if it did arise, were offered as a justification for a wide-ranging drug-testing program.

The Supreme Court, this time by a 5-4 vote, once again held that neither probable-cause nor reasonable suspicion were needed to test government employees in "sensitive" positions. Justice Kennedy wrote: "Our precedents have settled that, in certain limited circumstances, the Government's need to discover . . . latent or hidden conditions, or to prevent their development, is sufficiently compelling to justify the intrusion on privacy entailed by conducting such searches without any measure of individualized suspicion" (489 U.S. 656, 668).

The Court's opinion emphasized the job demands in the Customs Service that would be specially threatened by employees who used drugs. Thus, the Court noted that "the physical safety of these [Customs] employees may be threatened, and many may be tempted not only by bribes from the traffickers with whom they deal, but also by their own access to vast sources of valuable contraband seized and controlled by the Service" (id. at 669).

The reasonableness test adopted in *Skinner* and *Von Raab* requires courts passing judgment on drug-testing programs to balance the intrusion on tested individuals against the government interests served by the test. While this standard is easy to articulate, it has no clear meaning. In *Skinner* the standard justified the testing of employees in highly safety-sensitive positions, predicated on suspicious circumstances. The Court's deference to the FRA's safety concerns suggest that drug testing throughout the transportation industry and in other areas in which safety concerns are easily and plausibly invoked, such as fire departments and public utilities, will be upheld against Fourth Amendment challenges, at least so long as the testing program is required of employees in safety-related positions and no more intrusive than the urine testing in *Skinner*. *Von Raab* extends *Skinner's* permission for warrantless searches to situations in which there is no reason to believe that drug use has been a problem and to employees whose performance will not necessarily be adversely affected by drug use.

Justice Scalia's dissent in *Von Raab* suggests the potential scope of this case:

> [In] extending approval of drug testing to that category consisting of employees who carry firearms, the Court exposes vast numbers of public employees to this needless indignity. Logically, of course, if those who carry guns can be treated in this fashion, so can all others whose work, if performed under the influence of drugs, may endanger others—automobile drivers, operators of other potentially dangerous equipment, construction workers, school crossing guards. A similarly broad scope attaches to the Court's approval of drug testing for those with access to "sensitive information."
>
> Since this category is not limited to Service employees with drug interdiction duties, nor to "sensitive information" specifically relating to drug traffic, today's holding apparently approves drug testing for all federal employees with security clearances—or, indeed, for all federal employees with valuable confidential information to impart. . . . Moreover, there is no reason why this super-protection against harms arising from drug use must be limited to public employees; a law requiring similar testing of private citizens who use dangerous instruments such as guns or cars, or

who have access to classified information would also be constitutional" (489 U.S. 665, 686, 1989).

It seems likely that law enforcement agencies will see the Court as having approved drug testing for all employees who carry firearms. Many other agencies will take *Von Raab* as approving drug testing for all employees who have any access to "sensitive information." In addition, law enforcement agencies may attempt to justify drug-testing programs solely on the basis of a claimed need to assure the public that there are no drug users serving in their ranks.

Two other aspects of *Skinner* and *Von Raab* are worth noting. First, in neither case was the urine sample subject to visual observation. The need for reliable drug testing might have to be greater than it was in one or both of these cases to justify a drug-testing program that required an employee to urinate in the presence of an observer. Second, in each case only certain employees defined by the nature of their job responsibilities were required to provide urine samples. Agency-wide drug testing programs remain constitutionally suspect.

Applying the Reasonableness Standard

While *Skinner* and *Von Raab* opened the door to substantial drug testing, several cases that have since been decided in the Federal Courts of Appeals indicate that the courts will scrutinize the constitutionality of drug-testing programs and that lower court judges do not see *Skinner* and *Von Raab* as eliminating all constitutional barriers to governmentally mandated drug testing.

For example in *Harmon v. Thornburgh* (878 F.2d 484, D.C. Cir. 1989, Cert. denied 493 U.S. 1056, 1990), a case brought by the U.S. Department of Justice employees challenging that agency's drug-testing program, the D.C. Court of Appeals read *Von Raab* as "suggesting that the government may search its employees only when a clear, direct nexus exists between the nature of the employee's duty and the nature of the feared violation." Applying this standard, the court upheld random testing for employees with access to top secret classified information and suggested that the drug testing of drug prosecutors would be permissible. However, the court held that the government's interests in work force integrity, public safety, and protection of sensitive information did not, for Fourth Amendment purposes, make reasonable a plan for randomly testing employees in less sensitive positions, including Antitrust Division attorneys. The appellate court also rejected the department's plan to test all criminal prosecutors and all employees with access to grand jury materials. In a later case, a different panel of the D.C. Court of Appeals, in evaluating the U.S. Department of

Defense's drug-testing program for civilian employees, distinguished between laboratory personnel on one hand (random testing not allowed) and aviation workers, police guards, and drug counselors on the other (random testing allowed) (*National Federation of Federal Employees v. Cheney*, 884 F.2d 603, D.C. Cir. 1989, Cert. denied, 493 U.S. 1056, 1990). In a similar vein the Seventh Circuit Court required the Cook County Department of Corrections to limit its unannounced drug-testing program to employees with regular prisoner contact, with opportunities to smuggle drugs, or with access to firearms (*Taylor v. O'Grady*, 888 F.2d 1189, 7th Cir. 1989). The D.C. Circuit Court has, however, upheld the testing of mail van operators, not because of safety risks but on the rationale they are vulnerable to blackmail (*American Federation of Government Employees v. Skinner*, 885 F.2d 884, D.C. Cir. 1989, Cert. denied, 495 U.S. 923, 1990), and it has upheld the urine testing, without probable-cause, of a person who had been tentatively accepted for employment by the Department of Justice's Antitrust Division (*Willner v. Thornburgh*, 928 F.2d 1185, D.C. Cir. 1991).

Factors to Be Considered

In striking the balance mandated by *Skinner* and *Von Raab*, there appears to be an emerging consensus among federal courts reviewing drug testing by public employers about what makes a governmentally mandated program reasonable within the meaning of the Fourth Amendment.

First, the courts have been concerned with who gets tested and whether there is a reasonable basis for demanding that they do get tested. When drug-testing programs have been found unconstitutional, it has usually been because they targeted too wide a range of employees. In such cases, the remedy has typically been to narrow the program to employees whose drug use poses an actual or symbolic threat of harm to fellow employees, the public, or an agency's mission.

While few courts demand proof of significant employee drug use or drug-related impairment for postemployment testing, the employer must offer some reason why drug abuse by employees could impair the safety, integrity, or productivity of the operation; a threat to the employees' own health or safety or the moral desirability of a drug-free workplace is not enough. Employers have been found to lack the compelling safety interest that would justify random or routine testing of transportation maintenance custodians (*Bolden v. SEPTA*, 3rd Cir. April 1, 1991) or sanitation enforcement agents (*Watson v. Sexton*, 755 F. Supp. 583, S.D.N.Y. 1991).

An exception to this requirement of job-specific dangers may arise in heavily regulated industries like transportation, in which a reduced expectation of privacy on the part of all workers seems to obviate the need for an inquiry into the specific risks that drug abuse would pose to their work

(*IBEW v. Skinner*, 913 F2d 1454, 9th Cir. 1991). But those expectations of privacy are often reduced precisely because intensive screening, regulation, or supervision are thought to be necessary to protect the safety or integrity of the operation—which makes it difficult to assess the independent significance of privacy expectations in the judicial review of workplace drug-testing programs.

Second, the courts recognize three distinct but overlapping factors as justifying random, routine, or universal testing for whole job categories. The most important is the actual risk to safety or integrity posed by employee drug use, particularly to nonemployees, as, for example, in the case of workers at a nuclear power plant (*Ensor v. Rust Engineering Co.*, 704 F. Supp 808, E.D. Tenn. 1989, Aff'd 935 F.2d 269, 6th Cir. 1991). A second factor that reinforces the first is the special responsibility of the tested employees for the safety of those who might be endangered by their drug use—bus drivers are an example (*Holloman v. GCRTA,* 741 F. Supp. 677, N.D. Ohio, 1990, Aff'd 930 F.2d 918, 6th Cir. 1991). The third factor is the need to maintain public trust and confidence. For example, the district court in *O'Connor v. Police Commissioner of Boston* wrote, in upholding a drug-testing program for police cadets, "[P]ublic confidence in the police is a social necessity and is enhanced by procedures that deter drug use by police cadets" (557 N.E.2d 1146, 1150, Mass. 1990. See also: *Gauthier v. Police Commissioner of Boston*, 557 N.E. 2d 1374, Mass. 1990).

While there are cases that suggest that programs that mandate the testing of all employees within a particular category are more likely to survive constitutional scrutiny than those that randomly select individuals for testing, random testing has been allowed in situations in which it seems reasonable for deterrence or other reasons. It also appears that, although the Supreme Court in *Skinner* pointed to the absence of visual monitoring as a factor supporting the constitutionality of the program at issue in that case, monitoring seldom appears as a crucial factor, perhaps because visual monitoring of the urine sample collection process seldom seems to occur.

The reliability of testing techniques in detecting the presence of illegal drugs (or their metabolites) has been noted by some courts as a factor in their decisions, but little attention has been paid to whether the type of drugs tested for or the amount detected reflects a threat to safety, integrity, or productivity. Thus, by far the most common illicit drug revealed in workplace testing is marijuana, the adverse effects of which are comparatively slight and disputed. Even less attention has been paid to the preventive or deterrent value of the testing, that is, to whether a drug-testing program really reduces employee drug consumption. The courts seem surprisingly uninterested in the empirical research bearing on these questions.

Although some court decisions mention the fact that a positive drug test will not lead to the dismissal of an employee or will not be shared with law enforcement agencies as a factor supporting a testing program, by and large the courts have not expressed much concern about the consequences of positive test results. The judicial silence on these issues may result in part from the growing uniformity of public- and private-sector testing programs, promoted by statutes like the DFWA and OTETA, which impose stringent restrictions on the sanctions that can be imposed for positive test results and on the disclosure of those results. The private employers whose testing programs lack these restrictions are less likely to be subject to judicial scrutiny.

The Private Sector

Private businesses are not subject to the strictures of the Fourth Amendment unless their testing programs are mandated by law. Thus the factors that lead courts under the Fourth Amendment to approve or disapprove of drug-testing programs in the public sector will not in themselves validate or undermine the drug-testing programs that private businesses establish at their own initiative. The other two dichotomies that we have mentioned, the distinction between pre- and postemployment drug testing and the distinction between state and federal law, do play an important role here. Generally speaking, both public and private sectors have considerably more leeway in establishing preemployment drug-screening programs than they do in establishing postemployment drug-testing programs.

In the private sector, the potential limitations are greatest among the unionized segment of the work force. This is because the National Labor Relations Board has held that the institution of a drug-testing program for current employees constitutes a "material change" in the employees' working conditions that is subject to collective bargaining (*Johnson-Bateman Co.*, 295 N.L.R.B. No. 26, June 15, 1989), but it has reached the opposite conclusions with respect to preemployment programs (*Star Tribune*, 295 N.L.R.B. No. 63, June 15, 1989). This means that preemployment drug-testing programs may take whatever form management prefers, but postemployment testing of unionized employees is subject to negotiations that usually produce compromise programs, often restricting the testing of employees to cases of reasonable suspicion and almost always mandating treatment rather than discipline as the initial response to positive test results. Also, it is possible for employees in unionized industries to file grievances regarding certain characteristics of drug-testing programs. Arbitrators have struck down drug-testing programs on such grounds as (1) the testing procedures were not accurate, (2) a testing program was not within the employer's prerogative, and (3) the testing program was not reasonable given the lack of evidence of a workplace drug problem. But as unions and management agree on the details of such programs and as drug testing in the workplace becomes more common, such decisions are increasingly rare (Hopson, 1986; Veglahn, 1988; *Labor Relations Week,* 1989).

In the nonunionized sector, existing employees, but not job applicants, may benefit from the erosion that has been occurring in some jurisdictions in the "employment at will" doctrine; that is, the rule that gives employers wide latitude in dismissing employees for any reason that is not prohibited by law. This body of law is beginning to change so that in certain situations courts will hold that dismissals for certain reasons are against public policy. Given the national policy against drug use, employees to date have had little success in claiming that discharges based on positive drug tests violate public policy, but one court did indicate that a firing in contravention of a state statute regulating workplace drug testing would be against public policy (*Johnson v. Carpenter Technology Corp.,* 723 F. Supp. 180, D. Conn. 1989).

Private employers may be reluctant to fire employees who refuse to submit to drug testing if they will be held liable for that employee's unemployment compensation. A discharged employee is not eligible for unemployment compensation if she was fired for misconduct, but her refusal to obey an employer's rule is held to constitute misconduct if and only if that rule was reasonable as applied to her. Although no court has held that an employer's drug testing must conform to the Fourth Amendment to be reasonable, courts have found drug testing predicated solely on unsupported allegations to be unreasonable. Testing based on "suspicious behavior" has, however, been found reasonable (*Annotation* "Private Employee's Loss of Employment Because of a Refusal to Submit to a Drug Test as Affecting Right to Unemployment Compensation" 86 A.L.R. 4th 309, 1991).

In a related area, courts and unemployment boards generally uphold the denial of unemployment benefits to employees fired because of arrest or conviction for off-the-job drug possession, on the grounds that the employees have not become unemployed "through no fault of their own," as most applicable statutes require. Recent cases have also upheld denial of compensation to school teachers and job counselors on the grounds that drug possession is a form of misconduct incompatible with their responsibilities. Other cases have required compensation when the statutory exclusion covered only employees discharged for misconduct "in connection with . . . employment." A workplace drug test may reveal misconduct that warrants discharge without compensation. One recent decision found that a bus driver was not entitled to compensation after discharge for a positive drug-test result, since by coming into the office during his vacation to report an earlier accident, he violated a company ban on employees having drugs in their system while on the premises (*Shaw v. Unemployment Compensation Board of Review,* 539 A.2d 1383, Pa. Comwlth 1988. See also *Annotation* "Jobless Pay—Off-Duty Conduct" 35 A.L.R. 4th 691, Secs. 5,8, 1991 Supp.).

Employees and Applicants

The preemployment/postemployment distinction is important in the public sector as well, for it is a factor that may bear on the constitutionality of a drug-testing program. One reason relates to the property interest that an individual may be seen to have in the expectation of continued employment and the protection that due process gives such interests. Another reason relates to the reasonableness of a drug-testing program. One factor that might lead a court to find a preemployment drug-testing program reasonable whereas a postemployment program would not be is that an employer cannot observe an applicant at work and so has little basis apart from a drug test for determining whether his or her work might be impaired by drug use.

A pair of cases from the D.C. Circuit indicate the potential importance of the distinction. In *Harmon v. Thornburgh* (878 F.2d 484, D.C. Cir. 1989, Cert. denied 110 S. Ct. 865, 1990) the appellate court held that a drug-testing program for current Justice Department employees could not include, among others, the department's antitrust lawyers because there was an insufficient nexus between their work and drug use to justify the privacy invasion. (The same decision upheld the testing of prosecutors who handled drug cases.) In *Willner v. Thornburgh* (928 F.2d 1185, D.C. Cir. 1991) a different panel of the same court approved a program that required an applicant for a position with the department's Antitrust Division to submit to a drug test. An important rationale for this decision was that the Fourth Amendment precludes only unreasonable intrusions on privacy, and the fact that applicant drug testing is common in the private sector "is some indication of what expectations of privacy society is prepared to accept as 'reasonable' (id. at 1192-93)." If this rationale were generally accepted, it could eliminate the importance of the public-private distinction with respect to job applicants, as private-sector behavior unconstrained by the Fourth Amendment would ultimately determine what were reasonable expectations of privacy under the Fourth Amendment. At least some other courts, however, have relied on *Harmon* in job applicant cases and have not made this bootstrap argument (*Georgia Ass'n of Educators v. Harris*, 749 F. Supp. 1110, N.D. Ga. 1990).

State Law

The third distinction that we alluded to at the outset is between state and federal law. When federal law, including the valid regulations of federal administrative agencies, mandates drug testing, that testing is required, regardless of any state law to the contrary, so long as it is otherwise constitutional. A federal agency testing its own employees pursuant to federal law is similarly unaffected by state legal restrictions. However, private entities and state agencies may in particular states be barred by state law from engaging in drug testing in circumstances in which federal law and the U.S. Constitution pose no legal barriers.

State legal barriers may arise because identically worded state and federal constitutional provisions are interpreted differently by the state and federal supreme courts, because state constitutions may protect rights that are not explicitly protected in the U.S. Constitution, and because state legislatures may enact statutes that relate specifically to drug testing.

Ten states have explicit constitutional rights to privacy, and most other states have recognized an implicit right to privacy in their constitutions (Silverstein, 1989). California courts interpret their explicit constitutional provision to apply to private as well as public employers. California constitutional law requires a showing of "reasonableness" for preemployment drug testing and of "compelling interest" for postemployment testing. In 1987, a California appellate court affirmed a $485,000 jury award for wrongful discharge to a programmer for the Southern Pacific Railroad, who had been fired for refusing to provide a urine sample for drug testing. The court held that the railroad lacked a safety interest strong enough to justify testing. Not all states, however, would apply constitutional privacy provisions to private actions (The Alaska Supreme Court, for example, has held that its constitutional right to privacy only protects against state action and could not be violated by a private employer's drug-testing program. *Luedtke v. Nabors Alaska Drilling, Inc.*, 78 P.2d 1123, 1989) and, in another California case, a state appellate court held that preemployment drug and alcohol testing through urinalysis was not so intrusive as to violate that state's constitutional privacy protection (*Wilkinson v. Times Corp.*, 215 Cal. App. 3rd 1034, Cal. App. 1 Dist. 1989).

At least seven states have legislation that restricts the right of employers to order their employees to submit to mandatory urinalysis for purposes of identifying or deterring illegal drug use. Montana, Iowa, Vermont, and Rhode Island have banned all random or blanket testing of employees (without probable-cause or reasonable suspicion) and Minnesota, Maine, Connecticut, and Oregon permit random testing only of employees in safety-sensitive positions or otherwise limit the circumstances in which employees can be tested. These states also mandate confirmatory testing, certified laboratories, confidentiality of test results, and other procedural protections. Louisiana, Maryland, Nebraska, and Utah also regulate test procedures and protect the confidentiality of test results, but they do not limit the circumstances in which employees can be tested. In addition, several municipalities, including Boulder, San Francisco, and New York, have ordinances that restrict workplace drug testing for some employers. Municipal restrictions are valid to the extent that they do not conflict with applicable state or federal law.

Fearing that a patchwork of restrictive laws would deter employers, especially multistate employers, proponents of drug testing have sought to create national standards for drug testing through federal laws that preempt state and local legislation. With the enactment of OTETA, with a strong preemption provision, they have gained a major victory in the transportation field. Parts of the Vermont and Rhode Island statutes have already been held to be preempted by federal regulations; other state statutes explicitly defer to conflicting federal laws and regulations.

CONCLUSION

The scope of workplace drug testing is limited by certain state and federal constitutional restrictions, particularly in the public sector and in postemployment settings, but these limits are generous and allow a broad range of employees to be tested using a wide range of reliable methodologies. If there is a general limitation discernable, it is that the drug testing of public employees or of any employees pursuant to a governmentally mandated program violates the Constitution if the testing program appears directed at the general enforcement of the nation's drug laws and lacks a particularized occupational nexus. Even this principle, however, appears to be substantially relaxed in the case of job applicants, at least as a practical matter. Although there are a few states that legislatively protect certain workers from drug testing, most laws and regulations that regulate drug testing are important not for restricting who may be tested but for mandating testing in certain situations, for requiring protections against test error, and for restricting the consequences of positive findings. Indeed, the imposition of drug testing on a wide range of public and private workplaces by federal law and regulation has standardized testing programs and alleviated many of the early concerns about reliability and confidentiality. It is virtually impossible for an "innocent" employee to be fired or blackballed because of a false positive result in a program that complies with the DHHS guidelines.

Accuracy and confidentiality, however, remain concerns for nonunionized private employers not regulated by the DHHS guidelines. Except in states with restrictive legislation or constitutional provisions, private employers in industries unaffected by federal regulations are essentially free to test any employee at any time, without guarantees of the accuracy of the testing process and with few restrictions on the use or disclosure of the test results. For employers who invest little in training, have little concern with morale, and cannot afford confirmatory tests or treatment programs, a high probability that an employee uses illegal drugs may be reason enough to fire him. If such quick-and-dirty drug testing becomes widespread, it may provoke another round of restrictive state statutes, not to supersede federal guidelines, but to extend them to a wider range of workplaces.

New legislation may also come with new technologies of drug and performance testing, and such developments might also reopen constitutional issues that for the moment appear settled. For example, hair assays are less intrusive than urine testing and so might justify testing in situations that now fail to pass constitutional muster when the need for and intrusiveness of testing are balanced. At the same time, hair assays may raise new legal and constitutional problems due to their capacity to detect drug metabolites long after they have left the urine. The nexus between detected drug use and occupational impairment will be weaker than it is with urine testing, and the provisions of the Americans With Disabilities Act of 1991, which excludes current drug users but protects recovering addicts, might be more likely to be at issue when workers test positive.

Additional problems might also be posed with advances in performance testing. To the extent that new performance tests, such as tests of hand-eye coordination, can cheaply and accurately measure job-relevant psychomotor skills at the start of each workday, the apparent necessity of drug testing will diminish[1] and the relative intrusiveness of urine testing may appear to increase.

Ultimately, however, the legal future of drug testing is likely to turn less on the development of new technologies than it is on widespread social attitudes. The emerging judicial consensus in favor of drug testing appears to be built on four widely shared perceptions: (1) that drug abuse is one of the nation's most serious problems; (2) that drug-taking workers, at least in certain job categories, pose a threat to themselves, their coworkers, and the public and to the integrity and productivity of their operations; (3) that drug testing is reliable and accurate and can be protected from arbitrary and discriminatory implementation; and (4) that drug testing can be carried out in a way that minimizes intrusions on privacy and dignity. So long as judges continue to have these perceptions, courts are unlikely to interfere greatly with either legally mandated or private drug-testing programs.

A WORD ABOUT ETHICS

The fact that the law allows the government to test its employees in many circumstances and imposes few or no limits on applicant drug testing

---

[1]To the extent that drugs use substantially degrades job performance, performance tests will even serve some of the deterrence functions of chemical drug testing, for a worker using drugs can expect to fail the performance test and be sent home, losing a day's pay. Also not doing well on a performance test might serve to establish cause for a drug test.

or on drug testing in the private sector does not, however, mean that drug testing is a wise or proper thing to do. Policies that are legally permissible may be ethically wrong. We do not mean to canvass ethical issues here, for there is neither a body of authority to summarize nor a scientific consensus to restate. But we do wish to emphasize that, when a drug-testing program is challenged on ethical grounds, it is no answer to say, "But the law allows it." Similarly the fact that the law forbids drug testing in certain circumstances does not mean that testing in those circumstances would, apart from the legal violation, be ethically unjustified.

To give just one example, preemployment screening is ordinarily allowed without a strong nexus between revealed drug use and likely job performance. It does not follow that it is right to screen for drugs where no job-related nexus can be shown. The privacy of many is invaded to screen out a few whose drug use would have caused no harm had they not been screened out. The situation would be even more problematic if testing for non-job-related drug use disproportionately screened out members of a particular group and was known to do so. Indeed, in those circumstances even some job-relatedness might not be enough to ethically justify drug screening. At the same time, the lack of a job-related nexus does not necessarily mean that a drug-testing program is ethically wrong. If such testing programs discourage the use of drugs associated with non-job-related harms, this deterrent effect can form the basis for a coherent ethical argument supporting both applicant and employee drug testing. The strength of the argument from deterrence and its weight relative to the ethical case against generalized drug screening are matters that can be and have been disputed.

An interesting feature of the different ethical stances that can be maintained toward ethically problematic policies, like some preemployment drug screening, is that an evaluation of their persuasive force depends in large measure on empirical judgments. If widespread preemployment drug screening offended few people, discouraged many people from using dangerous drugs, did not systematically disadvantage people of a particular social status, and had a strong job nexus, then the ethical status of generalized screening programs would, for most people, be different from what it would be if the characteristics of the screening program were just the reverse. Thus empirical research is important not only to develop more effective drug-testing programs or to tell organizations whether proposed programs make economic or safety sense. It is also important to inform the serious ethical conversation that should take place whenever there is a proposal to institute, cancel, or substantially change a program of workplace drug testing.

REFERENCES

Hopson, E.S.
  1986   Alcohol and drug abuse cases in arbitration. Pp. 275-290 in W. Dolson, ed., *Annual Labor and Employment Law Institute*. Littleton, Colo.: Fred B. Rothman & Co.
Labor Relations Week
  1989   Workplace drug testing: evolving law and employer practice. *Labor Relations Week* (suppl) 9:3-32
Silverstein, M.
  1989   Privacy rights in state consitutions: models for Illinois? *University of Illinois Law Review* 215-296.
Veglahn, P.A.
  1988   What is a reasonable drug testing program?: insight from arbitration decisions. *Labor Law Journal* 39:688-695.

C

Biographical Sketches

CHARLES O'BRIEN is chief of psychiatry at the Philadelphia Veterans Affairs Medical Center, professor and vice chairman of psychiatry at the University of Pennsylvania, and director of the University of Pennsylvania Addiction Research Center. He is board certified in both neurology and psychiatry, and his research interests include the psychopharmacology of addiction and the development of new behavioral and pharmacological treatments for addiction, including alcoholism using controlled clinical trials. Involved in delivering general psychiatric and substance abuse treatment, he also directs training for medical students, fellows, and residents. He has authored more than 260 publications in the area of addictive disorders and biological psychiatry. In 1988 he received the first annual Wikler award for excellence in drug abuse research from the National Institute on Drug Abuse, the MERIT award in 1992, and a Pacesetter research award from the National Institute on Drug Abuse in 1993. In 1991 he was elected to the Institute of Medicine. He has B.S., M.D., and Ph.D. degrees from Tulane University.

TERRY BLUM is professor of organizational behavior in the School of Management, Ivan Allen College of Management, Policy and International Affairs at Georgia Institute of Technology, where she has been a member since 1986. She received a Ph.D. in sociology from Columbia University in 1982, and formerly was adjunct assistant professor of sociology and biostatistics at Tulane University. She served 4 years as a member of the Alcohol

Psychosocial Review Committee of the National Institute on Alcohol Abuse and Alcoholism, was editor of the *Organizations and Occupations Newsletter* of the American Sociological Association, and served a 3-year term on the editorial board of *Social Forces.* Her current research is focused on the dynamics of referral patterns within employee assistance programs, the epidemiology of depression in the workplace, and the genesis and maintenance of human resource practices to deal with social problem issues.

ROBERT M. BRAY is a senior research psychologist at Research Triangle Institute in Research Triangle Park, North Carolina. Previously he was at the University of Kentucky. He has B.S. and M.S. degrees in psychology from Brigham Young University and a Ph.D. in social psychology from the University of Illinois, Urbana-Champaign. He is a member of the American Psychological Association, the Society for Personality and Social Psychology, and the American Public Health Association. His recent work has focused on substance use epidemiology and related problems in civilian and military populations, including those in the work force. He has directed the 1982, 1985, 1988, and 1992 Worldwide Surveys of Substance Abuse and Health Behaviors Among Military Personnel and has been coordinator of analytic reports for the 1988 and 1990 National Household Surveys on Drug Abuse. He is currently directing the Washington, D.C., Metropolitan Area Drug Study, a 4-year comprehensive project of the prevalence, correlates, and consequences of drug abuse in household and nonhousehold populations (including people who are homeless, institutionalized, adult offenders, juvenile offenders, clients entering treatment programs, and new mothers).

JAMES H. DWYER is associate professor of preventive medicine with joint appointments in the Atherosclerosis Research Institute and the Institute for Prevention Research at the University of Southern California School of Medicine. He has a B.S. in mathematics from Pepperdine University and a Ph.D. in psychology (statistics) from the University of California, Santa Cruz. He has been a visiting scientist at the University of Bern (Switzerland) and the Institute for Epidemiology (Berlin). The major focus of his substantive research is the relation between diet and atherosclerosis, but he serves as a coinvestigator and consultant on large community trials aimed at the prevention of drug abuse. He is the principal investigator on several National Institute of Health and state-supported research grants. In addition to numerous articles, he is the author of *Statistical Models for the Social and Behavioral Sciences* and one of the editors of *Statistical Models for Longitudinal Studies of Health.*

BRYAN S. FINKLE is research professor of pharmacology-toxicology in the College of Pharmacy and the Department of Pathology in the College of

Medicine, University of Utah Health Sciences Centers. He is also a consultant in medico-legal toxicology and preclinical new drug development. He has a Ph.D. from the School of Medicine, University of Utah. From 1973 to 1983, he was director of the Center for Human Toxicology at the University of Utah and from 1983 to 1989 was director of the Department of Pharmacological Sciences at Genentech Inc. He has been a consultant to the National Institute on Drug Abuse and other government and private agencies involved with the toxicology of drug abuse. He is past president of the International Association of Forensic Toxicologists and of the Forensic Sciences Foundation, past vice-president of the American Academy of Forensic Sciences and a member of several state, national, and international organizations of forensic scientists and toxicologists. He has also served on committees of the Pharmaceutical Manufacturers Association. He is the recipient of the Stas Medal, awarded by the German Society of Toxicology and Chemistry, and the Rolla Harger Award, the highest honor given by the American Academy of Forensic Sciences Toxicology Section.

MARIAN W. FISCHMAN is professor of behavioral biology in the Department of Psychiatry and codirector of the Division on Substance Abuse at the College of Physicians and Surgeons of Columbia University. She is also a research scientist and director of the Substance Use Research Center at the New York State Psychiatric Institute. She has a B.A. from Barnard College, an M.S. in psychology from Columbia University, and a Ph.D. in biopsychology from the University of Chicago. Her research has focused on the determinants and consequences of substance use and misuse and the implications of drug use for workplace performance, with special emphasis on stimulant drugs, alcohol, and marijuana. With her colleagues, she has developed important new approaches to evaluating, understanding, and treating the effects of drugs of abuse. She has served on a number of drug abuse advisory boards, including the Board of Scientific Counselors of the Addiction Research Center, Advisor to World Health Organization (Division of Mental Health), the Scientific Advisory Panel of the Ciba Foundation, the Scientific Advisory Board of National Families in Action, and as chair of the Scientific Advisory Board of the American Council on Drug Education. She is a member of numerous professional organizations and is a fellow of the American Psychological Association, the College on Problems of Drug Dependence, and the American College of Neuropsychopharmacology. She is the author or coauthor of more than 100 papers covering various aspects of drugs of abuse, including their behavioral and physiological effects, as well as possible treatment approaches, and has lectured extensively, internationally as well as nationally, on these subjects.

BRADLEY K. GOOGINS is founder and director of the Boston University

Center on Work and Family, a multidisciplinary research organization, formed under the aegis of the School of Management and the Graduate School of Social Work. The center works to bring new solutions and perspectives to family and work life issues. He received B.A. and M.S.W. degrees from Boston College and a Ph.D. in social policy and research from the Heller School, Brandeis University. He is also associate professor at the Graduate School of Social Work at Boston University and a recent National Kellogg fellow (1989-1992). His recent research funded by the National Institute on Alcohol Abuse and Alcoholism and the National Institute on Drug Abuse has focused on several areas relevant to employee assistance programs including supervisor training, the role of social supports, and assessment practices. He has published extensively on work/family issues, employee assistance programs, and workplace substance abuse. His recent work includes *Work/ Family Conflicts: Private Lives—Public Responses*, *Linking the Worlds of Family and Work*, *Family Dependent Care and Workers' Performance*, and *Balancing Job and Homelife Study*.

DANIEL LANIER, JR., is a visiting professor at the Florida State University, School of Social Work, and is also director of EAP HealthCare Institute. He was formerly assistant director of the United Auto Workers International Union-General Motors (UAW-GM) National Human Resource Center. Previously, he was associate director of the employee assistance program for General Motors Corporation. Before joining General Motors, he held a number of executive-level human service management positions as a senior officer in the U.S. Army Medical Service Corps. He received a B.S. from North Carolina Agricultural and Technical State University, an M.S.W. from the University of North Carolina at Chapel Hill, and a Ph.D. from Case Western Reserve University. He is the immediate past president of the Employee Assistance Professionals Association and was formerly chairman of the Employee Assistance Certification Commission. He is a Certified Employee Assistance Professional. He is also an adjunct profession at Western Michigan University. He has written numerous articles and professional publications, including, as coauthor, a best selling series of handbooks on employee assistance programming.

WAYNE E.K. LEHMAN is a research scientist with the Institute of Behavioral Research at Texas Christian University and was previously with the Behavioral Research Program at Texas A&M University. He has a B.A. in psychology from Heidelberg College and a Ph.D. in psychology from Texas Christian University. His research centers on substance abuse issues, primarily in the area of drugs in the workplace. His current research program includes development of employee drug use measures and performance issues related to drug use in work settings. He is currently directing a large-scale, multisite project involving employee surveys of substance use and its impact on organizations. He is a member of the American Psychological Society and the Society for Industrial/Organizational Psychology.

RICHARD O. LEMPERT is the Francis A. Allen Collegiate professor of law, professor of sociology, and acting chair of the sociology department at the University of Michigan. He is a fellow of the American Academy of Arts and Sciences, past chair of the National Research Council's Committee on Law and Justice, and a former editor of the *Law and Society Review*. He has also served on National Research Council committees and panels on tax compliance, on statistical evidence and the courts, and on DNA technology in forensic science. His research interests include informal justice, the jury system, the law of evidence, and uses of scientific evidence. He is the author (with Stephen Saltzburg) of *A Modern Approach to Evidence* and (with Joseph Sanders) of *An Invitation to Law and Social Science*.

COLLINS E. LEWIS is associate professor of psychiatry in the Department of Psychiatry at Washington University School of Medicine. He received a B.A. in biological sciences from Rutgers University and an M.D. from Harvard University Medical School. He also received an M.P.H. from the Harvard University School of Public Health. His interests center on the effect of comorbidity on problem drinking with particular emphasis on antisocial personality. He is the author of numerous publications and several invited book chapters. He has served on the National Institute on Alcohol Abuse and Alcoholism initial review group and is currently on the National Institute of Mental Health's special projects review committee. He is currently on the editorial board of *The Journal of Employee Assistance Program Research* and is a member of the Research Society on Alcoholism and the International Society for Biomedical Research on Alcoholism.

ELAINE MCGARRAUGH is research associate for the Committee on the Impact of Needle Exchange and Bleach Distribution Programs, National Research Council, and production editor with the Commission on Behavioral and Social Sciences and Education, National Research Council. For the past 9 years she has worked on numerous National Research Council and Institute of Medicine studies that looked at the treatment and prevention of alcohol and illicit drugs. Prior to joining the National Research Council, she was the educational director at an adolescent inpatient drug rehabilitation center. She has a B.S. from McMurry College.

JEFFREY A. MIRON is professor of economics at Boston University and research associate at the National Bureau of Economic Research. He received a B.A. in economics from Swarthmore College in 1979 and a Ph.D.

in economics from the Massachusetts Institute of Technology in 1984. From 1984 to 1990, he served on the faculties of the University of Michigan and the Sloan School of Management at the Massachusetts Institute of Technology. He has served as consultant to the Federal Reserve Board on several occasions. In 1988 he was awarded an Olin Fellowship from the National Bureau of Economics, and in 1989 he received a Sloan Foundation Research Fellowship. He has published extensively in professional journals on such topics as the theory and practice of monetary policy, the quality of government statistics, the seasonal fluctuations in aggregate activity, the seasonality of births, and the economics of illegal drugs.

KEVIN R. MURPHY is a professor of psychology at Colorado State University. He has a B.A. in psychology from Siena College, an M.S. from Rensselaer Polytechnic Institute, and a Ph.D. from Pennsylvania State University, both in industrial/organization psychology. He is a fellow of the American Psychological Association and of the American Psychological Society and serves as associate editor for the *Journal of Applied Psychology*. He is a member of the editorial boards of *Human Performance*, *Personnel Psychology*, *Journal of Vocational Behavior*, and *International Journal of Selection and Assessment*. He has published extensively in a number of areas, including performance appraisal, psychological measurement, drug testing, and integrity testing. His most recent book, *Honesty in the Workplace*, examines a variety of techniques for reducing counterproductive behavior in the workplace, including programs aimed at reducing substance abuse.

MICHAEL D. NEWCOMB is professor of counseling psychology and chairperson of the Division of Counseling and Educational Psychology at the University of Southern California. He is also a research psychologist and codirector of the Substance Abuse Research Center in the psychology department at the University of California, Los Angeles. He received a Ph.D. in clinical psychology from UCLA and is a licensed clinical psychologist in the state of California. He is a fellow in several divisions of the American Psychological Association and also fellow in the American Psychological Society. He is principal investigator on several grants from the National Institute on Drug Abuse. He has published over 100 papers and book chapters and is the author of *Consequences of Adolescent Drug Use* (with Bentler), *Drug Use in the Workplace*, and *Sexual Abuse and Consensual Sex: Women's Developmental Patterns and Outcomes* (with Wyatt and Riederlie). He has served on several journal editorial boards, including the *Journal of Personality and Social Psychology*, *Archives of Sexual Behavior*, *Journal of Addictive Diseases*, and *Journal of Child and Adolescent Substance Abuse*. His research interests include the etiology and consequences of adolescent drug abuse; structural equation modeling, methodology, and multivariate analysis; human sexuality; health psychology; attitudes and affect related to nuclear war; and cohabitation, marriage, and divorce. He has served on several national review and advisory committees for such groups as the National Research Council, the National Institute on Drug Abuse, the National Institute of Mental Health, the Office of Substance Abuse Prevention, and various research centers.

JACQUES NORMAND is a study director at the National Research Council of the National Academy of Sciences in Washington, D.C. He is currently directing a study on the impact of needle exchange and bleach distribution programs on the incidence of HIV and drug use behavior among intravenous drug users. Prior to joining the National Research Council in 1991, he held research psychologist positions in both the private and public sectors. In that capacity, he was responsible for the development, validation, and implementation of various personnel selection and organizational intervention programs. He has published in various professional research journals and has spoken at numerous professional meetings on personnel evaluation issues. He has also served as a consultant to the National Institute on Drug Abuse and acts as an ad hoc reviewer of applied drug-use research manuscripts for various professional journals. He has also served as a technical advisor on the National Institute on Drug Abuse's Technical Review Meeting on Research Methods in Workplace Settings and recently completed a 4-year term as a full member of the Drug Abuse Epidemiology and Prevention Research Grant Review Committee at the National Institutes of Health. He has a B.A. from McGill University and M.S. and Ph.D. degrees from the Illinois Institute of Technology.

PATRICK M. O'MALLEY is research scientist at the Institute for Social Research at the University of Michigan. He has a B.S. degree from the University of Massachusetts at Amherst in psychology and a Ph.D. in psychology from the University of Michigan. Since 1975, he has been a codirector of the Monitoring the Future project, an ongoing study of the lifestyles and values of American youth. This study, which involves annual national surveys of secondary school students in grades 8, 10, and 12 and young adults through age 35, provides the nation with annual reports on trends in the use of psychoactive drugs, including alcohol, tobacco, and illicit drugs. Since 1987 he has been a member of the Drug Abuse Epidemiology and Prevention Research Review Committee for the National Institute on Drug Abuse. He has published extensively on the use and abuse of psychoactive drugs and is senior author of a major report on the role of minimum drinking age laws in alcohol use by young Americans.

ADRIAN M. OSTFELD is the Anna M.R. Lauder professor of epidemiology and public health and of medicine at the Yale University School of Medicine and a senior member of the Institute of Medicine. He is a former member of the National Advisory Council on Aging and the American Society for Clinical Investigation. Most of his research has been concerned with the epidemiology of cardiovascular disease and of aging. He is author or coauthor of 10 books and 230 papers and book chapters on these subjects, and editor emeritus of the *American Journal of Epidemiology*, as well as an editorial board member or member emeritus of seven journals.

ANDREW M. WEISS is professor of economics at Boston University. He received a B.A. from Williams College and a Ph.D. from Stanford University. He was a research economist with Bell Laboratories and Bell Communications Research, and a visiting professor at Tel Aviv University in 1991 and 1992. His research interests center on the role of imperfect information in economic and social processes. His research has recently focused on integrating recent developments in neuropsychology with modern techniques of economic analysis to gain a better understanding of individual responses to addictive substances. He has written numerous articles in professional journals and has lectured at major universities and professional associations in the United States, Japan, Great Britain, Israel, Germany, Czechoslovakia, France, Italy, Canada, Argentina, and Uruguay. He is a fellow of the Econometric Society. His recent book, *Efficiency Wages*, was published jointly in the United States and Great Britain.

M. DONALD WHORTON is vice president of ENSR Consulting and Engineering, the environmental consulting division of American NuKEM, an integrated environmental services company in Alameda, California. He is a physical epidemiologist specializing in occupation and environmental health issues. He is a member of the Institute of Medicine and has served or is serving on other Institute of Medicine and National Research Council committees. He is a fellow of the American College of Environmental and Occupational Medicine, chairman of its Occupational Medical Practices Committee, and a fellow of the American Public Health Association.

Index